A Practical Guide
to
ECG Interpretation

A Practical Guide
to
ECG Interpretation

Ken Grauer, M.D., F.A.A.F.P.

Professor
Department of Community Health and Family Medicine

Assistant Director
Family Practice Residency Program
University of Florida, College of Medicine
Gainesville, Florida

ACLS National Affiliate Faculty

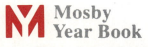

Mosby
Year Book

St. Louis   Baltimore   Boston   Chicago   London   Philadelphia   Sydney   Toronto

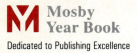
Mosby
Year Book

Dedicated to Publishing Excellence

Editor: Don Ladig
Developmental editor: Jeanne Rowland
Project manager: Mark Spann
Production editor: Stephen C. Hetager

Illustrations: Mark Swindle, George Wassilchenko
Cover Illustration: © George Wassilchenko

Printed in the United States of America

Mosby—Year Book, Inc.
11830 Westline Industrial Drive
St. Louis, Missouri 63146

Library of Congress Cataloging-in-Publication Data

Grauer, Ken.
    A practical guide to ECG interpretation / Ken Grauer.
        p.   cm.
    Includes bibliographical references and index.
    ISBN 0-8016-2159-3
    1. Electrocardiography.   I. Title.
    [DNLM: 1. Electrocardiography—programmed instruction.   WG 18
G774pa]
RC683.5.E5G665   1991
616.1'207547—dc20
DNLM/DLC
for Library of Congress   91-25668
                                                             CIP

CL/VH   9   8   7   6   5   4   3   2

TO MY FATHER

Samuel Grauer

without whom this book would not have been possible

About the Author

Ken Grauer, M.D., F.A.A.F.P., is a professor in the Department of Community Health and Family Medicine, College of Medicine, University of Florida, and assistant director of the Family Practice Residency Program in Gainesville. He is board certified in family practice, and is a National ACLS Affiliate Faculty member and contributor to the American Heart Association ACLS Textbook. Dr. Grauer is the principal author of the following books and teaching resources: *Clinical Electrocardiography: A Primary Care Approach* (Medical Economics Books, 1986; second edition in press by Blackwell Scientific Publications), *ACLS: Certification Preparation and Comprehensive Review* (C.V. Mosby, 1987; third edition in press by Mosby–YearBook), *ACLS: Mega Code Review Study Cards* (C.V. Mosby, 1988), and *ACLS Teaching Kit: An Instructor's Resource* (Mosby–Year Book, 1990). He has lectured widely and is primary author of numerous articles on cardiology for family physicians, including an "ECG of the Month" series that was published for over six years in several primary care journals. Dr. Grauer has become well known throughout Florida and nationally for teaching ACLS courses and ECG/dysrhythmia workshops to diverse medical audiences including nurses, paramedics, medical students, physicians in training, and physicians in practice. His trademark has always been the ability to simplify otherwise complicated topics into a concise, practical, and easy-to-remember format.

Acknowledgments

I am indebted to the following people whose contributions were instrumental to the preparation of this book:

Laura Gasparis (Vonfrolio), RN; **Dan Cavallaro,** REMT; and **Karen Hall,** MD, for reviewing the majority of the text and keeping me aimed at my target audience.

Kinsey Judkins-Waldron, RN, for her invaluable insight, unfailing support, and tremendously welcome 100%-biased positive feedback!

Holly Jensen, RN; Fred Langer, RN; Kevan Metcalfe, RN, BSN; Jane Scudder, RN; Ellie Green, RN; Katherine Littrell, RN, MSN, CCRN; Pam Schroeder, RN; and Geno Romano, MD, for their assistance in reviewing selected aspects of the text.

Marv Dewar, MD, JD, for his advice that made this book possible.

Whit Curry, Jr., MD, for allowing me to "pump his brain" on numerous occasions throughout the years on primary care questions about cardiology issues.

Don Ladig, Stephanie Manning, and Rick Weimer of Mosby–Year Book, Inc., for their encouragement, enthusiasm, and motivation, out of which this book was born. Terry Van Schaik, for making the birth possible.

Jeanne Rowland of Mosby–Year Book, Inc., for her special attention to every last detail, which enabled the book to come to fruition—and for always being there with an open ear and friendly encouragement.

Mark Swindle and George Wassilchenko, who must be the two best medical illustrators in existence.

Steve Hetager of Mosby–Year Book, Inc., for his patience in putting up with my multiple "just one more" corrections!

Jay and Jackie Katz of Resource Applications, for making it possible for me to teach nurses across the country.

Pat (and the crew at Sonny's) and Phil Heflin (and the crew at Chaucer's), for their great food and ever EXCELLENT service, and for providing me with a peaceful, pleasant, and inspiring environment for writing and reviewing much of the text.

Maria Alvarez and Cindy Freiberger—the best dance teachers I know—for their inspiration toward excellence in ballroom dancing, and who, together with Virginia Hungerford and all my friends at the Maria Alvarez Imperial Dance Studio, were instrumental in helping me to maintain my sanity (and still have fun by dancing) while working on this book.

Barney Marriott, MD, and **William P. Nelson,** MD, for teaching me more about ECGs than I can ever say.

The Cardiology staff at Alachua General Hospital (Burt Silverstein, MD; Steve Roark, MD; Mike Dillon, MD; and Gary Cooper, MD), for their tremendous support of me, and for teaching cardiology to our residents.

All of the other excellent cardiologists who have inspired me and from whom I have learned.

All those who have knowingly (and unknowingly) provided me with tracings through the years.

All the nurses, medical students, residents, and other paramedical personnel who have allowed me to learn by teaching them.

Ken Grauer

Consultants

Janell Bartley, LPN
BSN Student
Methodist College of Nursing
Omaha, Nebraska

Nancy Beck
ECG Technician
Electrocardiology & Echocardiology
Kaiser Permanente Medical Center
Vallejo, California

Toni Cascio, MN, RN, CCRN
Clinical Educator — Critical Care
Ochsner Foundation Hospital
New Orleans, Louisiana

Edward M. Geltman, MD
Associate Professor of Medicine
School of Medicine
Washington University
St. Louis, Missouri

Elizabeth M. Hoehne
Student
Deaconess College of Nursing
St. Louis, Missouri

Garland Hughes, MD
Intern
Department of Internal Medicine
University of Texas Southwestern Medical School
Dallas, Texas

Kelly McDonald, BSN, RN
Staff Nurse
St. Louis University Hospital
St. Louis, Missouri

Judy L. Myers, MSN, RN
Assistant Professor
School of Nursing
St. Louis University
St. Louis, Missouri

David P. Rardon, MD
Assistant Professor of Medicine
Indiana University School of Medicine
Indianapolis, Indiana

Susan B. Stillwell, MSN, RN, CCRN
Critical Care Consultant
Emtek Health Care Systems, Inc.
Tempe, Arizona

Stephen Stribling, MSN, RN, CCRN
Cardiovascular Clinical Nurse Specialist
Mississippi Baptist Medical Center
Jackson, Mississippi

Robert D. Wiens, MD, FACC
Professor of Internal Medicine
School of Medicine
St. Louis University
St. Louis, Missouri

How to Use this Book

Before how, we need to ask why. *Why another book on electrocardiography?*

The answer lies in the approach. Despite the hundreds of books already written on the topic, the need is still there for a comprehensive yet practical approach to electrocardiography for the beginning or novice student. **A Practical Guide to ECG Interpretation** has been written expressly with the needs of this audience in mind.

Our approach is different. We don't stress endless memorization of little-used (and all-too-easily-forgotten) facts. Instead we stress application of practical concepts encountered in the daily practice of most medical care providers.

Two unique teaching features are introduced and used repeatedly in our text: an *ECG Interpretation Pocket Reference* and schematic tracings. The beauty of the pocket reference is that it eliminates the need for (and the burden of) memorization. We encourage using it as you read through the book, and referring to it in your everyday practice after you complete the book. With time (and use), the content will become automatic, and you will find yourself referring to the pocket reference less often. If for any reason your practice situation takes you away from ECGs for a period of time, however, the pocket reference will be there when you come back and serve as a rapid refresher and welcome summary of the systematic approach to interpretation and the key core content.

Schematic tracings are used liberally throughout our book. These illustrations focus attention on the key leads to look at for the conditions being discussed. For example, diagnosis of bundle branch block can almost always be made from examination of just three leads: I, V_1, and V_6. To emphasize this point (and to train your eye to focus on these three key leads), we present numerous practice tracings that show complexes ONLY in these three leads.

Part One (Chapter 1) of our book opens with a brief *Philosophical Overview* of electrocardiography. We stress that the reader need not be a cardiologist (or even a physician) to obtain a high degree of proficiency in the art of interpretation. Knowledge and application of a systematic approach, awareness of the clinical setting, availability of a prior tracing, and common sense are the key ingredients to the successful electrocardiographer.

We then move to a brief *Review of Fundamentals* in an attempt to unify the knowledge base of our readers. Much of this material may be basic to those with prior experience. Nevertheless, this brief review is essential to the understanding of the balance of the book.

Part Two comprises the key core content of the book. We begin by presenting our *Systematic Approach* to interpretation (Chapter 2). There follows discussion of *Rate & Rhythm* (Chapter 3), the *PR Interval* (Chapter 4), the *QRS Interval* and *Bundle Branch Block* (Chapter 5), *WPW* (Addendum to Chapter 5), the *QT Interval* (Chapter 6), *Axis (and Hemiblocks)* (Chapter 7), *Chamber Enlargement* (Chapter 9), and *QRST Changes* (Chapter 10). Review exercises and *Putting It* (the Systematic Approach) *All Together* are presented in Chapters 8 and 11.

We hope most readers will want to read on to **Part Three:** *For Those Who Want to Know More.* The section begins with Chapter 12, *Infarction and Ischemia,* which many may feel is our most important chapter. In addition to emphasizing ECG diagnosis of acute infarction and ischemia, the coronary circulation is reviewed, clinical application of thrombolytic therapy (and the use of the initial ECG to determine which patients are most likely to benefit from this treatment) is stressed, and tips are included on recognizing silent infarction and diagnosing posterior and right ventricular infarction by ECG.

Chapter 13 introduces the *Five Essential Lists* in electrocardiography. Awareness of the contents of these lists (which are reproduced in the pocket reference) greatly facilitates the task of the interpreter. There follows discussion of *Electrolyte Disturbances* (Chapter 14) and *Pericarditis* (Chapter 15).

Part Four puts on *"Finishing Touches."* It includes chapters on *Recognizing Lead Misplacement* (Chapter 16), *When the Patient is a Child* (Chapter 17), *If the Patient has a Pacemaker* (Chapter 18), *What Can We Learn from Comparison Tracings?* (Chapter 20), and *Does the Computer Know Better?* (Chapter 21). We believe Chapter 19 *(When 12 Leads are Better than One)* will offer a real challenge to any reader actively involved in arrhythmia interpretation. Those who apply the principles put forth in this chapter will make a quantum leap in their ability to interpret cardiac arrhythmias.

We conclude our book with **Part Five:** *Putting Yourself to the Test.* A total of 45 basic review and challenge tracings for interpretation are included in Chapters 22 and 23. Each practice tracing is accompanied by a short clinical scenario to add realism. You are asked to systematically interpret these tracings, and then to compare your answers with the detailed explanations that follow. Clinical relevance is stressed. Accompanying each tracing are *Questions to Further Understanding*, which seek to bridge the gap from ECG theory to clinical (and practical) application. The book then closes with Chapter 24 *(Where Do We Go From Here?)*, which provides some parting advice.

> It is *NOT* essential to wait until the end of the book to do the practice tracings in Chapters 22 and 23. On the contrary, appreciation of clinical relevance may be enhanced by periodically trying your hand at a few of these basic review and challenge tracings as you read through the book. Use the pocket reference as needed along the way. Refer back to pertinent chapters in the text when questions arise. Then *Put Yourself to the Test* again after reviewing the relevant material or completing the text.

We hope you enjoy this book. *It was written with YOU in mind!*

Ken Grauer

Contents

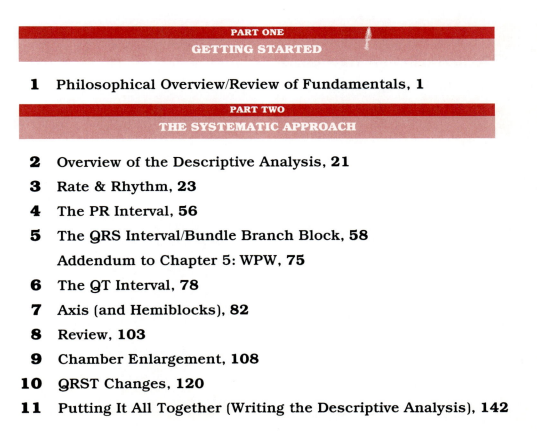

PART THREE

FOR THOSE WHO WANT TO KNOW MORE

PART FOUR

FINISHING TOUCHES

PART FIVE

PUTTING YOURSELF TO THE TEST

Abbreviations

We intentionally use numerous abbreviations throughout this book. We have chosen to do so because:

Abbreviations occupy a ubiquitous presence in the field of electrocardiography. They are part of the vernacular spoken by medical personnel, as well as the standard for written interpretations. Rare is the cardiologist who will meticulously (and legibly) write out intraventricular conduction defect, right atrial enlargement, or left ventricular hypertrophy each time these abnormalities occur. It's just so much easier (and clearer) to write IVCD, RAE, and LVH.

We feel that readability of our book is enhanced by using abbreviations instead of writing each term out.

Learning is facilitated by becoming accustomed to the terms and abbreviations used in everyday practice.

For clarification and reference, we've therefore listed the abbreviations you'll encounter throughout this book:

A

AV atrioventricular
AV block atrioventricular block
AV node atrioventricular (or junctional) node
AV nodal rhythm atrioventricular (or junctional) rhythm

B

BBB   bundle branch block

C

CCU   coronary care unit
ccw   counterclockwise
c/w   consistent with
cw   clockwise
CNS   central nervous system
COPD   chronic obstructive pulmonary disease
CSM   carotid sinus massage (= CSP)
CSP   carotid sinus pressure (= CSM)
CVA   cerebral vascular accident

D/E/F/G/H

ECG   electrocardiogram
ED   emergency department
EKG   electrocardiogram (i.e., from the German: "ElektroKardioGraph")
ETT   exercise tolerance (stress) test

I

ILBBB   incomplete left bundle branch block
IRBBB   incomplete right bundle branch block
IVCD   intraventricular conduction delay (defect)
IVS   interventricular septum

J/K

J point   junctional point (i.e., point marking the junction between the end of the QRS complex and the beginning of the ST segment)

L

LA   left atrium
LAA   left atrial abnormality
LA electrode   left arm recording electrode
LAD   left axis deviation
LAD artery   left anterior descending artery
LAE   left atrial enlargement
LAFB   left anterior fascicular block (= LAHB)
LAH   left anterior hemidivision (i.e., of the LBB)
LAHB   left anterior hemiblock
LAI   left atrial involvement (= LAA)
LBB   left bundle branch
LBBB   left bundle branch block

LCA left coronary artery
LGL syndrome Lown-Ganong-Levine syndrome
LL electrode left leg electrode
LPFB left posterior fascicular block (= LPHB)
LPH left posterior hemidivision (i.e., of the LBB)
LPHB left posterior hemiblock
LV left ventricle
LVE left ventricular enlargement (= LVH)
LVH left ventricular hypertrophy

M/N/O

MAT multifocal atrial tachycardia (= chaotic atrial mechanism)
NPT No prior tracing (is available for comparison)
NS ST-T Abns nonspecific ST-T wave abnormalities

P

PAC premature atrial contraction
PAT paroxysmal atrial tachycardia
PJC premature junctional contraction
PJT paroxysmal junctional tachycardia
PSVT paroxysmal supraventricular tachycardia
PVC premature ventricular contraction

Q

QT interval period from onset of Q wave until end of T wave
QTc the QT interval corrected for heart rate

R

RA right atrium
RA electrode right arm recording electrode
RAA right atrial abnormality
RAD right axis deviation
RAE right atrial enlargement
RAI right atrial involvement (= RAA)
RBB right bundle branch
RBBB right bundle branch block
RCA right coronary artery
RV right ventricle
RVE right ventricular enlargement (= RVH)
RVH right ventricular hypertrophy

S

SA block sinoatrial block
SA node sinoatrial node

SSS   sick sinus syndrome
SVT   supraventricular tachycardia

T

Ta wave   atrial T wave (i.e., wave of atrial repolarization)

U/V/W/X/Y/Z

VT   ventricular tachycardia
wnl   within normal limits
WPW syndrome   Wolff-Parkinson-White Syndrome

Philosophical Overview/Review of Fundamentals

PHILOSOPHICAL OVERVIEW

The most appropriate place to start a book on rapid interpretation of the 12-lead ECG is at the beginning—with the definition of an electrocardiogram. Simply stated, an ECG is "the graphic representation of the heart's electrical activity." It is nothing more, and nothing less.*

We feel that most of the time health care providers are disappointed with the ability of the ECG to provide the information they seek, it is because this basic definition is forgotten. All an ECG does is reflect the heart's electrical activity. It says nothing about the relation of this electrical activity to the clinical situation at hand. That's the job of the interpreter. An *identical* tracing may therefore be interpreted as strongly suggestive of acute infarction if it came from a middle-aged adult with new-onset chest pain, or as totally normal for a child or asymptomatic young adult. Moreover, a single ECG, viewed by itself, says nothing about whether any abnormalities found are new (acute) or old.

---

*The electrical activity of the heart originates at a cellular level. During the resting state, individual myocardial cells are said to be *polarized:* they are negatively charged on the cell interior and positively charged on the outside (surface) of the cell. With electrical stimulation of the cell, it becomes *depolarized* as the inherent negatively of the cell interior becomes positively charged. With organized spread of the wave of depolarization across the mass of cardiac cells, mechanical *contraction* of the heart muscle occurs. Some time later, depolarized myocardial cells return to their resting states (i.e., they again become negatively charged on their interior) during the process known as *repolarization*. Recording of these electrical events as the mass of cardiac cells in the atria and ventricles depolarize and repolarize produces the ECG.

Optimal ECG interpretation therefore requires:

1. **Clinical correlation,** including knowledge of the patient's *age* and the *reason* for obtaining the ECG in the first place (e.g., new-onset chest pain, assessment for chamber enlargement in a patient with hypertension, or simply "routine")

AND

2. Availability of a **prior tracing** for *comparison*. This becomes especially important when the current tracing shows abnormalities that may be acute.

COMPONENTS OF ECG INTERPRETATION

The *KEY* to ECG interpretation is *RESTRAINT*. The key to restraint is using a **systematic approach.** Doing so not only protects you from focusing on obvious abnormalities (and overlooking more subtle findings in the process), but also keeps you organized. Even without knowing the clinical significance of some of the findings detected, being systematic is invaluable in helping you recognize that something's amiss.

We have found it easiest to approach the art of ECG interpretation by dividing it into two principal components:

1. **Descriptive Analysis**
2. **The Clinical Impression**

Most errors in interpretation arise from failure to keep these two components SEPARATE in your mind!

Descriptive analysis is merely a statement of what is found on the ECG. It includes assessment of the tracing for *rate, rhythm, axis, chamber enlargement,* and *QRST changes.* Following a systematic approach makes it easy to list these findings without leaving anything out. We fully explore how to do this in Chapter 2.

The **clinical impression** is the heart of the interpretation. Based on the findings described, it results from consideration of the likely clinical significance (if any) of each of these findings. We summarize the essential core content of electrocardiography in the accompanying ECG pocket reference. Chapters 3 to 11 develop our approach to applying this information in formulating a clinical impression.

Before going any further, it's important to clarify what we mean by the complexes and waveforms we'll be describing. Thus the rest of this chapter is devoted to explanation and illustration of the normal ECG complex and its variations. Although these fundamentals need to be stated, they may already be familiar to many of you. If this is the case, feel free to read through this section briefly, *but please do NOT skip it entirely!*

REVIEW OF FUNDAMENTALS
The Normal Conduction Pathway

ECG complexes reflect the heart's electrical activity. This electrical activity begins in the sinoatrial (SA) node, which is the principal pacemaker of the heart. The SA node is found in the upper portion of the right atrium. *This is why the right*

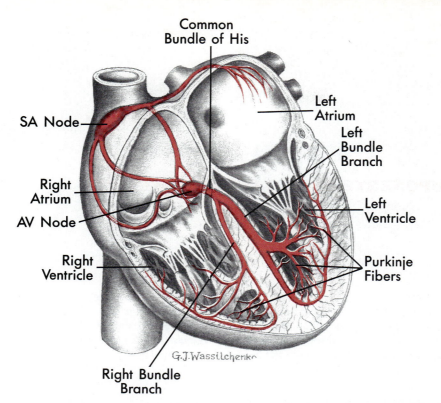

Common
Bundle of His

SA Node

Right
Atrium

AV Node

Right
Ventricle

Left
Atrium

Left
Bundle
Branch

Left
Ventricle

Purkinje
Fibers

G.J.Wassilchenko

Right Bundle
Branch

Figure 1-1.   The normal conduction pathway. The electrical impulse begins in the SA node and is transmitted to the AV node, bundle of His, bundle branches, and Purkinje fiber network.

atrium depolarizes before the left atrium (Figure 1-1). In adults, the normal SA node fires at between 60 and 100 beats/minute, which defines the limits of normal sinus rhythm (NSR).

Following discharge of the SA node, the electrical impulse is carried by specialized conduction fibers to the left atrium and through the right atrium to the atrioventricular (AV) node. The impulse is momentarily delayed at the AV node. It then enters the ventricular conduction system, which is made up of the bundle of His and the right and left bundle branches. From the bundle branches, the electrical activity is carried to the ventricular muscle itself by the network of specialized Purkinje fibers.

The speed at which the impulse travels through the specialized cells of the conduction system is much more rapid than travel over nonspecialized atrial or ventricular tissue. This is the reason a PVC* (premature ventricular contraction) is

---

*Ectopic impulses originate outside of the normal conduction pathway (i.e., these impulses do not arise from the SA node). They may arise from elsewhere in the atria, from the AV node, or from the ventricles. **PVCs** are *premature* ectopic impulses that arise early in the cardiac cycle (hence, "premature") from the ventricles; **PACs** arise early in the cycle from the atria; and **PJCs** arise early in the cycle from the AV node (i.e., the "junction").

Many different terms have been used to designate the premature impulses we describe above. Thus, PVCs are also known as premature ventricular "complexes," PVBs (premature ventricular beats), VPDs (ventricular premature depolarizations), etc. None of these terms are strictly correct, because they mix up ECG waveforms with mechanical and electrical events. Because of habit and extremely common usage, we favor the terms PVCs, PACs, and PJCs—but alert the reader to the existence of many other terms.

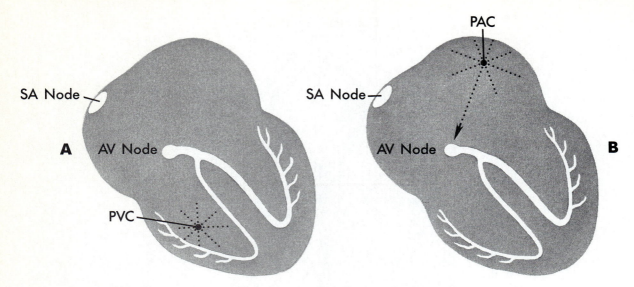

Figure 1-2. Ectopic impulses. **A,** PVCs are wide because they originate outside the ventricular conduction system and depolarize the myocardium slowly by spread of the impulse through nonspecialized ventricular tissue. **B,** PACs are narrow (provided they are not "blocked," or conducted with aberration or bundle branch block) because their origin is supraventricular, allowing them to travel over the normal conduction pathway.

wide—the ectopic focus originates outside the conduction system and is forced to travel over nonspecialized ventricular tissue. Depolarization of myocardium by a PVC therefore takes place much more slowly than it does for a supraventricular impulse that is able to follow the normal conduction pathway (Figure 1-2, *A*).

In contrast, PACs (premature atrial contractions) are usually narrow because they most often are conducted in a manner similar to normal beats (Figure 1-2, *B*). That is, once the atrial impulse arrives at the AV node, it is directed down the normal pathway of conduction—through the bundle of His, the bundle branches, and the Purkinje fiber network. The only exceptions to this are if the AV node is still completely refractory* and unable to conduct the PAC (i.e., if the PAC is "blocked") or if a portion of the ventricular conduction system is still refractory so that conduction is impaired (i.e., if conditions for aberrant conduction are present or if there is bundle branch block).

ECG Waveforms

Electrical events of the cardiac cycle are represented by waveforms on the ECG. Thus the **P wave** represents atrial depolarization, the **QRS complex** ventricular depolarization, and the **T wave** ventricular repolarization (Figure 1-3). Occasionally a **U wave** (thought to represent the terminal phase of ventricular repolarization) may also be seen after the T wave.

---

*The *refractory period* is the time during which myocardial cells are unable to respond to an electrical stimulus. Immediately following depolarization, cells are refractory. This is why a PAC that occurs very early in the cycle may be "blocked" (i.e., not conducted to the ventricles). Toward the end of the refractory period, the ventricular conduction system will have almost regained the ability to conduct normally. A PAC occurring during this time may be conducted with *aberration,* reflecting the fact that the normal conduction pathway has not yet fully recovered. The shape of aberrantly conducted beats depends on the path of conduction available at the time the impulse is generated.

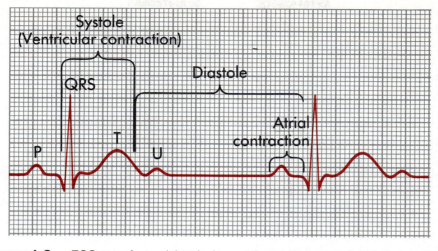

Figure 1-3.   ECG waveforms (electrical events) and the *approximate* timing of their mechanical counterparts.

Electrical events of the cardiac cycle are followed by their *mechanical* counterparts. The mechanical counterparts include contraction and relaxation of the cardiac chambers. Thus atrial contraction follows the P wave and ventricular contraction follows the QRS complex. The QRS complex therefore marks the approximate beginning of mechanical systole, which continues through the T wave. Diastole (with ventricular filling) then begins, culminating with atrial contraction (which follows the P wave). The QRS complex marks the onset of the next mechanical systole.

Intervals

Three key intervals are included within the cardiac cycle: the *PR interval*, the *QRS complex* itself (since the duration of this complex really is an interval), and the *QT interval* (Figure 1-4).

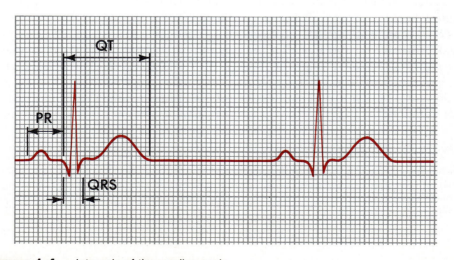

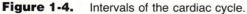

Figure 1-4.   Intervals of the cardiac cycle.

The **PR interval** comprises the time from the onset of atrial depolarization (beginning of the P wave) until the onset of ventricular depolarization (beginning of the QRS complex). A large part of this interval is represented by delay of the electrical impulse in the AV node. This delay serves the physiologic purpose of allowing the atria to contract and empty their contents into the ventricles (i.e., deliver the "atrial kick") prior to the onset of ventricular systole.

The **QRS interval** is the time it takes for ventricular depolarization. This interval may be prolonged with ventricular hypertrophy (since the electrical impulse needs more time to get through the thickened myocardium) or with a defect in conduction (such as bundle branch block or an intraventricular conduction defect).

The **QT interval** is the period from the beginning of ventricular depolarization (onset of the QRS complex) until the end of ventricular repolarization (end of the T wave). During the initial portion of this interval the heart is completely refractory to all premature stimuli. Partial refractoriness of the conduction system is seen during the latter portion of this interval. PACs occurring during this period of partial refractoriness may be conducted with aberration. Premature impulses (PACs or PVCs) occurring at a critical point (i.e., in the "vulnerable period") of the QT interval may predispose the patient to development of atrial or ventricular fibrillation (respectively).

Certain antiarrhythmic agents act by prolonging repolarization. This is especially true of the type IA antiarrhythmic drugs (quinidine, procainamide, and disopyramide). As a result, these drugs commonly prolong the QT interval. When they excessively prolong repolarization, they may predispose the patient to development of a potentially lethal arrhythmia known as *torsade de pointes.**

ST Segment Deviations

Two key segments must be considered in the analysis of any ECG: the *PR segment* and the *ST segment* (Figure 1-5).

The **PR segment** is the horizontal line from the end of the P wave until the onset of the QRS complex. *The PR segment is the baseline from which **ST segment deviations** are judged.* Deviations above this baseline are referred to as *ST segment elevation,* whereas those below it are referred to as *ST segment depression.* Although the PR segment is easy to identify in Fig. 1-5, this is not always the case. The presence of artifact, tachycardia, or a short PR interval may make determination of the PR segment baseline difficult.

ST segment deviations are sometimes described with respect to the J point. The **J point** is best thought of as the **j**uncture of the end of the QRS complex and the beginning of the ST segment. This point is sometimes marked by a notch. Elevation of this notch (i.e., of the J point) may thus be referred to as *J point elevation* (Figure 1-6). This is a common feature of the normal variant known as **early repolarization.**

Torsade de pointes is an unusual ventricular arrhythmia that was first described by the French physician Dessertene. The English translation of the term is "twisting of the points," and it aptly describes this type of ventricular tachycardia, in which positively directed QRS complexes alternate with negatively directed ones. As may be imagined, this is often an extremely difficult arrhythmia to treat clinically.

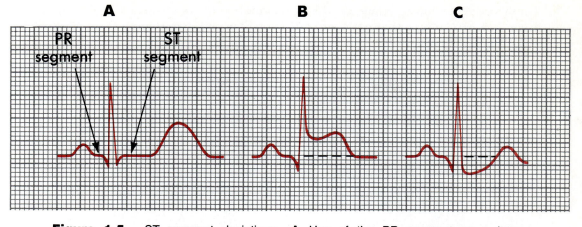

Figure 1-5. ST segment deviations. **A,** Use of the PR segment as a base-line. **B,** The ST segment is elevated with respect to the PR segment baseline. **C,** The ST segment is depressed with respect to the PR segment baseline.

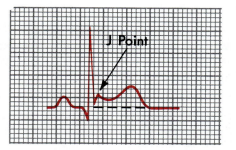

Figure 1-6. J point (ST) elevation. A prominent notch marks the takeoff of the ST segment.

QRS Nomenclature

The QRS complex is subject to great variability. As an aid to communication, a system has been developed that allows us to verbally describe the appearance of any QRS complex to persons who do not have the tracing in front of them. The six basic rules of the system are simple:

1. The first downward deflection of the QRS complex is termed a **Q** wave.
2. The first upward deflection is termed an **R** wave.
3. The downward deflection that follows an R wave is termed an **S** wave if it descends below the baseline.

These first three rules explain the QRS configuration of the examples shown in Figure 1-7. It can be seen that not every QRS complex necessarily has a Q wave, an R wave, and an S wave.

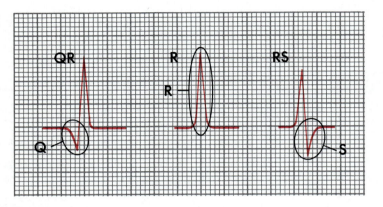

Figure 1-7.   QR, R, and RS complexes. Not every complex has a Q wave, an R wave, and an S wave. (For clarity, we have circled a Q wave, an R wave, and an S wave.)

4. Large deflections are denoted by capital letters. Smaller deflections (i.e., deflections that do not *exceed* 3 mm [3 little boxes]) are denoted by lower-case letters (Figure 1-8).

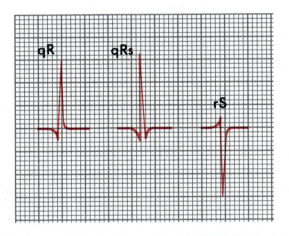

Figure 1-8.   qR, qRs, and rS complexes. Smaller deflections are denoted by lower-case letters.

5. If there is a second positive deflection, it is given a *prime* notation: **R′** or **r′** (depending on its size). A third positive deflection is termed an **R″** (or **r″**). Similarly, a second S wave (if present) is termed an **S′** or **s′** (Figure 1-9).

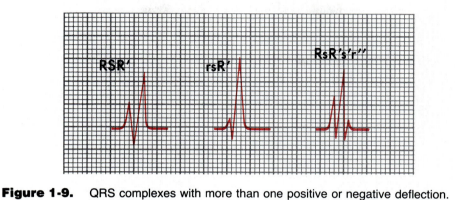

Figure 1-9.   QRS complexes with more than one positive or negative deflection.

6. When there is only a negative deflection, the configuration is called a **QS** complex. This is because we don't (can't) differentiate between a Q wave and a QS wave in the absence of an R wave (Figure 1-10).

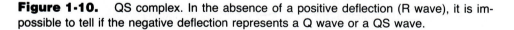

Figure 1-10.   QS complex. In the absence of a positive deflection (R wave), it is impossible to tell if the negative deflection represents a Q wave or a QS wave.

Practice using the system for QRS nomenclature to label the following complexes (Figure 1-11). Our answers can be found on the following page (Figure 1-12).

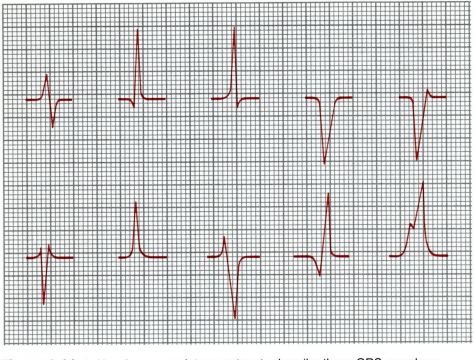

Figure 1-11.   Use the nomenclature system to describe these QRS complexes.

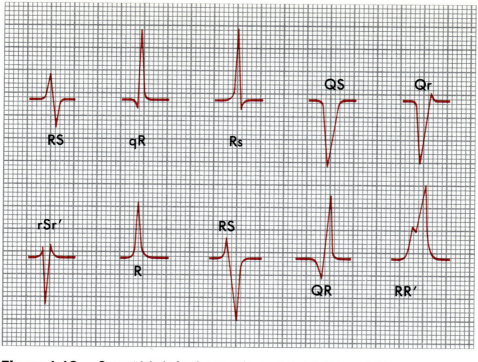

Figure 1-12.   Correct labels for the complexes shown in Figure 1-11.

The last complex in Figure 1-12 is deserving of special mention. Some clinicians may label this simply as an R wave because it is upright. We feel that designating it as an RR′ complex is more descriptive, since it has two definite peaks. The reason why it is not an RsR′ complex is that the downward deflection is extremely small and does not descend below the baseline.

Lead Systems

A standard ECG is recorded by viewing the heart's electrical activity from 12 leads. Each lead records the heart's electrical potential from its vantage point.* The reason so many leads are used is to provide as accurate a view as possible. If only one or two leads were used, certain changes might go unnoticed if they occurred in

---

*In order to understand the appearance of a particular QRS complex, it is important to appreciate the three basic principles of electrocardiography:
1. A wave of depolarization that approaches a monitoring electrode (lead) writes an *upward* (positive) deflection on the ECG.
2. A wave of depolarization that moves away from a monitoring electrode writes a *downward* (negative) deflection on the ECG.
3. A wave of depolarization that is perpendicular to a monitoring electrode writes an *equiphasic* (equally positive and negative) QRS complex.

(These principles will be applied in much greater detail in Chapter 7 when we discuss how to determine axis [the mean orientation of the heart's electrical activity].)

areas of the heart that were not viewed (i.e., monitored) by these particular leads. This is why rhythm interpretation from only one lead (as commonly occurs on telemetry units) is often a hazardous venture. The QRS complex may sometimes appear narrow in one lead (if part of the QRS lies on the baseline) when in fact it is grossly widened.

Realize that even more information could be obtained if the standard ECG routinely recorded *more* than 12 leads. However, doing so would require additional time for patient preparation, and usually won't add that much useful clinical information. Selection of 12 leads therefore represents a compromise that provides a time-efficient, multidimensional view of the heart's electrical activity. The 12 leads routinely recorded in a standard ECG are:

Leads I, II, and III
Leads aVR, aVL, and aVF
Leads V_1, V_2, V_3, V_4, V_5, and V_6

The *standard limb leads* are I, II, and III. These bipolar leads record the difference in electrical potential between the left arm (LA), the right arm (RA), and/or the left leg (LL) electrodes.

Einthoven's triangle* illustrates how the electrical potential for each of these leads is derived (Figure 1-13, *A*).

Fig. 1-13, *B*, simplifies the electrical relationship of the three standard limb leads that we derived from Einthoven's triangle. Thus, lead I is a lateral (leftward) lead that views the heart's electrical activity from a vantage point defined as 0°. Leads II and III are inferior leads that view the heart's electrical activity from vantage points of +60° and +120°, respectively.

Leads aVR, aVL, and aVF are *augmented limb leads.*† These unipolar leads record the difference in electrical potential between the respective extremity lead sites and a reference point with zero electrical potential at the center of the electrical field of the heart. As a result, the axis of each of the three unipolar augmented leads is a line from the electrode site (on the right arm, left arm, or left leg) to the center of the heart (Figure 1-13, *C*). Thus, lead aVL acts as a lateral (leftward) lead that records the heart's electrical activity from a vantage point that looks down from the left shoulder (at −30°). Lead aVF acts as an inferior lead; it records the heart's electrical activity from a vantage point that looks up from the left lower extremity (at +90°). Lead aVR is the most distant recording electrode. It looks down at the heart from the right shoulder. For practical purposes, it can almost always be ignored in the ECG analysis.

Figure 1-13, *D,* shows the effect of combining *B* and *C.* Thus, in the frontal plane, the lateral (or left-sided) leads are I and aVL, and the inferior leads are II, III, and aVF.

---

*Willem Einthoven was a Dutch physician who is thought of by many as the "father of electrocardiography." In 1902, he became the first person to record the heart's electrical current in an accurate and reproducible manner with his invention of the string galvonometer—the first ECG machine. The equilateral triangle that bears his name assumes that the heart lies at the center of the electrical field defined by the axes of the three standard limb leads. While not strictly true, Einthoven's theory is nevertheless still extremely useful, and it is from its concept that we have derived the hexaxial lead system that remains in use today.

†The reason leads aVR, aVL, and aVF are known as augmented leads is that these unipolar leads normally produce a relatively small electrical potential that is then magnified (i.e., *augmented*) approximately 50% by an internal alteration in the way the ECG machine is set up.

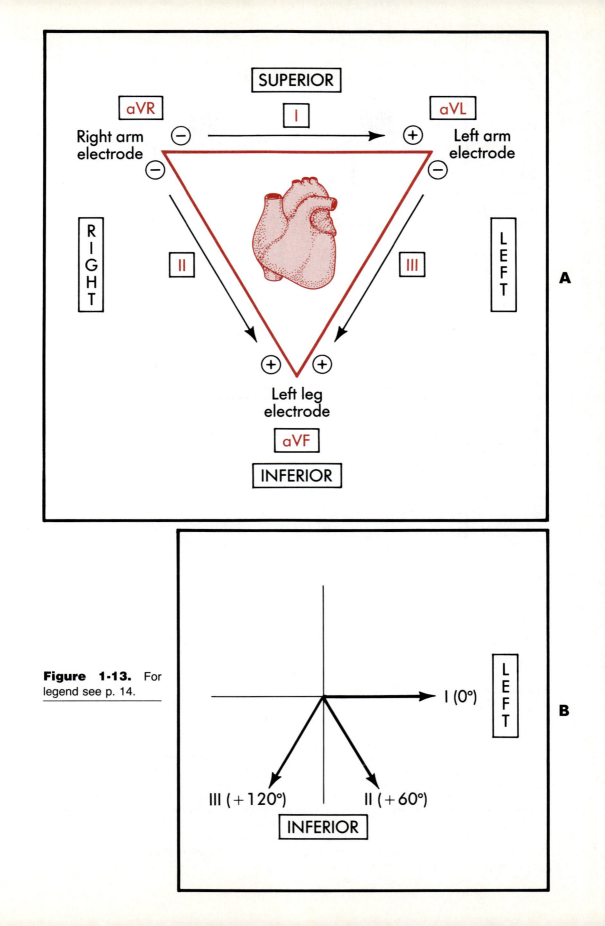

SUPERIOR

aVR

Right arm
electrode

aVL

Left arm
electrode

I

RIGHT

II

III

LEFT

A

Left leg
electrode

aVF

INFERIOR

Figure 1-13. For
legend see p. 14.

LEFT

I (0°)

B

III (+120°)

II (+60°)

INFERIOR

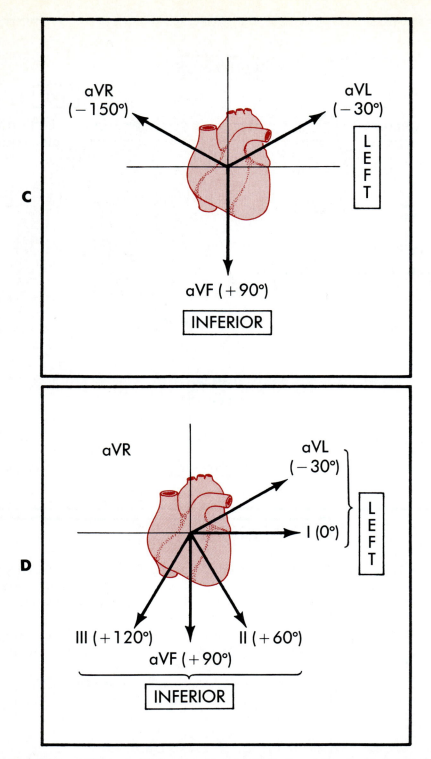

Figure 1-13, cont'd.   **A,** Einthoven's triangle. Derivation of the electrical potential for standard limb leads (I, II, and III) and augmented leads (aVR, aVL, and aVF) in the frontal plane. **B,** Electrical vantage points of the three standard limb leads. **C,** Electrical vantage points of the three augmented limb leads. **D,** Combined electrical vantage points of **B** and **C.** Leads II, III, and aVF are considered inferior leads; I and aVL are considered lateral leads. For practical purposes, the electrical activity from distant recording electrode aVR can usually be ignored in the ECG analysis.

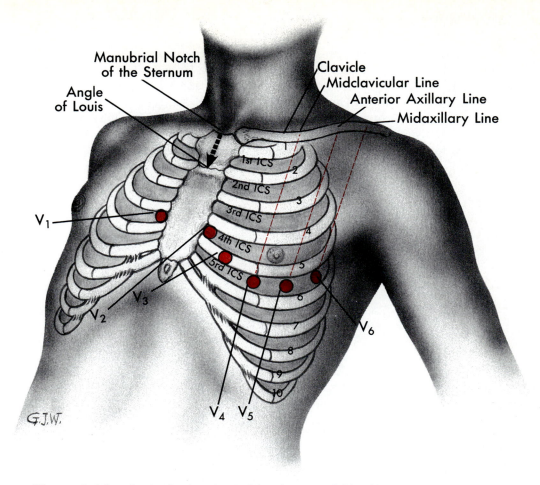

Figure 1-14. Anatomic placement of the six precordial leads.

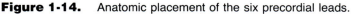

The six remaining leads are known as the *precordial leads*. These unipolar leads record the heart's electrical activity in the transverse (horizontal) plane. They are placed on the chest in reference to the following anatomic landmarks:

Lead V_1: at the fourth intercostal space,* just to the right of the sternum
Lead V_2: at the fourth intercostal space, just to the left of the sternum
Lead V_3: midway between leads V_2 and V_4
Lead V_4: in the midclavicular line, in the fifth intercostal space
Lead V_5: in the anterior axillary line, at the same level as lead V_4
Lead V_6: in the midaxillary line, at the same level as lead V_4

Placement of the precordial leads is shown in Figure 1-14.

*The key to accurately determining precordial lead placement is to first identify the angle of Louis. This can be done by lowering your finger from the manubrial notch of the sternum until it comes to lie on a small, horizontal ridge. The second intercostal space lies just below this point. Dropping down two additional intercostal spaces and moving just to the right will locate the reference position for lead V_1.

A schematic view of the areas of the heart recorded by the six precordial leads is shown in Figure 1-15. From this illustration it can be seen that leads V_1 and V_2 are septal leads, V_2, V_3, and V_4 are anterior leads, and V_4, V_5, and V_6 are lateral precordial leads. It can also be seen that the wall of the right ventricle (X in the figure) and the posterior wall of the left ventricle (Y in the figure) are areas of the heart not well visualized by the usual six precordial leads. Suggestions for assessing these "hard-to-get-at" areas are covered in Chapters 12 and 13.

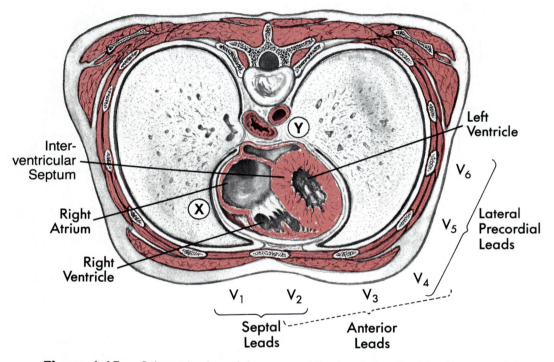

Figure 1-15.   Schematic view of the areas of the heart visualized by the precordial leads. Neither the right ventricular wall *(X)* nor the posterior wall of the left ventricle *(Y)* is well visualized by any of the usual six precordial leads.

Accurate placement of precordial leads on the chest is crucial. Placing a lead as little as one intercostal space too high or too low can dramatically alter QRS morphology and amplitude. In women, recording electrodes should be placed *under* the left breast, or similar errors in lead placement may occur.

Table 1-1 summarizes the basic lead groups, and the areas of the heart they represent.

Table 1-1
Basic Lead Groups

Inferior leads: II, III, aVF
Septal leads: V_1, V_2
Anterior leads: V_2 to V_4
Lateral leads:
   Lateral precordial leads: V_4 to V_6
   High lateral leads: I, aVL

12-Lead Orientation Systems

The two basic formats for displaying the 12 standard leads on an ECG are shown in Figure 1-16.

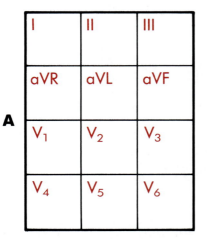

Figure 1-16. Horizontal **(A)** and vertical **(B)** orientation systems for displaying the 12 standard leads of an ECG.

The horizontal orientation system (Figure 1-16, *A*) was used much more in the past, when ECGs were obtained on a single-channel recorder and a representative portion of each lead was selected and then mounted by hand. Currently, three-channel recorders have become much more widely used. These newer machines most often utilize a vertical lead orientation (Figure 1-16, *B*). When a computerized ECG system is used, this orientation offers the distinct advantage of *simultaneous* recording of all three leads in a vertical column. We emphasize the importance of simultaneous recording later on.

Although all of our schematic illustrations and most of our example tracings in this book display a vertical (three-channel) orientation, we occasionally show ECGs with the older (horizontal) orientation so that you become accustomed to both systems.

PRACTICE

As a check on your understanding of basic principles, you may want to complete the following exercise.

Examine the ECG shown in Figure 1-17, taken from a 39-year-old man with chest pain.

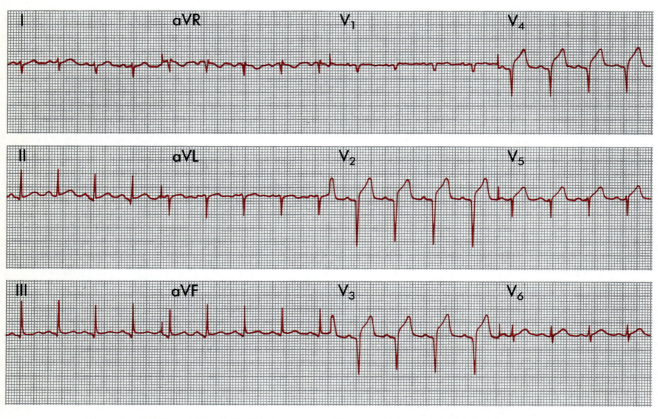

Figure 1-17.   12-lead ECG taken from a 39-year-old man with chest pain.

Questions on Figure 1-17

1. Does this ECG display a horizontal or vertical lead orientation?
2. Identify the three leads that look at the *inferior* portion of the heart. (Refer to Table 1-1, if necessary, as a reminder of the basic lead groups.)

    Is the configuration of the QRS complex in each of these three inferior leads similar? How would you describe the QRS complex by the QRS nomenclature system that we discussed and that was illustrated in Figures 1-7 through 1-12? Is the ST segment elevated or depressed in these leads?

3. Identify the *anterior* leads. Describe the QRS complex according to the nomenclature system. Is there ST segment elevation in these leads? If so, is the onset of the ST segment marked by a distinct J point, or is the transition from the end of the QRS complex to the ST segment more gradual?

4. Identify the two *high lateral* leads. Describe the QRS complex in these leads. Is there ST segment elevation?

(Our answers can be found on the following page.)

Answers to Figure 1-17

1. The ECG shown in Fig. 1-17 displays a vertical lead orientation, in which there is simultaneous recording of leads I, II, and III; aVR, aVL, and aVF; V_1, V_2, and V_3; V_4, V_5, and V_6.

2. Leads II, III, and aVF view the *inferior* portion of the heart. The QRS complex is similar in each of these three leads and displays a qR configuration. Although not at all obvious, there is an ever-so-slight amount of ST segment elevation in these leads.

3. The *anterior* leads are V_2, V_3, and V_4. A QS complex is seen in each of these three leads. There is marked ST segment elevation (of at least 3 mm, or 3 little boxes) above the PR segment baseline, but no distinct J point notching. Instead, the end of the QRS complex blends into the ST segment.

4. The *high lateral* leads are I and aVL. An rS complex is seen in each of these leads. There is no ST segment elevation.

As we will see in subsequent chapters, the ECG shown in Figure 1-17 is strongly suggestive of an acute anterior infarction.

Overview of the Descriptive Analysis

With review of fundamentals behind us, it's time to turn to the **descriptive analysis** portion of 12-lead ECG interpretation. The key to including all essential aspects of each interpretation is to use a systematic approach. We suggest the following:

Examine each ECG you encounter for:

1. **R**ate
2. **R**hythm
3. **A**xis
4. **H**ypertrophy
5. **I**nfarct

Slight modification of these key parameters completes the mnemonic for remembering our systematic approach (Figure 2-1):

R Ate   **R A**te

                                  R Hythm

R Hythm   **I** ntervals (PR/QRS/QT)

A xis

                                   A xis

H ypertrophy   **H** ypertrophy

                                   I nfarct (= **Q R S T** Changes)

I nfarct

Figure 2-1.   Mnemonic for systematic approach to ECG interpretation.

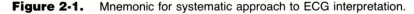

We routinely begin interpretation of each tracing by determining the heart **R**Ate and cardiac **R**Hythm. The sequence of these first two components should not be hard to remember. The second letter of r**A**te is an **A,** which prompts recall that after rate and rhythm comes **A**xis. The second letter of r**H**ythm is **H,** which prompts recall that after rate, rhythm, and axis comes **H**ypertrophy. The fifth (final) component is **In**farct. Thinking of Q waves as the essence of the ECG diagnosis of infarction should be enough to recall the mnemonic **Q**-R-S-T changes.

Note that according to the above mnemonic, assessment of **I**ntervals is accomplished *early* (under **R**hythm). This is a logical inclusion, since the P-QRS relationship (and the *PR interval*), and QRS duration (the *QRS interval*), are essential components of rhythm determination. For example, first-degree AV block is diagnosed by prolongation of the PR interval, and ventricular rhythms are suggested when there is QRS widening.

> *The importance of assessing intervals early cannot be overemphasized.* Failure to do so makes it all too easy to be "led down the garden path" of assessing a tracing for chamber enlargement and infarction — only to *retrospectively* find a short PR interval (from Wolff-Parkinson-White syndrome) or a bundle branch block pattern that invalidates the interpretation. *Checking for intervals early prevents this from happening!*

We devote the remaining chapters in Part Two to explaining the core content of the ECG pocket reference and developing each of the components of our systematic approach.

3

Rate & Rhythm

Comprehensive rhythm analysis extends beyond the scope of this book. We have discussed this subject in detail elsewhere *(see suggested readings at the end of this chapter)*. For practical purposes (and space constraints), *we only review the basics here.*

CALCULATION OF HEART RATE

The first step in rhythm analysis is calculation of heart rate. This is usually quite easy to do.

Electrocardiograms and rhythm strips are recorded on grid paper similar to that shown in Figure 3-1.

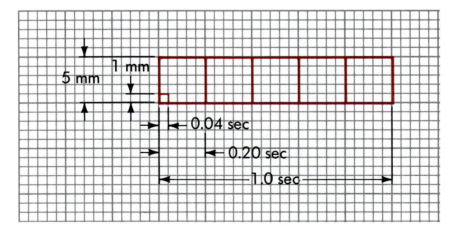

Figure 3-1. ECG grid paper. With the ECG machine set at the standard recording speed of 25 mm/second, the time required to record each little box is 0.04 second. Each little box is 1 mm in amplitude.

Note that this grid paper is made up of large and small boxes. Each little box is a square that measures one millimeter on each side. Each large box is a square that measures five little boxes (or 5 millimeters) on each side.

23

ECGs are recorded at a standard speed of 25 mm/second. This means that 25 little boxes (or five large boxes) of ECG paper will be used each second. It follows that the amount of time needed to record one little box = ⅟₂₅ second = 0.04 second.

Thus, in Figure 3-1 we see that time (in seconds) is displayed along the longitudinal axis of ECG grid paper while amplitude (in millimeters) is displayed vertically. Each little box represents 0.04 second in time and 1 millimeter in amplitude. The time required to record five little boxes (or one large box) is therefore 0.04 second × 5 = 0.20 second. It follows that the time required to record five large boxes is 0.20 second × 5 = 1.0 second.

Imagine that a QRS complex occurred each large box (Figure 3-2, *which also appears on p. 5 in the Pocket Reference*). This means that the **R-R interval** (i.e., the amount of time between each QRS complex) would be 0.20 second. With a QRS complex being recorded each 0.20 second, five QRS complexes would therefore be recorded each second (0.20 × 5). Since there are 60 seconds in a minute, the heart rate would be 300 beats/minute.

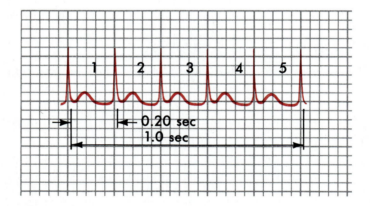

Figure 3-2.   A QRS complex occurs each large box. The R-R interval is therefore 0.20 second, and the heart rate is 300 beats/minute.

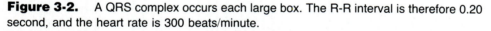

If it took twice as long (i.e., two large boxes, or 0.40 second) to record each QRS complex, the heart rate would be *half* as fast, or 150 beats/minute (300 ÷ 2). It follows that if it took three times as long to record each QRS, the heart rate would be one third as fast (300 ÷ 3 = 100 beats/minute); if it took four times as long to record each QRS (if the R-R interval was four large boxes), the heart rate would be 300 ÷ 4 = 75 beats/minute.

As an extension of this principle, we can develop an easy method for estimating heart rate:

If the rhythm is regular, heart rate can be estimated by dividing 300 by the number of large boxes in the R-R interval (Figure 3-3).

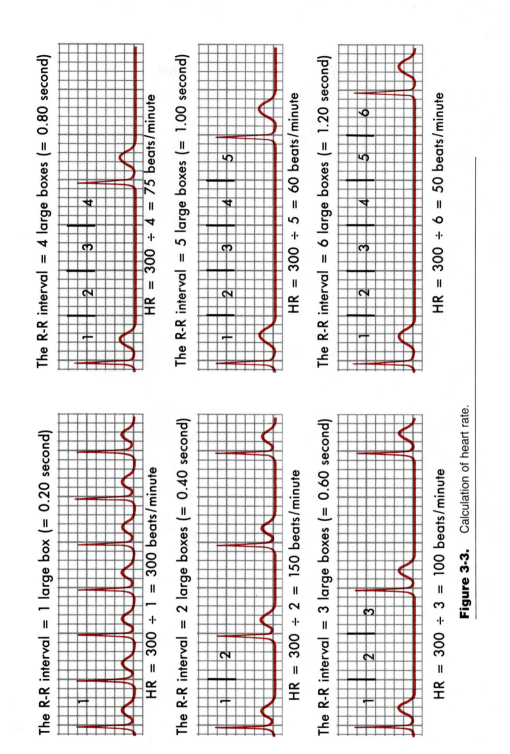

The R-R interval = 4 large boxes (= 0.80 second)

HR = 300 ÷ 4 = 75 beats/minute

The R-R interval = 5 large boxes (= 1.00 second)

HR = 300 ÷ 5 = 60 beats/minute

The R-R interval = 6 large boxes (= 1.20 second)

HR = 300 ÷ 6 = 50 beats/minute

The R-R interval = 1 large box (= 0.20 second)

HR = 300 ÷ 1 = 300 beats/minute

The R-R interval = 2 large boxes (= 0.40 second)

HR = 300 ÷ 2 = 150 beats/minute

The R-R interval = 3 large boxes (= 0.60 second)

HR = 300 ÷ 3 = 100 beats/minute

Figure 3-3. Calculation of heart rate.

The method works equally well for slow rates. Calculate the heart rate in Figures 3-4 and 3-5.

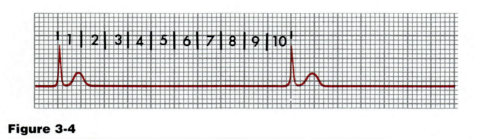

Figure 3-4

Answer to Figure 3-4

The R-R interval in Figure 3-4 is 10 large boxes. Therefore the heart rate is 300 ÷ 10 = 30 beats/minute.

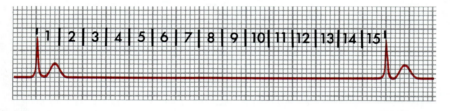

Figure 3-5

Answer to Figure 3-5

The R-R interval in Figure 3-5 is 15 large boxes. Therefore the heart rate is 300 ÷ 15 = 20 beats/minute.

What would you estimate the heart rate to be in Figure 3-6, *A* and *B,* in which the R-R interval does not come out to be an even number of large boxes?

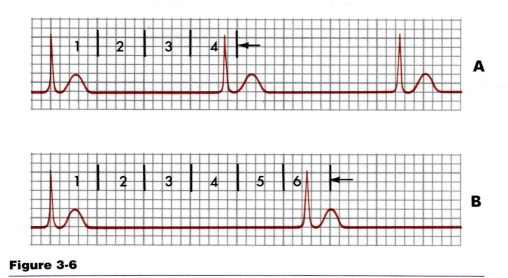

Figure 3-6

Answer to Figure 3-6, *A*

The rhythm is regular. The R-R interval is between three and four large boxes. If it were exactly three boxes, the heart rate would be 100 beats/minute; it if were four boxes, the heart rate would be 75 beats/minute. Since the R-R interval is closer to four boxes, the heart rate is about 80 beats/minute.

Answer to Figure 3-6, *B*

The R-R interval is between five and six large boxes. If it were exactly five boxes, the heart rate would be 60 beats/minute; if it were six boxes, the heart rate would be 50 beats/minute. Since the R-R interval is approximately midway between five and six boxes, the heart rate is about 55 beats/minute.

Note that use of this method for calculating heart rate depends on *regularity* of the rhythm. When the rhythm is slightly irregular, heart rate can be approximated by estimating the number of large boxes contained in the *average* cycle and dividing 300 by this number. With a greater degree of irregularity, it may be preferable to give a *range* for the heart rate.

For example, estimate the heart rate of the irregular rhythm shown in Figure 3-7.

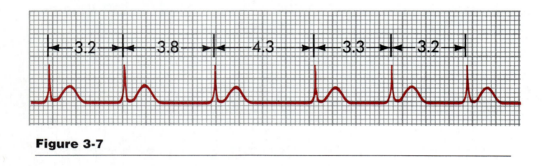

Figure 3-7

Answer to Figure 3-7

The rhythm is definitely irregular. Most R-R intervals are between three and four large boxes. This suggests that the heart rate ranges between 75 and 100 beats/minute.

There are many other methods for determining heart rate. Some calculate the number of beats in a finite period of time (such as 6 seconds) and then multiply this number by 10 to estimate the number of beats per minute. For simplicity, we favor the **rule of 300** that we have just discussed.

APPROACH TO RHYTHM ANALYSIS: THE FOUR QUESTIONS

Now that we can rapidly estimate heart rate, let's move on to rhythm analysis. The key components of rhythm analysis are best embodied by the four questions listed in Table 3-1, *which also appears on p. 5 in the pocket reference.*

Table 3-1
The Four Key Questions of Rhythm Analysis
1. Is the rhythm regular? 2. Are there P waves? 3. Is the QRS wide or narrow? 4. "Who's married to whom?" (i.e., *Is the P related to the QRS?*)

We illustrate application of the four-question approach to rhythm interpretation in the explained answers to the practice tracings that appear at the end of this chapter. For now we will simply emphasize that together with rate determination, these four items (assessment of the rhythm for regularity, identification of atrial activity, determination of QRS width, and recognition of the relation [if any] of P waves to the QRS complex) make up the framework for rhythm interpretation.

Accurate rhythm determination from a 12-lead ECG is not always easy. This is because one gets only a brief look (usually only a few beats) at any particular lead before that lead changes. P waves may be visible in some leads, but not in others. Even when P waves are present, P wave morphology changes each time the leads are changed (Figure 3-8).

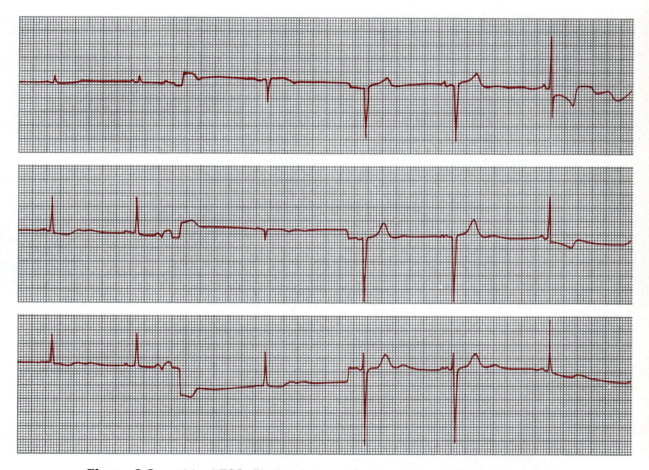

Figure 3-8. 12-lead ECG. Rhythm determination is sometimes difficult unless an accompanying rhythm strip is available. Because of the slow heart rate in this example, only one or two beats are seen in each lead before the lead is changed.

Fortunately, the rhythm in the majority of cases is sinus—the easiest rhythm to recognize. **Normal sinus rhythm (NSR)** is defined in *adults* as a regular rhythm with a heart rate between 60 and 99 beats/minute in which the PR interval is constant and the P wave is upright in lead II. All of these conditions are present in Figure 3-9.

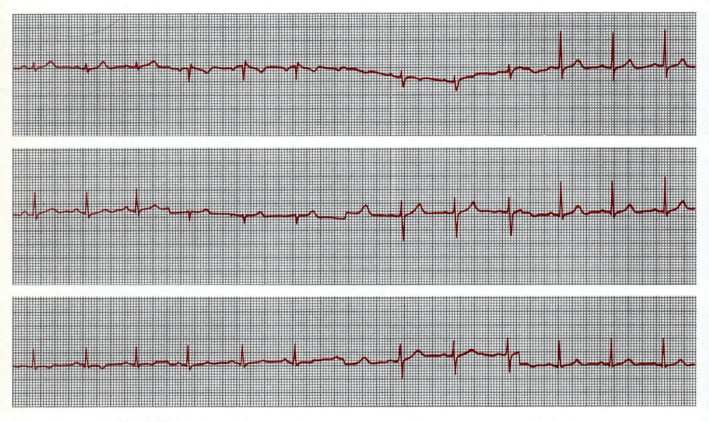

Figure 3-9.   The heart rate in this example is 80 beats/minute. There is NSR because the rhythm is quite regular, the PR interval is constant, and the P wave is upright in lead II.

Determinants of Sinus Rhythm

The most important point to emphasize in this section is that *by definition, the P wave will always be upright in lead II with sinus rhythm.* ***If the P wave is not upright in lead II, you DON'T have sinus rhythm!*** The *only* exceptions to this rule are if the patient has dextrocardia (in which the heart lies on the right side of the chest cavity) or if there has been an error in lead placement (e.g., lead reversal)—both extremely uncommon situations.

The reason why P waves are upright in lead II with sinus rhythm is that the orientation of the AV node with respect to the SA node should virtually always be parallel to this lead (Figure 3-10). Thus, if the electrical impulse originates at the SA node and travels down the normal conduction pathway toward the AV node, it will be viewed as approaching (i.e., positively) by lead II.

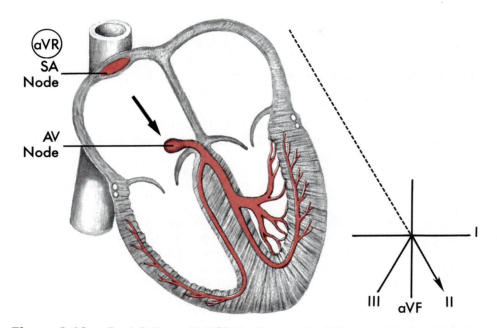

Figure 3-10. By definition, with NSR the P wave should be upright in lead II *(unless there is lead reversal or dextrocardia).*

Question

What would you expect the P wave to look like in lead aVR with NSR? (Hint: *Is the electrical impulse in Figure 3-10 being conducted toward or away from lead aVR?)*

Answer

As we discussed in Chapter 1, lead aVR views the heart from the right shoulder and is the most distant recording electrode. With normal conduction from the SA node to the AV node, the electrical impulse is thus conducted *away* from lead aVR. One might therefore expect that the P wave (as well as the QRS complex) will almost always be negative in lead aVR, since atrial (and ventricular) depolarization will be oriented away from this lead.

Other Rhythms with Sinus Mechanism

Strictly speaking, for **normal sinus rhythm (NSR)** to be present, not only must the heart rate be between 60 and 100 beats/minute, but the rhythm must be regular. When the P wave is upright in lead II and the PR interval is constant, but either the rate or regularity parameter is lacking, a sinus mechanism other than NSR is said to be present. This may include:

Sinus bradycardia—if the rhythm is regular and the rate slower than 60 beats/minute

Sinus tachycardia—if the rhythm is regular and the rate 100 beats/minute or faster

Sinus arrhythmia—if the rhythm is irregular but the mechanism is still sinus

These mechanisms may be combined. Thus, there may be sinus bradycardia and arrhythmia if the mechanism is sinus but the rate is slow (less than 60 beats/minute) and the rhythm irregular.

Escape Rhythms

The most common rhythm in otherwise healthy adults is NSR. However, the occurrence of a rhythm with sinus mechanism other than NSR does not necessarily imply an abnormal state. On the contrary, many individuals (especially runners) normally have resting sinus bradycardia (that may be marked) and/or sinus arrhythmia.

At times the sinus node may give up or falter in its function as the principal pacemaker of the heart. This may occur as the result of cardiac disease (from sick sinus syndrome or infarction of the SA node) or as a normal phenomenon (as when the rate of sinus node firing decreases during sleep or when an individual is put under anesthesia).

Question

What would you expect to happen in cases when the SA node fails to initiate the electrical impulse (Figure 3-11)?

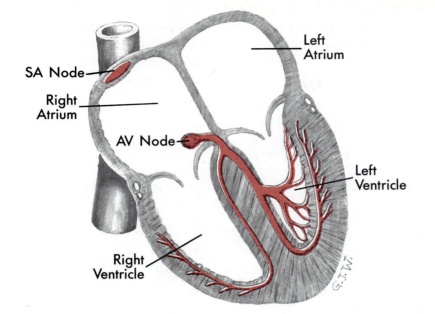

Figure 3-11. Where might the rhythm originate when the SA node gives up or fails in its pacemaking function?

Answer

If the SA node fails to initiate the electrical impulse, another *(escape)* pacemaker will hopefully assume the pacemaker function. Most often the escape focus will arise from the AV node, but it could also arise from elsewhere in the atria *(atrial escape rhythm)*. If neither the atria nor the AV node respond, an *idioventricular escape rhythm* may assume the pacemaker function.

Intrinsic rates of AV nodal and ventricular escape pacemakers tend to follow a logical sequence. Thus the usual AV nodal escape rate is between 40 and 60 beats/minute (or just below the limit for sinus bradycardia), and the usual idioventricular escape rate is 30 to 40 beats/minute (or just below the usual AV nodal escape rate).

The width* of the QRS complex may also provide information on the site of the escape pacemaker.

Question

What would you expect the QRS complex of an AV nodal pacemaker to look like? *(Should the QRS complex be wide or narrow? Should it look similar to the normally conducted QRS?)* How should the appearance and rate of an AV nodal escape pacemaker differ from those of an idioventricular pacemaker?

---

*QRS measurement is discussed in detail in Chapter 5. For now, suffice it to say that a QRS interval of up to 0.10 second is normal. Thus, for there to be QRS widening, the QRS complex must clearly be *greater* than *half* a large box (i.e., *greater* than 0.10 second) in duration.

Answer

Supraventricular rhythms are those in which the electrical impulse originates at or above the AV node (i.e., *at or above* the double dotted line in Figure 3-12).

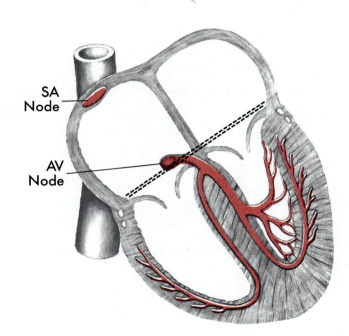

Figure 3-12.   Supraventricular rhythms originate at or above the double dotted line. Ventricular rhythms originate below the line.

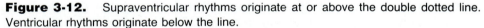

This includes all of the rhythms with sinus mechanism, atrial rhythms, and AV nodal rhythms. Supraventricular rhythms are all conducted to the ventricles over a similar conduction pathway (via the bundle of His and bundle branches). As a result, the QRS complex for all supraventricular rhythms should normally be narrow and look quite similar (if not identical) to the QRS complex with NSR.

Thus, under usual circumstances, an **AV nodal escape pacemaker** should be narrow, similar in appearance to the normally conducted QRS, and between 40 and 60 beats/minute. In contrast, an idioventricular pacemaker will usually have a slower rate (30 to 40 beats/minute) and manifest a wide, different-looking QRS complex (since the impulse originates in the ventricles, or below the dotted line in Figure 3-12).

Question

Can you think of one situation in which a supraventricular rhythm might manifest a wide QRS complex?

Answer

The QRS complex will be wide despite a supraventricular origin of the impulse if there is bundle branch block. In this case, the electrical impulse may arise normally from the SA node and be conducted normally to the AV node. After this point, however, conduction will be delayed because of a defect in the ventricular conduction system. Thus, the P wave and the PR interval may be normal, but the QRS complex will be widened.

Another situation in which the QRS complex will be wide despite a supraventricular origin of the impulse is aberrant conduction.

The P Wave in AV Nodal Rhythms*

Examine Figure 3-13. What would you expect the P wave to look like in lead II with an AV nodal rhythm? (Hint: *If the electrical impulse started in the AV node, would it travel toward or away from lead II to depolarize the atria?*)

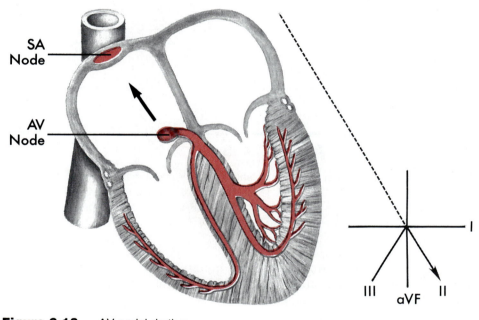

Figure 3-13.   AV nodal rhythm.

Answer to Figure 3-13

The P wave should be negative in lead II with AV nodal rhythm. This is because atrial depolarization is retrograde (i.e., occurs in a direction opposite from lead II).

---

*Two terms are in common use to describe the rhythm in this section: *AV nodal rhythm* and *junctional rhythm*. For practical purposes we treat these terms as synonyms and use them interchangeably.

Figure 3-14 is a *laddergram* that allows us to compare P wave morphology in lead II with NSR *(A)* and the three possibilities of an AV nodal (junctional) rhythm *(B, C,* and *D)*. A **laddergram** is an ideal teaching modality for illustrating the sequence of conduction and the mechanism of cardiac rhythms. Thus, with NSR (Figure 3-14, *A)*, the impulse begins in the SA node and sequentially travels through the atria (upper tier in the laddergram), the AV node (middle tier), and the ventricles (lower tier).

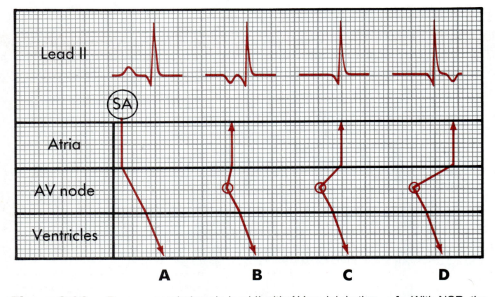

Figure 3-14.   P wave morphology in lead II with AV nodal rhythm.   **A,** With NSR, the P wave is upright in lead II. With AV nodal rhythm, the P wave in lead II will be negative and appear before the QRS **(B),** be hidden by the QRS **(C),** or appear after the QRS **(D).**

With AV nodal rhythm, onset of the impulse is in the AV nodal (middle) tier and travels backward *(retrograde)* to depolarize the atria as well as forward *(antegrade)* to depolarize the ventricles.

If retrograde atrial conduction is fast (i.e., faster than antegrade conduction to the ventricles), a negative P wave (with a short PR interval) will appear *before* the QRS complex in lead II (Figure 3-14, *B*). If retrograde atrial conduction is slow (i.e., slower than conduction to the ventricles), a negative P will occur *after* the QRS complex in lead II *(D)*. Most often, retrograde conduction to the atria takes approximately the same amount of time as antegrade conduction to the ventricles, in which case no P wave at all is seen in lead II *(C)*.

We summarize the essentials of escape rhythms in Table 3-2.

Table 3-2
The Essentials of Escape Rhythms

Usual rates (for *adults*) **of normal intrinsic pacemakers:**
   SA node: 60 to 100 beats/minute
   AV node: 40 to 60 beats/minute
   Ventricles: 30 to 40 beats/minute
Cause of escape rhythms: failure (or delay) in the sinus-initiated impulse
Usual appearance of escape rhythms:
   Atrial escape rhythm: narrow QRS complex preceded by a P wave; rate usually
      over 60 beats/minute*
   AV nodal escape rhythm: narrow QRS complex (which may or may not be preceded by an inverted P wave); rate usually between 40 and 60 beats/minute*
   Idioventricular escape rhythm: wide QRS complex not preceded by a P wave;
      rate usually between 30 and 40 beats/minute

*NOTE: It is sometimes difficult (if not impossible) to differentiate between an atrial escape rhythm and an AV nodal escape rhythm. Clinically this distinction is not important. Practically speaking, AV nodal escape rhythms are much more common.

A LIST OF COMMON ARRHYTHMIAS

We must again emphasize that space constraints prevent us from fully exploring the gamut of cardiac arrhythmias. Nevertheless, keeping in mind the basic principles we have covered thus far and having an appreciation of the major arrhythmias one is likely to encounter will often go a long way toward narrowing the differential diagnosis of rhythm analysis in 12-lead ECG interpretation.

In the hope of assisting in this task, we list, briefly describe, and schematically illustrate the most common arrhythmias below. (*All rhythm strips are taken from lead II.*)

Sinus Mechanism Rhythms/Arrhythmias (⇒ *the P Wave is Upright in Lead II)*

Normal Sinus Rhythm (NSR): regular rhythm; rate between 60 and 99 beats/minute (Figure 3-15, *A*)

Sinus Bradycardia: regular rhythm; rate below 60 beats/minute (Figure 3-15, *B*)

Sinus Tachycardia: regular rhythm; rate 100 beats/minute or faster (Figure 3-15, *C*)

Sinus Arrhythmia: sinus mechanism; irregular rhythm (Figure 3-15, *D*)

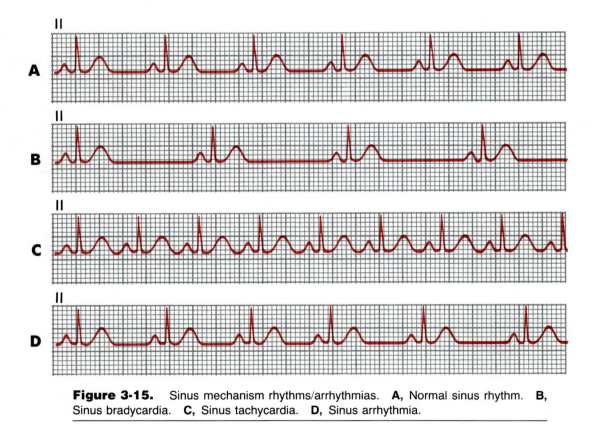

Figure 3-15. Sinus mechanism rhythms/arrhythmias. **A,** Normal sinus rhythm. **B,** Sinus bradycardia. **C,** Sinus tachycardia. **D,** Sinus arrhythmia.

Sinus arrhythmia is an exceedingly common normal finding in otherwise healthy, asymptomatic children and young adults.

Other Supraventricular (⇒ *Narrow QRS*) *Arrhythmias*

Atrial Fibrillation: irregularly irregular rhythm; no definite P waves. By definition, it is impossible to specify the rate of atrial fibrillation (since the rate of this irregularly irregular rhythm changes from beat to beat). We feel it best to describe atrial fibrillation as having one of the following:

A rapid ventricular response—if the rate averages over 120 beats/minute (Figure 3-16, *A*)

A controlled (moderate) ventricular response—if the rate averages between 70 and 110 beats/minute (Figure 3-16, *B*)

A slow ventricular response—if the rate averages less than 60 beats/minute (Figure 3-16, *C*)

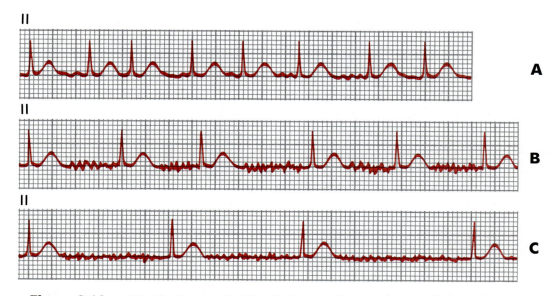

Figure 3-16.   Atrial fibrillation.   **A,** Atrial fibrillation with a rapid ventricular response. **B,** Atrial fibrillation with a controlled (moderate) ventricular response.   **C,** Atrial fibrillation with a slow ventricular response.

Although well-defined P waves are absent with atrial fibrillation, one will often see undulations in the baseline. These undulations are known as "fib waves," and result from the chaotic activity of atria that are fibrillating. In Figure 3-16, fib waves are coarse in *B,* and much finer (less evident) in *A* and *C*. Depending on the lead that is monitored, there are times when fib waves will not be evident at all. In such cases, diagnosis of atrial fibrillation must be made by recognition of an irregularly irregular rhythm in the absence of P waves.

Atrial Flutter: regular atrial rate that is most often close to 300 beats/minute; characteristic *sawtooth* pattern (especially in the inferior leads). Most commonly there is a 2:1 ventricular response (atrial rate about 300 beats/minute ⇒ ventricular rate about 150 beats/minute); less commonly there is a 4:1 ventricular response (ventricular rate about 75 beats/minute)—though other ratios or an irregular ventricular response may also be seen.

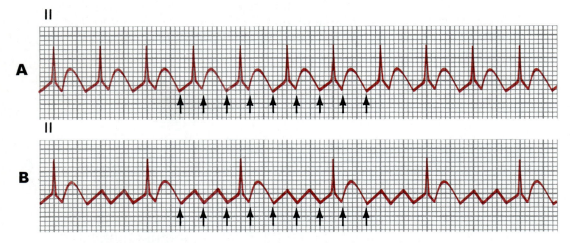

Figure 3-17.   Atrial flutter.   **A,** Atrial flutter with a 2:1 ventricular response (atrial rate ≈300 beats/minute, ventricular rate ≈150 beats/minute). *Flutter activity (arrows) appears as negative deflections that precede and immediately follow each QRS complex.*   **B,** Atrial flutter with a 4:1 ventricular response (atrial rate ≈300 beats/minute, ventricular rate ≈75 beats/minute). *Note how much easier it is to identify the sawtooth pattern of the flutter waves (arrows) with the slower ventricular response shown in* **B.**

Diagnosis of atrial flutter is easy when flutter waves are as obvious as they are in Figure 3-17, *B*. It may be much harder to diagnose when flutter waves are less evident in the lead being monitored. For this reason, it is often helpful to obtain a 12-lead ECG so as to allow the interpreter to select the lead in which flutter waves are seen best.

PSVT (Paroxysmal SupraVentricular Tachycardia): regular supraventricular tachycardia at a rate of 150 to 240 beats/minute without obvious atrial activity (Figure 3-18, *A*), although subtle notching or a negative deflection representing retrograde atrial activity may sometimes be seen at the tail end of the QRS complex. The rhythm often has a sudden onset (i.e., it is "paroxysmal"). It commonly occurs in otherwise healthy young adults, as well as in older individuals who do have underlying heart disease.

Formerly this rhythm was known as PAT or PJT (paroxysmal atrial or junctional tachycardia), but this older terminology implies more than we really know about the mechanism of the arrhythmia. In most cases in adults, PSVT is a *reentry* tachycardia that involves the AV node (Figure 3-18, *B*). This means that the electrical impulse is caught in a cycle that continuously circulates around the AV node. It "reenters" the AV node with each revolution at the same time as it divides into a branch that is conducted to the ventricles (to produce a QRS complex). The cycle (and the tachycardia) continues until the reentry pathway is interrupted (by drugs, vagal maneuvers, or spontaneously).

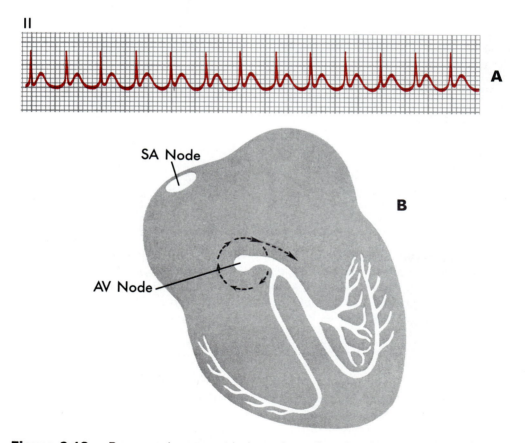

Figure 3-18. Paroxysmal supraventricular tachycardia. **A,** PSVT at a rate of 200 beats/minute. *There is a regular, supraventricular tachycardia without identifiable atrial activity.* **B,** The mechanism of PSVT is usually *reentry* that involves the AV node. The impulse continues to circulate around the AV node until the reentry pathway is interrupted (by drugs, vagal maneuvers, or spontaneously).

Junctional (AV Nodal) Rhythms: regular supraventricular rhythms in which the P wave in lead II is negative (preceding or following the QRS) or absent (Figure 3-14).

> **AV Nodal Escape Rhythm**—when the junctional rate is between 40 and 60 beats/minute and the rhythm arises because the SA node is delayed or fails in its pacemaking function (Figure 3-19, *A*)
>
> **Accelerated Junctional Rhythm**—when the junctional rate speeds up to between 61 and 99 beats/minute and takes over the pacemaking function (Figure 3-19, *B*)
>
> **Junctional Tachycardia**—when the junctional rate speeds up to over 100 beats/minute and takes over the pacemaking function (Figure 3-19, *C*)

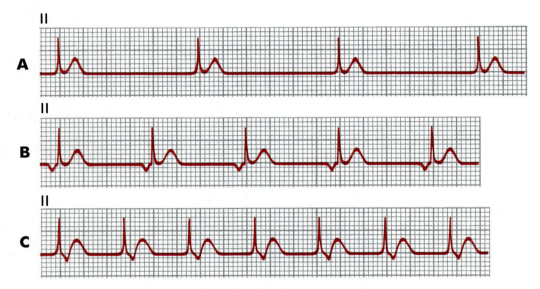

Figure 3-19.   Junctional (AV nodal) rhythms.   **A,** AV nodal escape rhythm at a rate of 50 beats/minute. In this example, *there is no evidence of atrial activity.*   **B,** Accelerated junctional rhythm at a rate of 75 beats/minute. In this example, *the P wave is negative and precedes the QRS complex, with a short PR interval.*   **C,** Junctional tachycardia at a rate of 110 beats/minute. In this example, *the P wave is negative and follows the QRS complex.*

Accelerated junctional rhythm and junctional tachycardia are relatively uncommon arrhythmias. The clinical settings in which they most commonly occur are digitalis toxicity and acute inferior infarction.

Premature Beats

Premature beats are beats that interrupt the underlying rhythm by occurring *earlier than expected*. They are of three types:

PACs (premature *atrial* contractions)—when the underlying rhythm is interrupted by an early beat arising from somewhere in the atria other than the SA node (Figure 3-20, *A*). Most often the impulse is conducted with a narrow QRS complex that is identical in appearance to that of normal sinus-conducted beats.

PJCs (premature *junctional* contractions)—when the underlying rhythm is interrupted by an early beat arising from the AV node (Figure 3-20, *B*). Most often the impulse is conducted with a narrow QRS complex that is similar or identical in appearance to that of normal sinus-conducted beats.

PVCs (premature *ventricular* contractions)—when the underlying rhythm is interrupted by an early beat arising from the ventricles (Figure 3-20, *C*). PVCs are wide and have an appearance quite different from that of normal sinus-conducted beats.

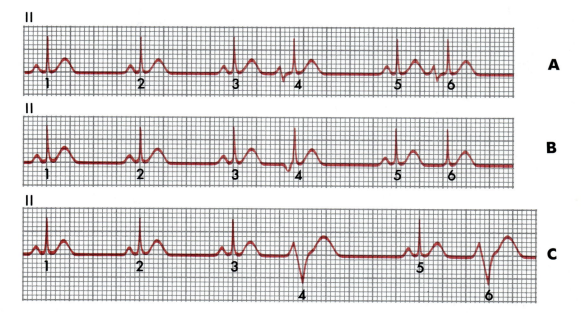

Figure 3-20. Premature beats. **A,** Sinus rhythm with PACs. *The fourth and sixth beats are preceded by premature P waves that are different in appearance from the normally conducted sinus beats. Note that the QRS complex that follows each of these PACs is narrow and identical in appearance to that of the sinus-conducted beats.* **B,** *Sinus rhythm with PJCs. The fourth and sixth beats are PJCs. The fourth beat is preceded by a negative P wave, with a short PR interval. There is no identifiable atrial activity associated with the sixth beat.* **C,** *Sinus rhythm with PVCs. The fourth and sixth beats are wide and very different in appearance from the normally conducted sinus beats. They are not preceded by P waves.*

Premature supraventricular beats (i.e., PACs or PJCs) are sometimes "blocked" (i.e., not conducted to the ventricles), or conducted with aberration (Figure 3-21). In the latter case, the QRS complex may be wide and quite different in appearance from normal sinus-conducted beats. Differentiation between premature supraventricular beats and PVCs extends beyond the scope of this chapter, and we will not treat the subject further here. Morphologic characteristics that are helpful in this differentiation are discussed in Chapter 19.

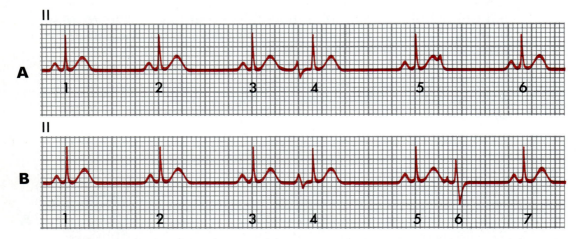

Figure 3-21. **A,** Sinus rhythm with PACs. The fourth beat is preceded by a premature P wave that conducts normally. A very early PAC notches the T wave that follows the fifth beat. This PAC is *blocked* (i.e., it does not conduct to the ventricles), and is therefore not followed by a QRS complex. **B,** Sinus rhythm with PACs. The fourth beat is preceded by a premature P wave that conducts normally. A somewhat earlier PAC immediately follows the T wave of the fifth beat. This PAC conducts with ***aberration*** (i.e., the associated QRS complex is wider and looks different from the normally conducted beats.)

As we have already implied, PACs may be quite similar in appearance to PJCs, since both of these premature beats usually have a narrow QRS complex and may be preceded by a negative P wave in lead II. Clinical implications of these two types of premature beats are identical. Practically speaking, *PACs are much more common than PJCs.*

Clinically the importance of distinguishing between PVCs and PACs or PJCs is that PVCs are much more likely to warrant treatment, especially when they occur in an emergency care setting. This is because PVCs may precipitate potentially life-threatening arrhythmias such as ventricular tachycardia or ventricular fibrillation. In contrast, neither PACs nor PJCs need to be treated, as long as the patient remains asymptomatic.

The question of whether PVCs also need to be treated in less acute settings has become highly controversial, and extends beyond the scope of this book. *The tendency is to reserve the treatment of chronic PVCs for patients who are symptomatic.*

Ventricular (⇒ *Wide QRS*) Arrhythmias

Ventricular rhythms are usually regular (or fairly regular) rhythms that arise from a focus in the ventricles. As a result, the QRS complex is wide and very different in appearance from that of normal sinus-conducted beats. Ventricular rhythms may arise as *escape* rhythms (if supraventricular pacemakers fail), or as *usurping* rhythms (when they override the preexisting supraventricular rhythm). Atrial activity is absent, unrelated to the QRS complex, or retrograde.

Idioventricular Escape Rhythm—when the ventricular rate is between 30 and 40 beats/minute (Figure 3-22, *A*).

AIVR (Accelerated IdioVentricular Rhythm)—when the ventricular rate is over 50 beats/minute, but less than 110 to 120 beats/minute. This is usually an escape rhythm (Figure 3-22, *B*).

Ventricular Tachycardia—when the ventricular rate is over 120 to 130 beats/minute. This is always a usurping rhythm (Figure 3-22, *C*).

Ventricular Fibrillation—a totally disorganized, chaotic ventricular rhythm. There is no meaningful perfusion with ventricular fibrillation (Figure 3-22, *D*).

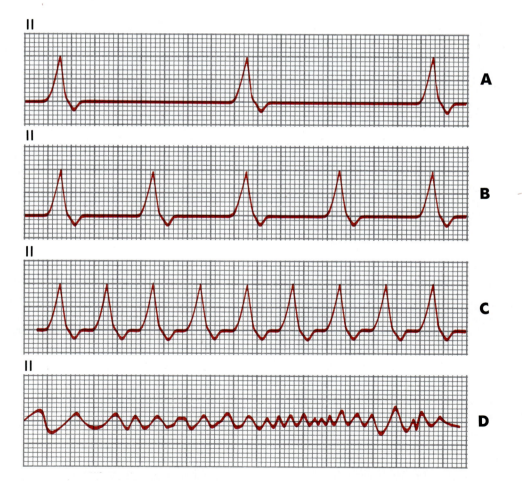

Figure 3-22.   Ventricular arrhythmias.   **A,** Idioventricular escape rhythm at 38 beats/minute.   **B,** Accelerated idioventricular rhythm (AIVR) at 75 beats/minute.   **C,** Ventricular tachycardia at 150 beats/minute.   **D,** Ventricular fibrillation.

The preceding list of arrhythmias is not complete. We do not even list the AV blocks, the concept of AV dissociation, or rhythms such as atrial tachycardia or MAT (multifocal atrial tachycardia), and we do no more than mention the concept of aberration. Nevertheless we hope that providing this basic structure will assist in differentiating among the most common arrhythmias seen on the 12-lead ECG. (Use of the 12-lead ECG in interpreting more difficult cardiac arrhythmias is discussed in Chapter 19.)

PEARLS IN RHYTHM ANALYSIS

Before closing this chapter with a series of review exercises on rhythm interpretation, let us emphasize the key points to our approach.

1. As with 12-lead ECG interpretation, the key to rhythm analysis is to have a systematic approach. The system we suggest is based on asking four questions:
    a. Is the rhythm regular?
    b. Are there P waves?
    c. Is the QRS wide or narrow?
    d. If P waves are present, are they related to the QRS complex?

    It doesn't matter which of these questions is asked first (and we often alter the sequence in which we analyze these points), as long as each of the questions is addressed with each rhythm that is interpreted.

2. The best lead to look for P waves on a 12-lead ECG is lead II. If the P wave is upright in this lead, and the PR interval is fixed (constant), practically speaking the mechanism of the rhythm must be sinus! Assessing the regularity of the rhythm and its rate will determine the type of sinus mechanism (NSR, bradycardia, tachycardia, and/or arrhythmia).

    Realize that the guidelines given for rate apply to adults only (and may be quite different in children).

    Finally, we defer discussion of the upright P wave with a short or long PR interval until Chapter 4.

3. If the P wave is not upright in lead II, some mechanism other than sinus is operative. Sometimes the answer will be obvious from inspection of lead II (as when the characteristic sawtooth pattern of atrial flutter or the negative P waves of junctional rhythm are seen). At other times, the overall irregular irregularity of the rhythm and complete absence of P waves in all 12 leads will suggest atrial fibrillation. More complex rhythm analysis extends well beyond the scope of this book.

4. Next to lead II, we find lead V_1 the most helpful for visualizing atrial activity. If atrial activity is not seen in either of these leads, search for it in the remaining 10 leads before assuming it is absent.

5. If the QRS complex is narrow in all 12 leads (i.e., not *greater* than half a large box), the rhythm is supraventricular.

6. If the rhythm is fast or normal, upright P waves are not apparent in lead II, and the QRS complex is wide, there are three possibilities:
   a. The rhythm is still supraventricular but some type of bundle branch block or conduction defect is present. (We discuss this in detail in Chapter 5).
   b. The rhythm is supraventricular and there is aberrant conduction.
   c. The rhythm is ventricular tachycardia. This is by far the most common cause of a regular, wide complex tachycardia in which normal sinus P waves are absent.

These three possibilities make up the first of our lists. Note how we have prioritized the entities in this list (Table 3-3) for emphasis.

Table 3-3
Causes of a Regular, Wide Complex Tachycardia
1. Ventricular tachycardia 2. VENTRICULAR TACHYCARDIA 3. **VENTRICULAR TACHYCARDIA** 4. SVT with preexisting bundle branch block 5. SVT with aberrant conduction

PRACTICE

Interpret the following rhythm strips (Figures 3-23 to 3-38). All are taken from lead II. Write your answers out (using the systematic four-question approach of Table 3-1) *before* looking at our answers.

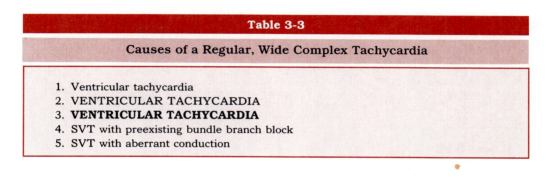

Figure 3-23

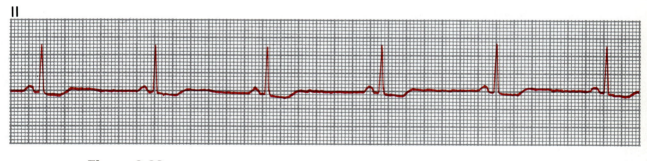

Figure 3-24

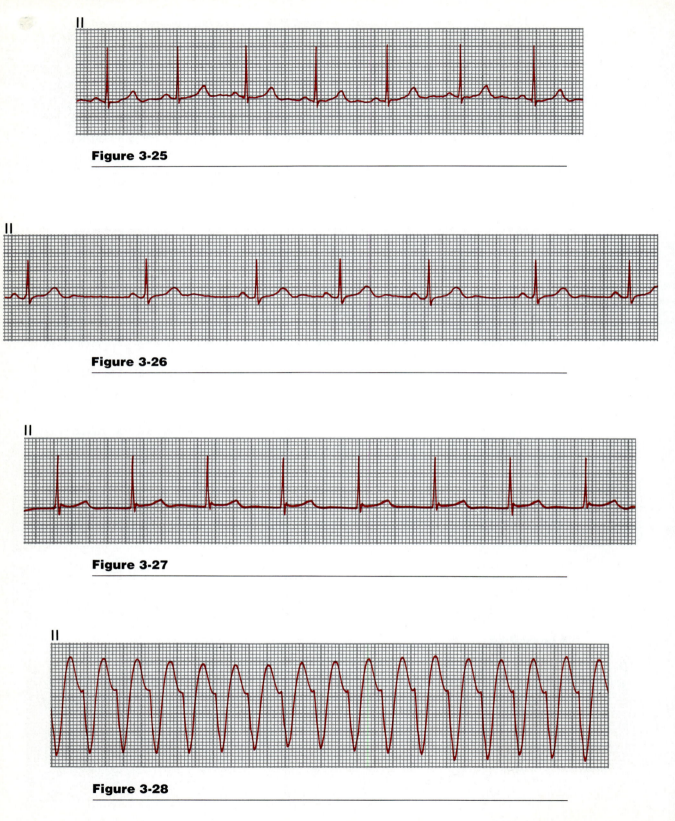

Figure 3-25

Figure 3-26

Figure 3-27

Figure 3-28

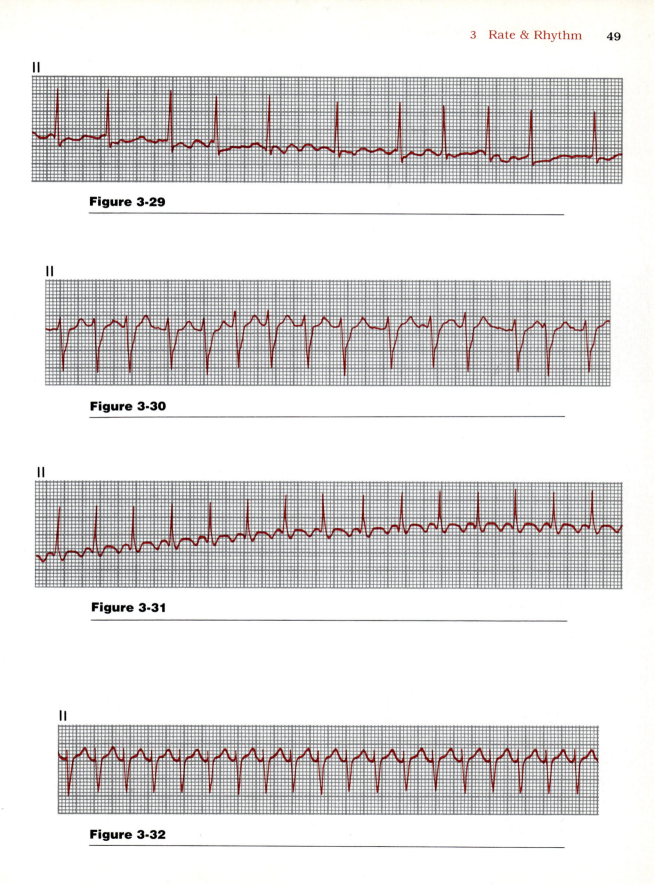

Figure 3-29

Figure 3-30

Figure 3-31

Figure 3-32

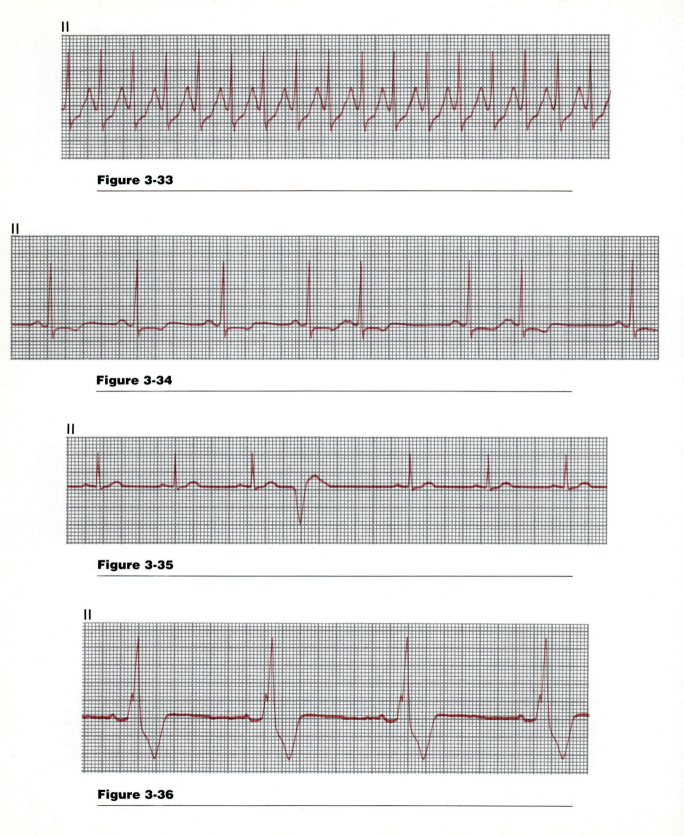

II

Figure 3-33

II

Figure 3-34

II

Figure 3-35

II

Figure 3-36

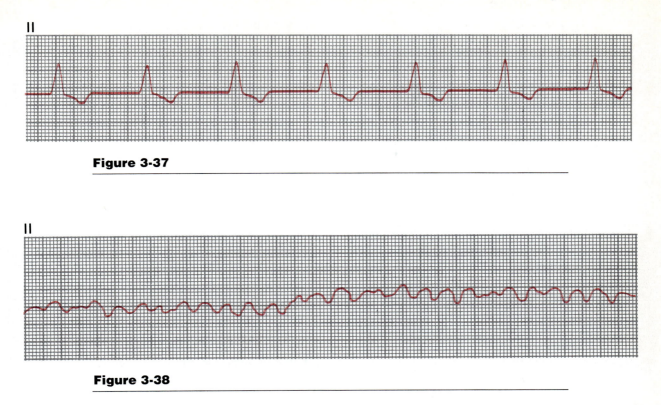

Figure 3-37

Figure 3-38

ANSWERS TO PRACTICE TRACINGS

Figure 3-23: The rhythm is regular at a rate of just under 50 beats/minute. Upright P waves precede each QRS complex, with a constant PR interval. The QRS complex is narrow. This is *sinus bradycardia*.

Figure 3-24: The rhythm is regular, at a rate of about 115 beats/minute. The QRS complex is narrow (i.e., it is not *greater* than half a large box). Atrial activity is absent. This is an AV nodal rhythm. Because the rate is over 100 beats/minute, we call this *junctional tachycardia*.

Figure 3-25: The rhythm is regular, at a rate of 75 beats/minute. Upright P waves precede each QRS complex, with a constant PR interval. The QRS complex is narrow. This is *normal sinus rhythm (NSR)*.

Figure 3-26: The rhythm is not regular, but varies from beat to beat. Nevertheless, the QRS complex is narrow and upright P waves precede each QRS complex, with a constant PR interval. Thus, the mechanism of the rhythm is sinus. Because the rate is slow as well as variable, this is *sinus arrhythmia and bradycardia*. The heart rate varies between 45 and 65 beats/minute (since the R-R interval varies between about seven and just less than five large boxes).

Figure 3-27: The rhythm is regular, at a rate of 72 beats/minute. The QRS complex is narrow. Atrial activity is absent. This is an AV nodal rhythm. Since the rate is faster than usual for an AV nodal escape rhythm (which is usually between 40 and 60 beats/minute in adults), but less than the 100 beats/minute definition of "tachycardia," we call this an *accelerated junctional rhythm.*

Figure 3-28: This is a regular, wide-complex tachycardia in which definite atrial activity cannot be identified. The rate is just over 150 beats/minute. As suggested by Table 3-3, *ventricular tachycardia* should always be assumed as the etiology until proven otherwise.

Figure 3-29: The rhythm is irregularly irregular, and no regular (repetitive) atrial activity can be identified. The QRS complex is narrow. The rhythm is *atrial fibrillation with a controlled ventricular response* (since most R-R intervals are between 2½ and four large boxes, corresponding to a rate between 80 and 120 beats/minute). The coarse undulations of the baseline are "fib waves."

Figure 3-30: Once again the rhythm is irregularly irregular. Definite (repetitive) atrial activity is absent. Thus the rhythm is again *atrial fibrillation,* this time with a *rapid ventricular response* (since the rate is consistently over 110 to 120 beats/minute).

Note that "fib waves" are less prominent in this example than they were in Figure 3-29. Note also that the QRS complex appears to be wide in this example. This probably reflects underlying bundle branch block. Despite QRS widening, the gross, irregular irregularity of the rhythm strongly suggests that the rhythm is atrial fibrillation rather than ventricular tachycardia.

Figure 3-31: This is a regular, supraventricular tachycardia at a rate just under 150 beats/minute. Although one might consider sinus tachycardia and PSVT in the differential diagnosis, the rhythm is actually *atrial flutter.* The arrows below suggest atrial activity ("flutter waves") at a rate of about 300 beats/minute, which would make the rhythm *atrial flutter with a 2:1 AV response.*

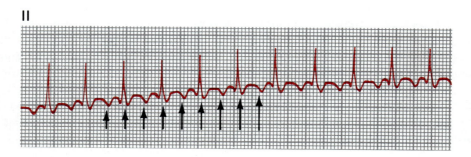

The rhythm shown in Figure 3-31, with arrows suggesting atrial (flutter) activity at a rate of about 300 beats/minute.

In our experience, atrial flutter is by far the most commonly overlooked arrhythmia. This is because flutter activity is often even more subtle than it is in

Figure 3-31. *Whenever a patient has a regular, supraventricular tachycardia at a rate close to 150 beats/minute, strongly consider atrial flutter in the differential diagnosis.* A clue to the presence of atrial flutter in this example is, in addition to the rate, the fact that normal sinus activity is absent. If one construes the upright deflection preceding each QRS complex in Figure 3-31 as a P wave, the PR interval is too short to have been conducted by the normal pathway. And, if the negative deflection preceding each QRS complex in Figure 3-31 reflects atrial activity, the mechanism of the rhythm still couldn't be sinus because the P wave would have to be upright in lead II for sinus rhythm to be present.

The tracing below shows the effect of a vagal maneuver (in this case, **carotid sinus massage)** on the arrhythmia. Application of firm pressure to the area of the carotid sinus (at the angle of the jaw) for 3 to 5 seconds transiently increases vagal tone, which may transiently slow the ventricular response by increasing the degree of "block" at the AV node. The result is a decrease in the rate of AV conduction from 2:1 to 4:1. Note how much easier it is to be sure of flutter activity when there is 4:1 AV conduction *(see small arrows).*

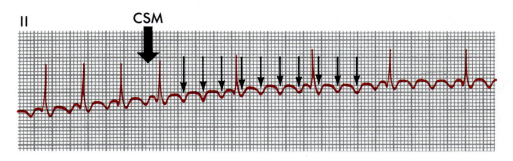

Application of **CSM (carotid sinus massage)** to the rhythm shown in Figure 3-31 decreases the rate of AV conduction from 2:1 to 4:1. This allows atrial activity to become more evident *(small arrows),* and confirms the rhythm to be atrial flutter.

Although CSM will not convert atrial flutter to sinus rhythm, it often confirms the diagnosis, allowing the treating clinician to confidently use appropriate therapy (drugs or cardioversion).

Figure 3-32: This is a regular, supraventricular tachycardia at a rate just under 200 beats/minute. Once again, the diagnostic possibilities should include atrial flutter, sinus tachycardia, and PSVT.

In this example, calculation of the heart rate provides an important clue to the etiology of the rhythm. Sinus tachycardia in adults rarely exceeds 150 to 160 beats/minute, so it is unlikely in this case. Similarly, with *untreated* atrial flutter, the ventricular response is almost always between 140 and 160 beats/minute (reflecting 2:1 AV conduction at the usual atrial rate of approximately 300 beats/minute). This leaves PSVT as the most likely diagnosis for the rhythm shown in Figure 3-32.

Figure 3-33: The rhythm is regular, at a rate of 160 beats/minute. The QRS complex appears to be narrow in this lead, although it is not completely possible to be sure where the QRS complex ends and the ST segment begins from this one monitoring lead. *A full, 12-lead ECG would be needed to verify that the QRS complex is truly narrow (and to rule out the possibility of ventricular tachycardia).*

If other leads confirmed that the QRS complex is narrow, we would again be left with three diagnostic possibilities: atrial flutter, PSVT, and sinus tachycardia.

In Figure 3-33, the upright deflection preceding the QRS complex may well be a P wave. If this were the case, the rhythm would be sinus tachycardia. However, if instead of being a P wave, this upright deflection was really the T wave, the rhythm would be PSVT. Finally, one cannot completely rule out the possibility that the rhythm is atrial flutter (with flutter waves hiding within the ST segment). *Thus, it is not really possible to be certain of the etiology of this tachyarrhythmia from the single monitoring lead shown in Figure 3-33.*

Figure 3-34: The underlying rhythm is sinus, at a rate of 65 beats/minute. This can be determined from observing the first four beats in the tracing. The fifth beat is early, and is preceded by a P wave with a slightly different morphology from normal. This is a PAC. The sixth beat is again sinus, and the seventh, another PAC. The last beat in the tracing is sinus.

Thus, the rhythm is *sinus with PACs*. Note that the QRS complex is narrow and identical in morphology for all of the beats in this tracing.

Figure 3-35: The underlying rhythm is sinus, at a rate of 65 to 70 beats/minute. The fourth beat is early, wide, and very different in morphology from the sinus-conducted beats. It is a PVC. The last three beats in the tracing are sinus.

Thus the rhythm is *sinus with a PVC*.

Figure 3-36: The rhythm is fairly regular, at a rate in the low 40s. Despite the fact that the QRS complex is wide, the mechanism of the rhythm is sinus because upright P waves precede each QRS complex, with a constant PR interval. Thus, the rhythm is *sinus bradycardia*. A bundle branch block is present.

Figure 3-37: The rhythm is regular, at a rate of 60 beats/minute. The QRS complex is wide. Atrial activity is absent. Thus, this is a ventricular rhythm. Since the ventricular rate is faster than one would usually expect, we call this an *accelerated idioventricular rhythm (AIVR)*.

A question that often arises is whether the rhythm in Figure 3-37 could be junctional with a preexisting bundle branch block or with aberrant conduction. Although either of these explanations is possible, they are both much less common than AIVR. Thus, unless there is clinical evidence to the contrary, it is best to assume that the rhythm in Figure 3-37 is AIVR.

Figure 3-38: This is ventricular fibrillation. It is a totally disorganized, chaotic ventricular rhythm. *With luck, you won't see this on any of the 12-lead tracings you'll be asked to interpret!*

This concludes our chapter on rhythm interpretation. We would like to again emphasize that comprehensive rhythm analysis extends beyond the scope of this book. We also acknowledge that a number of the examples we chose to present in the review exercises (Figures 3-23 through 3-38) were somewhat difficult (if not downright tricky). Our purpose was *not* to trick you. Instead, our goal was to reinforce the basic concepts involved in rhythm interpretation, and to demonstrate how application of these basic concepts can facilitate interpretation of the most common arrhythmias.

The majority of rhythms in the remainder of this book will be sinus in mechanism. However, to keep you "honest," we'll occasionally slip in a few other arrhythmias.

SUGGESTED READINGS

Grauer K and Cavallaro D: ACLS: certification preparation and a comprehensive review, ed: 2, St Louis, 1987, The CV Mosby Company.

Grauer K and Cavallaro D: ACLS: Mega Code review/study cards, St Louis, 1988, The CV Mosby Co.

4

The PR Interval

As we emphasized in Chapter 2, assessment of intervals *early* in the process of systematic analysis is critical. Failure to do so makes it all too easy to overlook Wolff-Parkinson-White (WPW) syndrome or QT prolongation, or to misdiagnose infarction or ischemia when the correct diagnosis is bundle branch block.

We therefore suggest that assessment of intervals be done immediately after rhythm analysis. The three key intervals to consider are the PR interval, the QRS interval, and the QT interval. In this chapter we discuss the PR interval. The QRS and QT intervals follow in Chapters 5 and 6.

MEASUREMENT OF THE PR INTERVAL

As we discussed in the section on intervals in Chapter 1, the PR interval is the period from the onset of atrial depolarization (beginning of the P wave) until the onset of ventricular depolarization (beginning of the QRS complex).

The best lead to measure the PR interval in is lead II. In adults, if the P wave is upright in this lead (i.e., if there is sinus mechanism), the PR interval is considered normal if it is between 0.12 second and 0.21 second.

DETERMINING IF THE PR INTERVAL IS ABNORMAL

A large part of the PR interval is normally made up of the delay of the impulse in passing through the AV node. If the PR interval is short (i.e., less than 0.12 second), it may be because the impulse has avoided passage through the normal conduction pathway. This can occur when there is an accessory pathway (as in WPW, which we discuss in the addendum to Chapter 5).

If the PR interval is long (i.e., clearly *greater* than 0.21 second), we say that **1° AV block** is present. All atrial impulses are still conducted with this form of AV block—they simply take longer to travel through the normal conduction pathway. This differs from 2° and 3° AV blocks, in which not all atrial impulses are conducted.

In general, we do *NOT* spend a lot of time precisely measuring the PR interval. Practically speaking, it matters little whether the PR interval is 0.15 or 0.18 second, since both measurements are within the normal range. We feel it suffices in either case to simply state that the PR interval is "normal." Furthermore, we don't believe in applying the term "borderline 1° AV block" when the PR interval is between 0.19 and 0.20 second. This is because the *isolated* finding of 1° AV block (in the absence of other cardiac pathology) has virtually no clinical significance (or impact on prognosis). A "borderline" call of a clinically insignificant finding would therefore be of even less importance. Finally, because the PR interval may normally be as much as 0.21 second (especially in elderly individuals), we tend not to call 1° AV block unless the PR interval is *at least* 0.22 second. Table 4-1 *(which also appears on p. 11 in the pocket reference)* summarizes this information.

Table 4-1
Assessing the PR Interval

1. Verify that the patient is in sinus rhythm (by verifying that the P wave is upright in lead II). Measurement of the PR interval means little in the absence of a sinus mechanism.

2. If there is a sinus mechanism and the PR interval in lead II is:
   - < 0.12 second ⇒ The PR is short
   - 0.12 to 0.21 second ⇒ The PR is normal
   - ≥ 0.22 second ⇒ The PR is long (= 1° AV block)

   > *Thus, the* **PR interval** *is* **short** *if it is less than 3 little boxes and* **long** *if it is clearly more than a large box!*

3. Precise measurement of a PR interval that falls within the normal range is not necessary. Clinically it suffices to say that the PR interval is "normal."

4. The limits given above do not necessarily hold true for children (for whom lesser degrees of PR prolongation are abnormal).

5

The QRS Interval/Bundle Branch Block

The QRS interval represents the time it takes for ventricular depolarization. Normally this process is complete in no more than 0.10 second in adults. As may be expected, depolarization of the thinner ventricles of children takes less time, so that the upper normal limit for QRS duration in children is correspondingly less.

There are two principal causes of QRS prolongation: left-ventricular thickening or hypertrophy (i.e., LVH) and abnormalities in conduction (bundle branch block, intraventricular conduction delay, hemiblocks, or Wolff-Parkinson-White syndrome). Ventricular hypertrophy sometimes produces QRS prolongation because of the longer time required for the electrical impulse to travel through a thicker ventricle. Abnormalities in conduction produce QRS prolongation by altering the sequence of ventricular depolarization and/or the ability of specialized conduction tissue (such as the bundle branches) to conduct.

MEASUREMENT OF THE QRS INTERVAL

Practically speaking, QRS duration can be measured in any of the 12 leads of a standard ECG. There is no lower limit of normal. All one is concerned with is whether QRS duration is normal or prolonged. As was the case for PR interval assessment, it matters little whether the QRS measures out to 0.07, 0.08, or 0.10 second, since all of these values are within the normal range. Thus, if the QRS appears "narrow," we don't feel there is value in precisely measuring its duration. Simply say the QRS is normal, and move on.

Realize that sometimes the QRS complex may appear narrow in one lead, but in reality be quite wide. This is because a portion of the QRS complex may be *equiphasic,* or *isoelectric* (lie on the baseline). For this reason, it is essential to always examine *all* 12 leads in assessing QRS duration. Use the lead in which the QRS appears to be longest. Measure from the onset of the Q wave (or the onset of the R if there is no Q) until the termination of the QRS complex. Since a large box on ECG grid paper represents 0.20 second, *this means that for there to be QRS widening, the QRS complex must clearly be GREATER than half of a large box in duration* (i.e., >0.10 seconds).

58

This information is summarized in Table 5-1 *(which also appears on p. 12 in the pocket reference).*

Table 5-1
Assessing QRS Duration

1. QRS duration can be measured from any of the 12 leads of a standard ECG.
2. All that matters is whether the QRS is normal or wide. Precise measurement of a QRS complex that is clearly of normal duration is unnecessary.
3. Judge QRS prolongation from the lead where the QRS appears to be longest.
4. If the QRS is:
   ≤0.10 second ⇒ The QRS is normal
   >0.10 second (i.e., clearly *GREATER* than half a large box) ⇒ The QRS is wide
5. The limits given above do not hold true for children (for whom lesser degrees of QRS prolongation are abnormal).

IF THE QRS IS WIDE

If the QRS complex is wide, we suggest you *short-circuit* your systematic approach and immediately branch to the algorithm shown in Figure 5-1 *(which also appears on p. 13 in the pocket reference).*

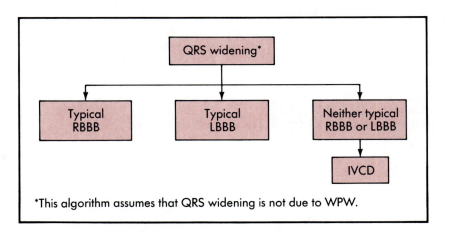

Figure 5-1.   Algorithm for assessment of QRS widening.

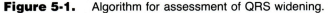

Evaluation of QRS widening is the *ONLY* situation in which we suggest you vary from the systematic approach. Our reasons for suggesting this are:

1. To save time
2. To improve diagnostic accuracy

As we will soon see, the presence of bundle branch block often makes diagnosis of chamber enlargement, infarction, and ischemia quite difficult. Recognition of the cause of QRS widening *early* in the process alerts the interpreter to this possibility, and may prevent misinterpretation of Q waves and ST segment changes that can be explained by the bundle branch block.

Thus, if the QRS is wide, determine why *before* going any further. By far, the easiest way to approach the bundle branch blocks is to accept only three possible explanations for the wide QRS*:

1. The QRS is wide because of *typical* **RBBB.**
2. The QRS is wide because of *typical* **LBBB.**
3. If the QRS is wide, but *neither* typical RBBB nor typical LBBB is present, there is **IVCD** (intraventricular conduction delay).

Diagnosis of bundle branch block can be made from examination of the three *KEY* leads. The three KEY leads are **I**, **V₁**, and **V₆**. Practically speaking, these are the *ONLY* three leads you need to look at to diagnose RBBB and LBBB!

Leads **I** and **V₆** are *left*-sided leads. Most of the time they will look quite similar to each other with RBBB and LBBB, but sometimes they may show subtle differences. This is why it is essential to always look at *both* of these leads. Lead aVL is also a left-sided lead, and it will also usually resemble what is seen in leads I and V₆. However, you *don't* need to look at lead aVL to diagnose the bundle branch blocks.

Lead **V₁** is a right-sided and anterior lead. For practical purposes in understanding the bundle branch blocks, it is easiest to think of lead V₁ as a *right*-sided lead. Even though leads V₂ and V₃ often closely resemble lead V₁, you *don't* need to look at them to diagnose the bundle branch blocks. Figure 5-2 schematically shows these relationships.

---

*This algorithm assumes that QRS widening is not due to WPW.

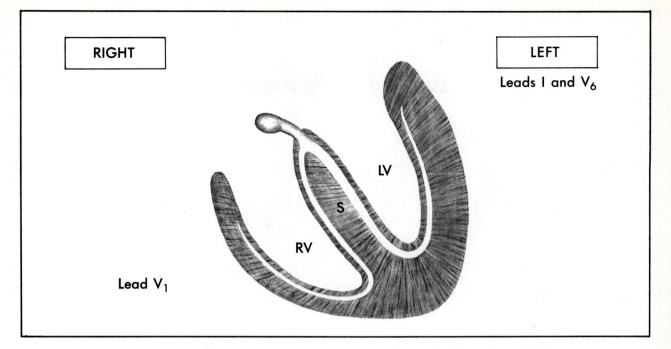

Figure 5-2.   Schematic representation of the three KEY leads for diagnosing the bundle branch blocks. Lead V₁ is a *right*-sided lead, while leads I and V₆ are *left*-sided leads. *S,* Interventricular septum; *RV,* right ventricle; *LV,* left ventricle.

With normal conduction, the first part of the ventricles to be activated is the *left* side of the septum. The electrical impulse then traverses the septum to activate the other side. Shortly thereafter, the left and right ventricles are simultaneously activated. Because the left ventricle is normally so much larger and thicker than the right ventricle, its electrical activity predominates over the electrical activity of the right ventricle (Figure 5-3).

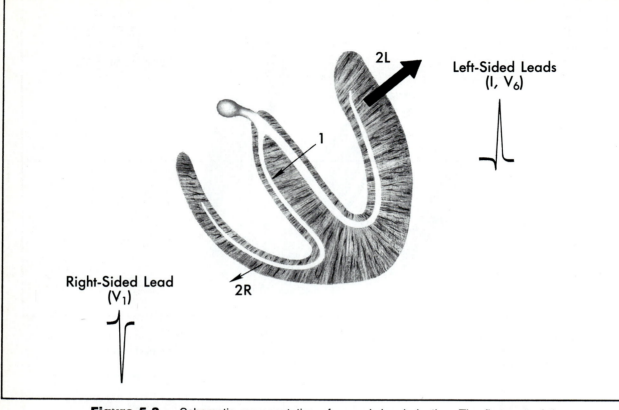

Figure 5-3.   Schematic representation of normal depolarization. The first part of the ventricles to be activated is the *left* side of the septum *(arrow 1)*. Shortly thereafter, the left and right ventricles are simultaneously activated *(arrows 2L and 2R,* respectively). Because the left ventricle is so much larger than the right venticle, its electrical activity predominates.

Note that the QRS complex in the left-sided leads of Figure 5-3 is predominantly upright. This is usually the case, because the left ventricle is normally so much larger and thicker than the right ventricle that overall electrical activity is seen as being directed toward the left. In contrast, the QRS complex in right-sided lead V_1 is predominantly negative in Figure 5-3. This is because right-sided leads see the overall process of ventricular activation as predominantly moving *away* from the right (i.e., toward the left).

There is often a small initial r wave in lead V_1. This reflects the fact that this right-sided lead sees the electrical impulse coming toward it as the septum is depolarized. Similarly, leads I and V_6 often demonstrate a small initial q wave, reflecting the fact that electrical activity initially moves *away* from the left as the septum is depolarized. Because it is so common to see small q waves in left-sided leads, they are often called *normal septal q waves.*

TYPICAL RBBB

Right bundle branch block (RBBB) reflects an alteration of the *terminal* portion of ventricular activation. The initial portion of ventricular activation is for the most part unaffected (Figure 5-4, *A*). Following activation of the septum, the left ventricle is activated (Figure 5-4, *B*). But because of the block, right-ventricular activation will be delayed until *after* the left ventricle has already depolarized (Figure 5-4, *C*). As a result, *terminal electrical activity in the ECG is directed toward the right* (i.e., toward lead V_1) *and away from the left* (i.e., away from leads I and V_6).

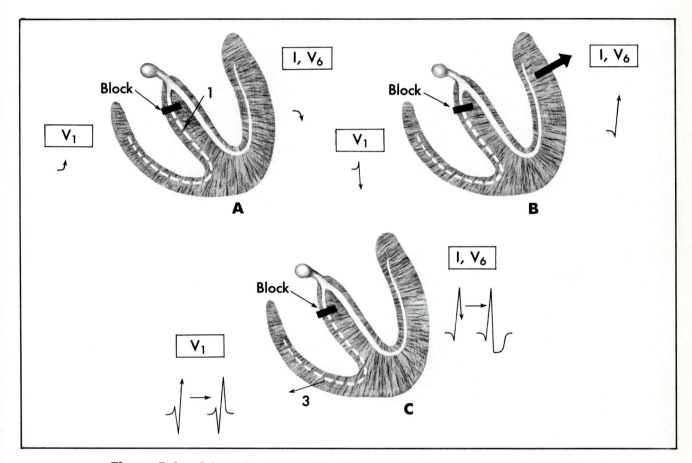

Figure 5-4.   Schematic representation of ventricular activation in RBBB. **A,** The initial portion of ventricular activation (septal activation, represented by arrow 1) is for the most part unaffected in RBBB. **B,** The left ventricle is then activated. Because of the block, right-ventricular activation is delayed and left-ventricular depolarization occurs alone. **C,** The right ventricle is finally activated. *Because the right ventricle is activated alone, terminal electrical activity with RBBB is directed toward the right (i.e., toward lead V_1) and away from the left (i.e., away from leads I and V_6).*

Clinically, typical RBBB is diagnosed by the following (Figure 5-5):

QRS widening of *at least* 0.11 seconds
An rSR′ or rsR′ in lead V₁
A wide terminal S wave in leads I and V₆. The QRS is usually predominantly positive in left-sided leads with RBBB. There may or may not be an initial small q wave. The key to the diagnosis is the finding of a *wide terminal S wave* in these leads.

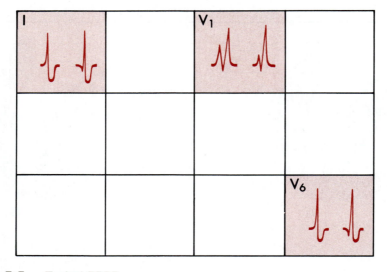

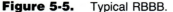

Figure 5-5.   Typical RBBB.

It can be seen from Figure 5-4 that the reason for the tall R′ in lead V₁ is the *terminal* delay in right-ventricular activation. The last portion of ventricular depolarization is thus directed to the right (i.e., toward lead V₁), and results in production of a tall R′ wave. Because the right ventricle depolarizes alone, it is able to produce a large deflection (the R′) despite the relatively small size of this chamber.

Similarly, the wide terminal S wave in left-sided leads I and V₆ results from the fact that the last portion of ventricular activation is directed *away* from the left (i.e., *toward* the right). The reason the S wave is wide is that conduction through the right ventricle is much slower in RBBB. As a result of the conduction defect, right-ventricular activation has had to take place by spread of the impulse through nonspecialized myocardial tissue—a much slower process than conduction over an intact bundle branch.

To emphasize the importance of focusing on the three KEY leads (I, V₁, and V₆) for diagnosis of the bundle branch blocks, we have omitted the other nine leads from Figure 5-5, as well as from many of the other schematic tracings used in this chapter.

TYPICAL LBBB

In contrast to RBBB, left bundle branch block (LBBB) reflects an alteration in conduction of the *initial* portion of ventricular activation. As a result, the initial direction of ventricular activation with LBBB is changed so that septal activation begins on the right and moves toward the left (Figure 5-6, *A*). The electrical impulse then travels down the intact right bundle branch and spreads across the ventricular septum to activate the left ventricle. Practically speaking, it is easiest to think of the process of ventricular activation in LBBB as being primarily directed to the left (Figure 5-6, *B*).

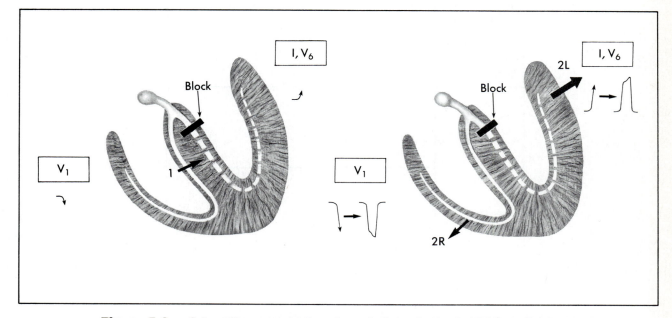

Figure 5-6.   Schematic representation of ventricular activation in LBBB. **A,** The initial direction of ventricular activation is altered with LBBB. As a result, the septum is activated from right to left *(arrow 1)*. **B,** The electrical impulse then travels down the intact right bundle branch *(arrow 2R)* and spreads across the ventricular septum to activate the left ventricle *(arrow 2L)*. *Practically speaking, it is easiest to think of the process of ventricular activation in LBBB as being primarily directed to the left.*

Because LBBB alters the initial portion of ventricular activation, and because Q waves are normally inscribed during this initial period, interpretation of Q waves is much more difficult in LBBB. It is therefore much more difficult to diagnose infarction when this conduction disorder is present. In contrast, RBBB does *not* affect the initial period of ventricular depolarization. As a result, it is not as difficult to diagnose infarction in the presence of RBBB.

Clinically, typical LBBB is diagnosed by the following (Figure 5-7):

QRS widening of *at least* 0.12 second.

An upright (monophasic) **QRS complex in leads I and V$_6$.** The QRS may be notched. There should *not* be any q wave in either lead I or lead V$_6$.

A predominantly negative QRS complex in lead V$_1$. There may or may not be an initial small r wave in lead V$_1$. (That is, *lead V$_1$ may show either a QS or an rS complex.*)

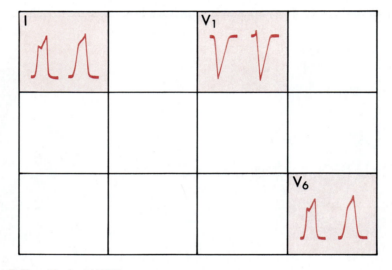

Figure 5-7.   Typical LBBB.

Thus, the conduction defect in **LBBB** alters the *initial* sequence of ventricular depolarization (and therefore affects Q wave development). It produces a predominantly *leftward* direction of ventricular activation, which explains why the QRS complex is upright in left-sided leads I and V$_6$, and predominantly negative in right-sided lead V$_1$. *The small, normal septal q waves that are often seen in leads I and V$_6$ are absent in LBBB.*

IVCD

Intraventricular conduction delay (IVCD) is a much more difficult conduction defect to characterize than either RBBB or LBBB. This is because IVCD often reflects a combination of several pathophysiologic processes including infarction, fibrosis, and ventricular hypertrophy, as well as a component of bundle branch block. This is why many patients with IVCD have some type of underlying heart disease such as prior infarction or cardiomyopathy.

Clinically, diagnosis of IVCD can be simplified by saying it is present if:

The QRS complex is wide (i.e., ≥ 0.11 second)

Neither typical RBBB nor typical LBBB is present. At times the QRS complex may resemble typical RBBB or LBBB in one or two of the key leads. As long as the typical morphology for RBBB or LBBB is missing in one or more of the key leads, we favor labeling the conduction defect as IVCD.

Diagnosis of the bundle branch blocks is summarized in Figure 5-8 *(which also appears on p. 14 of the pocket reference).*

	Lead V₁	Leads I and V₆	QRS duration
Typical RBBB	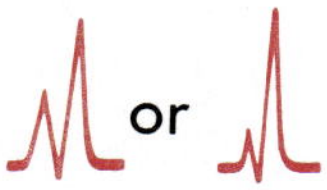 or	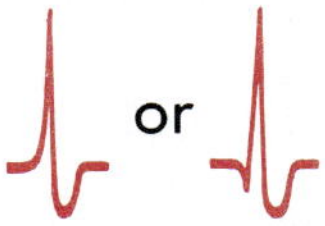 or	≥0.11 sec
Typical LBBB	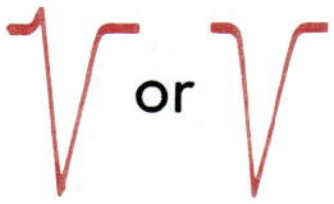 or	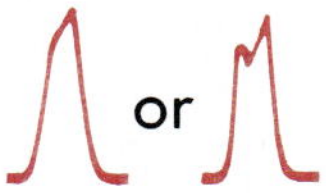 or	≥0.12 sec
IVCD	Neither typical RBBB nor LBBB morphology in the three key leads		≥0.11 sec

Figure 5-8.   Diagnosis of typical RBBB, typical LBBB, and IVCD.

In addition to the application of QRS morphology in diagnosing the type of conduction defect on a 12-lead ECG, attention to QRS morphology in the three KEY leads may prove invaluable in determining the etiology of wide-complex tachycardias. We discuss this application in detail in Chapter 19.

TYPICAL SECONDARY ST SEGMENT AND T WAVE CHANGES WITH RBBB AND LBBB

RBBB and LBBB each alter the sequence of ventricular depolarization. This is why they produce the alterations in QRS morphology that we have just discussed. As a direct result of this altered sequence of activation, these conduction defects also produce an alteration in the sequence of ventricular repolarization. This is known as a **secondary ST-T wave change.** It is *secondary* to (i.e., the direct result of) the conduction defect itself. As such, it is a normal, expected finding with bundle branch block, and does not reflect ischemia or infarction.

It is easy to determine if the ST-T wave changes seen with either RBBB or LBBB are the normal *(secondary)* changes one would expect to see with the conduction defect. All one has to do is remember the following rule:

Orientation of the ST segment and T wave with typical RBBB and LBBB is opposite to that of the last QRS deflection in each of the three KEY leads.

Expected ST-T wave changes with IVCD are harder to anticipate, and unfortunately will not always obey this rule.

Application of the rule for anticipating the normal (secondary) ST-T wave changes with typical RBBB and typical LBBB is illustrated in Figure 5-9 *(which also appears on p. 15 of the pocket reference).*

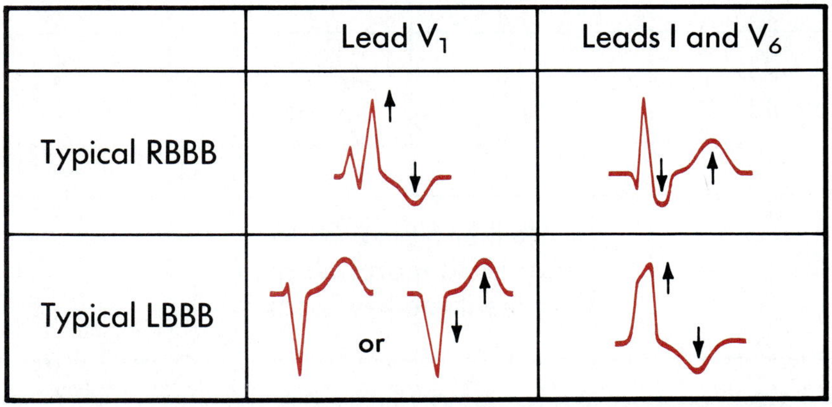

	Lead V$_1$	Leads I and V$_6$
Typical RBBB		
Typical LBBB	or	

Figure 5-9.   Typical secondary ST-T wave changes of RBBB and LBBB. The ST segment and T wave are oriented *opposite* to the direction of the last QRS deflection in these conduction defects.

Thus, with typical RBBB, the last QRS deflection is *upright* in lead V$_1$ (an R′). As a result, the ST segment and T wave are normally negative in this lead with RBBB (Figure 5-9). Similarly, the last QRS deflection in leads I and V$_6$ is negative in RBBB (the wide terminal S wave). As a result, the normal, expected secondary ST-T wave change in these leads is an upright T wave.

This same line of reasoning explains why the typical secondary changes of LBBB are an upright T wave in lead V$_1$ and a negative ST segment and T wave in leads I and V$_6$.

Deviation from the above ST-T wave changes in any of the key leads in typical RBBB or LBBB indicates a **primary ST-T wave change** and suggests ischemia and/or infarction may be occurring.

REVIEW—HOW GOOD ARE YOU AT DIAGNOSING BBB?

To check your mastery of the concepts we have covered thus far on assessing the causes of QRS prolongation, examine the following three simulated tracings (Figures 5-10, 5-11, and 5-12). Imagine that the QRS complex is wide in each case. For each tracing, indicate:

1. If the conduction defect suggests typical RBBB, typical LBBB, or IVCD
2. If normal secondary changes of bundle branch block are present in the key leads, or if there are primary changes

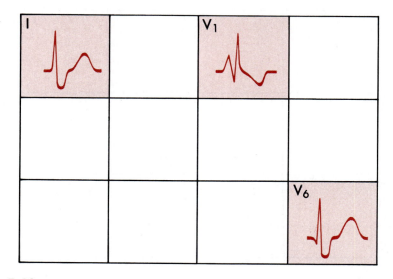

Figure 5-10.

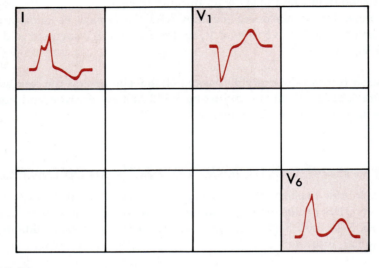

Figure 5-11.

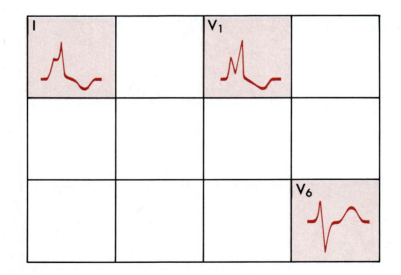

Figure 5-12.

Answers

Figure 5-10: QRS morphology in the three key leads (I, V_1, and V_6) is typical of RBBB. An rSR′ is seen in V_1, and a wide terminal S wave is seen in both leads I and V_6. Typical ST-T wave changes are present, since the ST-T wave is oriented opposite to the direction of the last QRS deflection in each of these leads. Thus, Figure 5-10 illustrates a typical, uncomplicated RBBB.

Figure 5-11: QRS morphology in the three key leads is typical of LBBB. A QS is seen in lead V_1, and a monophasic R wave is seen in leads I and V_6. (The R wave is notched in lead I.) Typical secondary ST-T wave changes are seen in leads I and V_1, but *NOT* in lead V_6. Normally with LBBB, one would expect the ST segment and T wave to be negative in this lead. Instead they are upright. Thus, Figure 5-11 illustrates a LBBB with a primary T wave change in lead V_6 (that suggests the possibility of underlying ischemia!).

Figure 5-12: QRS morphology in lead I suggests LBBB. However, the rsR′ in lead V_1 and wide terminal S wave in lead V_6 are not consistent with this diagnosis. QRS morphology in leads V_1 and V_6 instead suggests RBBB—but the QRS appearance in lead I is not consistent with RBBB (since there is no terminal S wave). Thus, neither typical LBBB nor typical RBBB is present—which means that the diagnosis is IVCD.

In this particular example, ST-T wave changes do obey the expected rule for secondary changes of bundle branch block (the ST-T wave is oriented opposite to the last deflection of the QRS complex)—but this will *not* always be the case with IVCD.

CLINICAL PEARLS ON DIAGNOSIS OF THE BUNDLE BRANCH BLOCKS

Much confusion surrounds ECG diagnosis of the bundle branch blocks. We conclude this chapter with the following section in the hope of relieving some of this confusion. Many of the following points are subtle and/or of a rather advanced nature. They will probably make a lot more sense if read (or reread) after completion of this book.

Will there always be a neat rSR′ (or rsR′) in lead V_1 with RBBB?

No. The shape of the QRS complex in lead V_1 may vary greatly with RBBB (Figure 5-13, *which also appears on p. 14 of the pocket reference*).

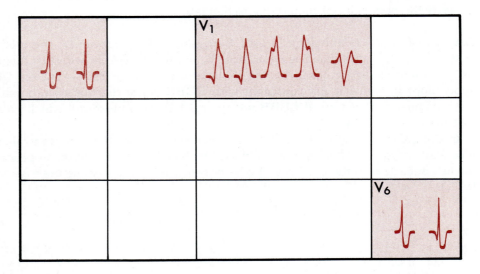

Figure 5-13.   Examples of variations of QRS morphology in lead V_1 in RBBB.

For example, after an anteroseptal infarction, one is likely to see a qR (or a QR) in lead V_1. You can still diagnose complete RBBB if:

The QRS complex is at least 0.11 second
There are terminal wide S waves in both leads I and V_6

We call the variations of QRS morphology in lead V_1 *RBBB-equivalent patterns* when (if) the other two criteria for diagnosing RBBB (QRS widening and wide terminal S waves in leads I and V_6) are met.

What is incomplete RBBB?

Incomplete RBBB is said to be present if QRS morphology is typical of RBBB (i.e., if there is an rsR′ or rSr′ in V_1 and a terminal S wave in leads I and V_6), but the QRS complex is *less* than 0.11 second.

Incomplete RBBB is a common clinical finding. It is often present in patients with COPD, right ventricular hypertrophy (RVH), or certain types of congenital heart disease (especially atrial septal defect), or as a normal variant in otherwise healthy, normal adults.

Is there also an incomplete LBBB?

Technically, yes. Practically speaking, we suggest you forget about looking for (or thinking about) incomplete LBBB.

Can you diagnose myocardial infarction in the presence of bundle branch block?

Yes—but it is usually *much* harder to recognize acute or old MI in the presence of conduction abnormalities. We emphasize the following points:

It is hardest to diagnose infarction in the presence of LBBB. Most of the time, you will *not* be able to say anything about the possibility of acute or old MI if there is LBBB. One exception is that if you see a Q wave in either lead I or lead V_6, it is likely that the patient has had an infarction at some time. Another is that if primary ST-T wave changes are present, there may be ischemia and/or ongoing infarction.

A deep QS complex is *normally* seen with LBBB. You *cannot* diagnose anterior infarction by this finding!

It is somewhat easier to diagnose MI in the presence of complete RBBB. This is because RBBB will often not mask Q waves in the same way that LBBB does.

Q waves suggestive of infarction may or may not be seen with IVCD.

Even if Q waves suggestive of myocardial infarction are seen in patients with a conduction abnormality, it is often exceedingly hard to date the infarction. Thus, one should always consider the possibility of recent or acute MI with development of *new* LBBB, RBBB, or IVCD.

Can you diagnose chamber enlargement in the presence of bundle branch block?

Diagnosis of atrial abnormality (LAA or RAA) is unaffected by LBBB, RBBB, or IVCD. In contrast, diagnosis of ventricular enlargement tends to be much more difficult in the presence of bundle branch block. We emphasize the following points:

Practically speaking, it is probably best not to even bother trying to diagnose RVH if LBBB, RBBB, or IVCD is present.

LVH may be suspected in the presence of RBBB if the R wave is tall in a lateral lead (i.e., if the R in aVL is ≥ 12 and/or the R in V_5 or V_6 is ≥ 25).

LVH is probably present with LBBB or IVCD if the S wave is *very* deep in any of the anterior leads (i.e., if the S wave in lead V_1, V_2, or V_3 is ≥ 30).

What is the clinical significance of bundle branch block?

The answer depends on the clinical setting in which the conduction defect occurs. When complete RBBB or LBBB is found in otherwise asymptomatic adults in an ambulatory setting, the clinical implication may be minimal other than to increase the likelihood that the patient has some type of underlying heart disease. The chance of developing complete AV block (and requiring a permanent pacemaker) is quite small when bundle branch block is detected in asymptomatic individuals.

On the other hand, acute development of bundle branch block is potentially a much more serious disorder. If it is associated with acute myocardial infarction, the chance of developing complete AV block is substantial, and prophylactic pacing may be required.

As we implied a moment ago, diagnosis of acute myocardial infarction is often much more difficult in the presence of bundle branch block. Clinically, the problem arises when a patient presents with new-onset chest pain, bundle branch block on ECG, and no prior tracing for comparison. Without the availability of a prior tracing, it may be impossible to tell if the conduction defect is new or old. And, in the presence of bundle branch block, it may not be possible to diagnose acute infarction by ECG. In such cases, it may be prudent to admit the patient to the hospital until the clinical situation can be clarified.

Addendum to Chapter 5: WPW

There is one exception to the simplified algorithm we presented in Figure 5-1 *(on pocket reference p. 12)* for assessment of QRS widening. This exception is the Wolff-Parkinson-White (WPW) syndrome. Although admittedly uncommon (with an estimated incidence of 2 per 1000 in the general population), WPW seems to occur just often enough to cause problems for the unwary.

There are three characteristic findings in WPW:

1. QRS widening
2. A delta wave
3. A short PR interval

Each of these findings is illustrated by Figure 5-14 *(which also appears on p. 16 of the pocket reference)*.

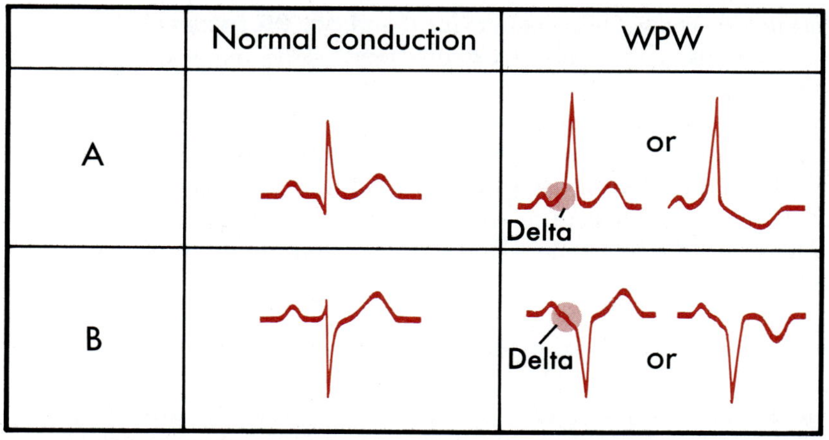

	Normal conduction	WPW
A		Delta ... or
B		Delta ... or

Figure 5-14. The characteristic findings in WPW (short PR interval, QRS widening, and delta wave), compared with normal conduction. **A** shows the usual appearance of WPW in leads where the QRS complex is predominantly upright, while **B** shows the appearance when the QRS complex is predominantly negative.

As we discussed in Chapter 4, a large part of the PR interval is normally made up of the delay in the impulse in passing through the AV node. In WPW, there is an *accessory* pathway (AP) that bypasses the AV node (Figure 5-15).

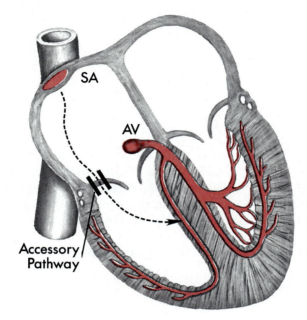

Figure 5-15.   Schematic representation of conduction over the accessory pathway in WPW. The usual conduction pathway (through the AV node) is bypassed. The AP is shown on the right side of the heart in this illustration, but it may also occur on the left side, anteriorly, or posteriorly.

Conduction across the accessory pathway occurs much more rapidly than conduction across the usual channel (i.e., through the AV node, the bundle of His, and bundle branch system). This accounts for the **short PR interval.** It also explains the other name for this syndrome—***preexcitation***—since ventricular activation begins *sooner* than expected. Once across the accessory pathway, however, conduction slows down dramatically. This is because the impulse now has to pass through non-specialized myocardial tissue. The result is a **delta wave,** seen as a slurring of the initial portion of the QRS complex (Figure 5-14). Because conduction through non-specialized myocardial tissue is so much slower than conduction over the usual pathway (through the AV node, bundle of His, and bundle branch system), there is **QRS widening.**

Recognition of WPW is important for two main reasons:

1. Patients with WPW are highly susceptible to certain cardiac arrhythmias. This is because the accessory pathway provides a ready-made re-entry circuit that allows continued transmission of the impulse from atria to ventricles. ECG diagnosis and treatment of the tachyarrhythmias associated with WPW extend beyond the scope of this book. Suffice it to say that many of the drugs used to slow down and treat reentry tachycardias in normal individuals are contraindicated in WPW because they paradoxically facilitate conduction over the accessory pathway.

2. WPW may mimic many other electrocardiographic findings. Failure to recognize WPW as the cause of the ECG abnormality may result in costly and unnecessary diagnostic and therapeutic intervention.

In days gone by, it was said that "he [she] who knows syphilis [and all of its clinical manifestations] knows medicine." We affectionately think of WPW as the electrocardiographic equivalent of syphilis. Like syphilis, **WPW is the GREAT mimic!** As shown in Figure 5-14, *B,* delta waves may be negative. When this occurs, they seem to produce Q waves that often mimic myocardial infarction. Figure 5-14, *A,* shows how QRS amplitude may be increased by conduction over the accessory pathway. This may simulate either LVH or RVH. *A* and *B* also show how the ST segment and T wave may be altered by WPW, sometimes producing changes that mimic ischemia or infarction. Finally, QRS widening itself may simulate LBBB, RBBB, or IVCD.

WPW is the perfect example of a condition that often goes overlooked because it catches the interpreter off guard. Adherence to a systematic approach offers several safeguards that should prevent this from happening. The PR interval is short. The QRS complex is widened. Detection of either of these findings should prompt the interpreter to ask why (and consider WPW as the cause). WPW often produces a tall (or relatively tall) R wave in lead V_1. Consideration of the common causes of a tall R wave in lead V_1 is the fourth of our lists (which we will discuss in Chapter 13)—and WPW is the first condition that should be ruled out whenever a predominant R wave is seen in lead V_1 (see *Table 13-5 on p. 39 of the pocket reference*).

We close by emphasizing that WPW is *not* a common electrocardiographic abnormality—but it is one that you will definitely see from time to time. Recognition is not hard if a systematic approach is followed. And to keep you honest, we'll sneak in a case (or two) in practice exercises presented later on in this book.

The QT Interval

MEASUREMENT OF THE QT INTERVAL

The QT interval is the period from the beginning of ventricular depolarization until the end of ventricular repolarization. The interval is measured from the onset of the Q wave until the termination of the T wave (Figure 6-1, *A*).

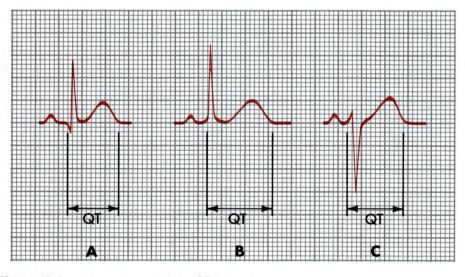

Figure 6-1.   Measurement of the QT interval.

If there is no Q wave, the QT interval is measured from the onset of the R wave until termination of the T wave (Figure 6-1, *B* and *C*).

All 12 leads of the standard ECG should be scanned when you are assessing for QT duration. Ignore leads in which it is hard to clearly define the end of the T wave. Measure the QT in the lead where this interval appears longest.

DETERMINING IF THE QT INTERVAL IS ABNORMAL

The QT interval may be short, normal, or prolonged. Although a short QT interval may suggest hypercalcemia, it is often quite difficult clinically to distinguish between a QT interval that is normal and one that is short. We therefore suggest not concerning yourself at all with QT shortening.

Practically speaking, then, one really only cares if the QT is "normal" or prolonged. As long as one can make this distinction, it matters little what the precise QT interval is.

The QT interval changes with heart rate. It also depends on the age and sex of the patient. You may sometimes see references to a **QTc.** The **c** in this case indicates that the QT interval that you measure has been *corrected* for the patient's heart rate. Corrections are made with respect to what the QT interval should be if the heart rate was 60 beats/minute.

For example, the upper limit of normal for the QT interval at a heart rate of 60 beats/minute is approximately 0.43 second. However, a QT interval that measures 0.43 second would be clearly prolonged if the heart rate was 90 beats/minute.

At this faster heart rate, the actual QT interval should measure no more than 0.37 second. That is, the QTc (corrected QT) for a QT interval that measures 0.37 second at a heart rate of 90 beats/minute is 0.43 second.

Realize that many ECG textbooks carry detailed tables that indicate the upper limits of normal for the QT interval at any given heart rate, depending on the patient's age and sex. *Life need not be so difficult.* QT lengthening can be determined in most cases by applying the following simple guideline:

> *The QT interval is probably prolonged if it exceeds HALF of the R-R interval.*

This method works well when the heart rate is 100 beats/minute or less. QT interval prolongation is much more difficult to determine at faster heart rates. Application of the method is illustrated in Figure 6-2 *(which also appears on p. 18 of the pocket reference).*

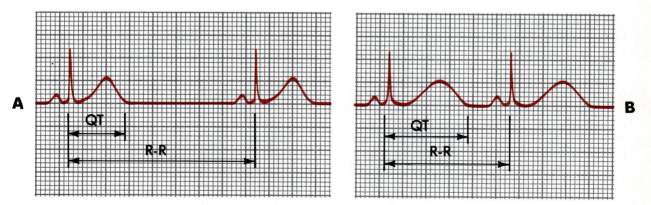

Figure 6-2.   Determining QT prolongation. **A,** The QT interval is clearly normal, since the QT is much less than half the R-R interval. **B,** The QT is obviously prolonged. It far exceeds half the R-R interval.

Table 6-1 *(which also appears on p. 17 of the pocket reference)* reviews the essentials for assessing the QT interval.

Table 6-1
Assessing the QT Interval

1. Measure the QT interval from the onset of the Q wave (or the onset of the R wave if there is no Q) until the termination of the T wave.
2. Select a lead where you can clearly see the T wave.
3. Select the lead in which the QT interval appears to be longest.
4. Precise measurement of the QT interval is not necessary. Practically speaking, one only cares if the QT is normal or prolonged. In general, when the heart rate is under 100 beats/minute:
    If the QT is less than half the R-R interval⇒ The QT is normal
    If the QT is clearly more than half the R-R interval⇒ The QT is prolonged
    If the QT is about half the R-R interval ⇒ The QT is "borderline"

As a check of your ability to apply the method for determining QT prolongation, examine the following three examples (Figures 6-3, 6-4, and 6-5). For each, indicate whether it is likely that the QT is prolonged. Assume that the heart rate is well under 100 beats/minute in each example.

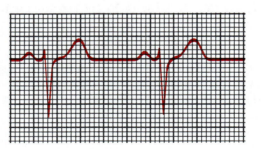

Figure 6-3

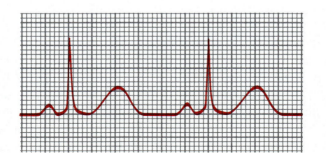

Figure 6-4

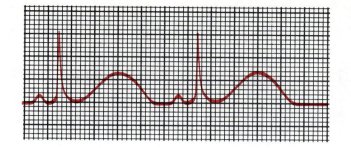

Figure 6-5

Answers

Figure 6-3: The QT appears to be normal. It is clearly less than half the R-R interval.

Figure 6-4: The QT is "borderline." It is approximately half the R-R interval.

Figure 6-5: The QT is prolonged. It is clearly more than half the R-R interval.

CLINICAL SIGNIFICANCE OF QT PROLONGATION

Common causes of QT prolongation are shown in Table 6-2.

Table 6-2
Common Causes of QT Prolongation

1. **Drugs**
    Type IA antiarrhythmic agents (i.e., quinidine, procainamide, disopyramide)
    Tricyclic antidepressants
    Phenothiazines
2. **"Lytes"** (i.e., electrolytes)
    Hypokalemia
    Hypomagnesemia
    Hypocalcemia
3. **CNS catastrophe**
    Stroke
    Intracerebral or brainstem bleeding
    Coma
4. Bundle branch block or IVCD
5. Ischemia or infarction

The causes of QT prolongation make up the second of our lists. *(The Essential Lists are discussed in detail in Chapter 13.)* As indicated in Table 6-2, bundle branch block, IVCD, ischemia, and infarction may all lengthen the QT interval. However, the presence of any of these conditions will usually be obvious on the ECG. The point to remember is that if the QT interval is prolonged in the absence of QRS widening, ischemia, or infarction, think "Drugs/Lytes/CNS" as the cause!

7

Axis (and Hemiblocks)

The mean QRS axis may be defined as the average direction (orientation) of the heart's electrical activity. Calculation of axis is dreaded by many beginning interpreters, but this need *NOT* be the case. *Calculation of axis can be easy!*

PRACTICAL CONSIDERATIONS: HOW IMPORTANT IS AXIS?

Although calculation of axis is important in diagnosis of the hemiblocks, and may contribute to diagnosing RVH, pulmonary embolus, or dextrocardia, and to suspecting lead misplacement, it otherwise provides only limited clinical information.*

Practically speaking, it is rarely important to be precise in axis calculation. Thus, it matters little clinically whether the axis is $+25°$ or $+27°$ (or $+45°$ for that matter). Ballpark estimation will usually suffice, and we feel it rarely worth spending more than a few moments on axis calculation.

Rather than simply saying that an axis is "normal" or "abnormal," however, a *rough* estimation of the axis in degrees is preferable. For example, a patient who previously had an axis of $+10°$ (which is normal) and now has an axis of $+80°$ (which is also normal) has undergone a considerable change in axis (of $70°$!). This potentially significant right axis shift would have gone undetected had the interpreter simply reported the axis as "normal" in each case. Clinically, a right axis shift of this degree may suggest development of RVH, left posterior hemiblock (LPHB), or pulmonary embolus. Comparable left axis shifts sometimes suggest development of LVH or left anterior hemiblock (LAHB).

CALCULATION OF AXIS: BASIC PRINCIPLES

There are numerous ways to calculate axis. There are also numerous opinions on the definition (and meaning) of various axis deviations. No uniform consensus

---

*An additional important clinical use of axis determination that we do not discuss in this chapter is in helping to determine the etiology of a wide-complex tachycardia. We illustrate this application in Chapter 19.

exists. We simplify calculation of axis by endorsing the **2-lead and quadrant approach.** The method is quick, easy to understand, fairly accurate, and unlikely to confuse the beginning or novice interpreter. By the end of this chapter, you should be able to approximate axis in seconds!

The two KEY leads for axis determination are leads I and aVF. Lead I is located at 0°, and lead aVF at +90° (Figure 7-1).

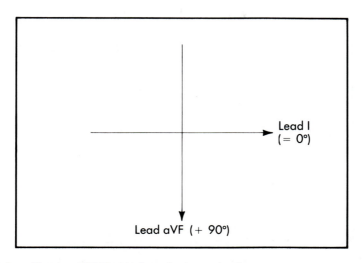

Figure 7-1.   The two KEY leads for axis determination.

We find it easiest to define axis deviations by quadrants. Thus, the axis is said to be **normal** if it is between 0° and +90°. There is **right axis deviation (RAD)** if the axis is between +91° and +180°, and **left axis deviation (LAD)** if between −1° and −90° (Figure 7-2).

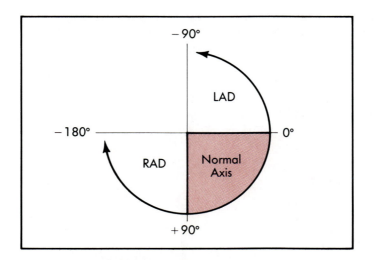

Figure 7-2.   Axis definition by quadrants.

One quadrant remains unnamed by this approach. This quadrant comprises axis deviations between +180° and +270° (i.e., between −90° and −180°). Because it is *impossible to determine* if axis deviations residing in this quadrant represent marked RAD or LAD, we call the quadrant **indeterminate.** It has also been colorfully labeled by some as **"no-man's land"** (Figure 7-3).

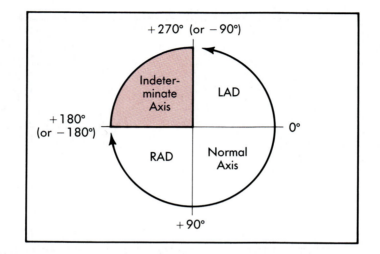

Figure 7-3.   Indeterminate axis is defined as an axis between +180° and +270° (i.e., between −90° and −180°).

CALCULATING NET QRS DEFLECTION

Axis determination is based on calculating the **net** QRS deflection in various key leads. Simply stated, *the mean QRS axis is oriented most toward the lead with the greatest net positive QRS deflection.*

Estimating net QRS deflections is easy. One merely adds up the number of little boxes in the R wave (positive deflection), and subtracts the number of little boxes in the Q and S waves (negative deflections).

Apply this principle to Figure 7-4. Which QRS complex in this figure has the greatest net positive deflection? Which has the greatest net negative deflection? Does one of the complexes have a net deflection of zero?

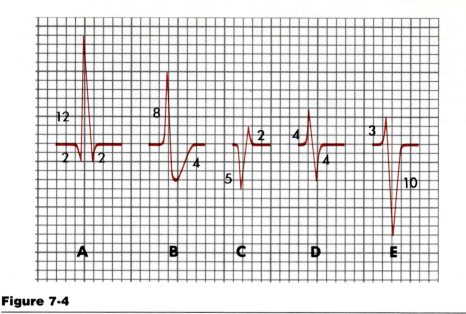

Figure 7-4

Net deflections of the QRS complexes shown in Figure 7-4 are as follows:

Net deflection of A:
= −**2** (for the q wave) + **12** (for the R wave) *and* −**2** (for the s wave) = +**8**

Net deflection of B:
= +**8** (for the R wave) *and* −**4** (for the S wave) = +**4**

Net deflection of C:
= −**5** (for the Q wave) *and* +**2** (for the r wave) = −**3**

Net deflection of D:
= +**4** (for the R wave) *and* −**4** (for the S wave) = **0**

Net deflection of E:
= +**3** (for the R wave) *and* −**10** (for the S wave) = −**7**

Thus, the greatest net positive QRS deflection in Figure 7-4 is *A*. The greatest net negative deflection is *E*. Complex *D* has a net deflection of zero.

If the QRS complexes shown in this figure reflected the appearance of different monitoring leads, the mean QRS axis would be closest to *A* (which has the greatest net positive QRS deflection) and furthest from E (which has the greatest net negative deflection. The mean QRS axis would be *perpendicular* to (90° away from) *D,* because the net QRS deflection is *equiphasic* (i.e., *isoelectric,* or equally positive and negative) in this lead.

Calculating net QRS deflections by counting the number of boxes in the components of the QRS complex is not completely accurate. Rather than the *number* of boxes in a deflection, it is really the *area* contained within each deflection that should be calculated. For example, the S wave in complex *B* of Figure 7-4 is obviously wider than the R wave of this complex. Technically one should account for this. If one did, the net QRS deflection would come out to less than +4 (and probably close to a net deflection of zero). Practically speaking, however, fairly accurate axis determination is usually possible simply by estimating the *relative* amplitude of each deflection rather than by strict counting of boxes or calculation of the area contained within each deflection. Application of this "eyeball technique" makes the task of axis determination infinitely simpler—and this is the method we endorse here.

ESTIMATING AXIS WHEN THE AXIS IS NORMAL

Apply the two-lead "eyeball" method to estimate the mean QRS axis for the following three examples (Figures 7-5, 7-6, and 7-7). The axis is within the normal range (i.e., between 0° and 90°) in each case. *Approximate the axis on the basis of the **relative** net deflection of the QRS complex in leads I and aVF.*

Note that we have intentionally excluded the grid from these examples because we want you to get used to **"guesstimating"** relative net deflections (i.e., mentally subtracting negative deflections from the positive deflection). Also note that we have omitted the appearance of the QRS complex for the remaining 10 leads from these tracings. This is because leads I and aVF are the *ONLY* leads essential for axis estimation when the axis is normal.

Application of the **Two-Lead Eyeball Method** is easier than it may sound, especially when the axis is normal.

All we ask you to do is:

Look at leads I and aVF.

"Guesstimate" the relative net deflection in these leads.

"Guesstimate" the axis in degrees.

Keep in mind that:

Lead I lies at 0° and lead aVF lies at 90°.

If the approximate size (i.e., net deflection) of lead I is about the same as that for lead aVF, then one would expect the axis to lie about midway between these leads (or close to +45°). We often give a range for our answer (i.e., *"The axis lies between +40° and +50°").*

If the net deflection of lead I looks a lot greater than that for lead aVF, then the axis should lie closer to lead I (i.e., between 0° and +40°, depending on how much larger the net deflection in lead I looks to be).

If the net deflection of lead aVF looks a lot greater than that for lead I, then the axis should lie closer to lead aVF (i.e., between +50° and +90°, depending on how much larger the net deflection in lead aVF looks to be).

You may find it helpful to:

Use the simplified axis diagram next to each tracing to remind you of the location of leads I and aVF.

Remember:

All you are doing is approximating.

It really doesn't matter if your guesstimate is 5°, 10°, or even 20° different from ours—*as long as you are in the "ballpark"!!!*

Now estimate the axis for Figures 7-5, 7-6, and 7-7.

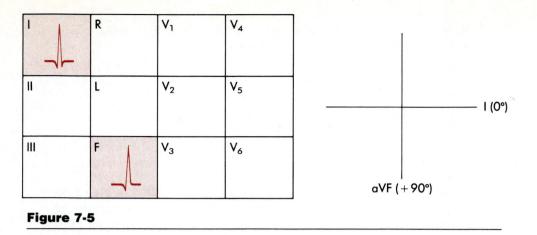

Figure 7-5

Answer to Figure 7-5

The net QRS deflection is positive and approximately equal in leads I and aVF. We estimate the mean QRS axis to be between +40° and +50°.

Note how easy it is to arrive at this estimate when we draw out our answer on the simplified axis diagram below. The thin arrows on the diagram represent the relative net deflection for leads I and aVF, while the thick arrow represents our approximation of the mean axis.

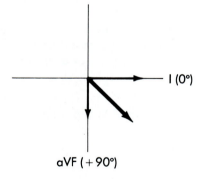

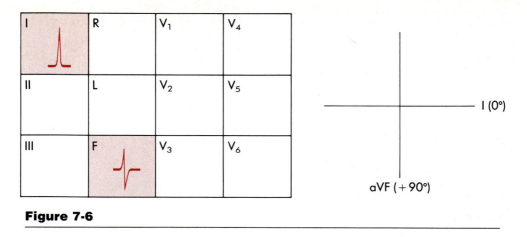

Figure 7-6

Answer to Figure 7-6

The QRS deflection in lead I is all positive (an R wave). In contrast, the QRS complex in lead aVF is equiphasic (equal parts positive and negative). ***The mean QRS axis lies perpendicular to (90° away from) a lead that is equiphasic.*** This means that the axis should be at 0°.

We indicate these relationships on our simplified axis diagram below. The mean QRS axis is oriented toward lead I (at 0°), and lies 90° away from equiphasic lead aVF. This puts the axis right at 0°.

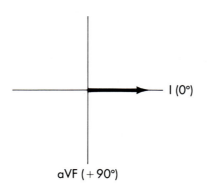

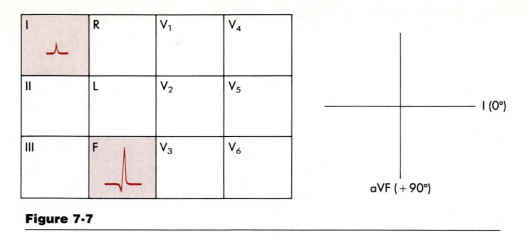

I	R	V₁	V₄
II	L	V₂	V₅
III	F	V₃	V₆

Figure 7-7

Answer to Figure 7-7

The net QRS deflection is largely positive in lead aVF. It is only minimally positive in lead I. The mean QRS axis will therefore be oriented much closer to lead aVF. We estimate the axis to lie somewhere between +70° and +85°.

Let us review how we arrived at this answer. If the relative net deflections of lead I (at 0°) and lead aVF (at +90°) were equal, the axis would lie midway between these two leads, or at about +45° (i.e., within a range of +40° to +50°). We can confidently say from looking at Figure 7-7 that the net deflection of lead aVF is larger than that of lead I. As a result, we know that the axis must lie closer to lead aVF than to lead I (or somewhere between +50° and +90°). Since the net deflection of lead aVF in Figure 7-7 looks quite a bit larger than that of lead I, the axis must lie much closer to lead aVF. Judging from the relative net deflections that we drew for leads I and aVF in the diagram below, we would estimate that the axis probably lies somewhere between +70° and +85°.

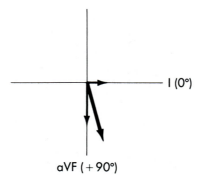

RAPID DETERMINATION OF AXIS DEVIATIONS

From the previous exercise, it should be apparent that when the net QRS deflection of lead I is positive, the axis will lie somewhere in the *left* hemisphere (i.e., between +90° and −90°). We illustrate this concept in Figure 7-8.

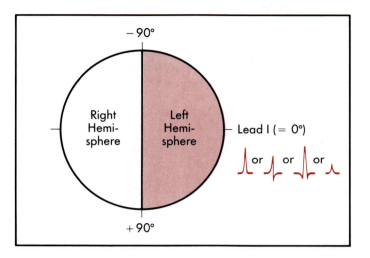

Figure 7-8.   If the net deflection of lead I is positive, the QRS axis will lie somewhere in the left hemisphere (from +90° to −90°).

Similarly, if the net QRS deflection of lead aVF is positive, the axis will lie somewhere in the inferior hemisphere (i.e., between 0° and +180°). We illustrate this in Figure 7-9.

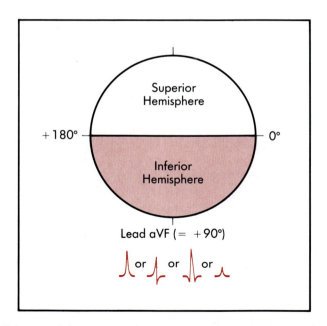

Figure 7-9.   If the net deflection of lead aVF is positive, the QRS axis will lie somewhere in the inferior hemisphere (from 0° to +180°).

Therefore, the *ONLY* way one can possibly have a normal mean QRS axis (i.e., an axis between 0° and +90°) is if the net QRS deflection in *both* leads I and aVF is positive.

From this deduction we extrapolate the following essential principle of rapid axis determination:

> *The ONLY leads one needs to look at to determine if the axis is normal are leads I and aVF.* **If the net QRS deflection is positive in BOTH of these leads, the mean QRS axis is normal.**

Examine the following three examples (Figures 7-10, 7-11, and 7-12). Indicate whether the mean QRS axis is normal. If so, approximate the axis in degrees. If the axis is not within the normal range, indicate the type of axis deviation (i.e., LAD or RAD).

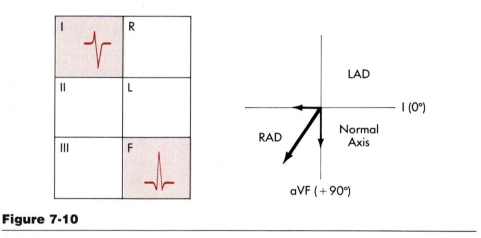

Figure 7-10

Answer to Figure 7-10

We know at a glance that the mean QRS axis is *not* normal, because the net QRS deflection is not positive in both leads I and aVF. The axis must lie in the inferior hemisphere, since the net deflection in lead aVF is positive. However, the net deflection of lead I is negative. This means that the axis must lie in the right hemisphere. There is RAD.

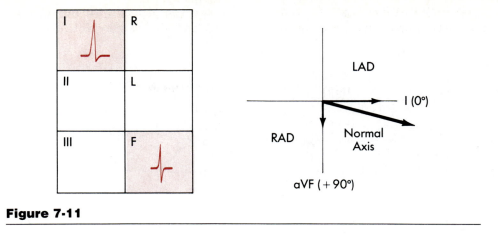

Figure 7-11

Answer to Figure 7-11

The net QRS deflection in both leads I and aVF is positive. Therefore the QRS axis must be normal. Since the relative net deflection in lead I is a good bit more than the net deflection in lead aVF, the axis probably lies somewhere between $+15°$ and $+30°$.

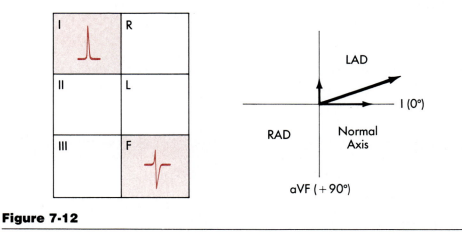

Figure 7-12

Answer to Figure 7-12

Since the net QRS deflection in lead I is positive, the axis must lie in the left hemisphere. The net negative deflection of the QRS complex in lead aVF, however, places the axis in the superior hemisphere. There must be LAD.

Question: What type of axis deviation would you expect if the net deflection of the QRS complex was negative in both leads I and aVF (Figure 7-13)?

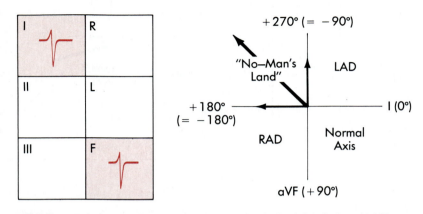

Figure 7-13. The net QRS deflection is negative in both leads I and aVF.

Answer to Figure 7-13

Since the net QRS deflection in lead I is negative, the axis must lie in the right hemisphere. Since the net deflection in lead aVF is also negative, the axis must lie in the superior hemisphere. This puts the axis in *"no-man's land"* (i.e., the axis is indeterminate).

Table 7-1 *(which also appears on p. 20 of the pocket reference)* summarizes these concepts.

Table 7-1		
Rapid Determination of Axis Deviation		
	NET QRS deflection	
	Lead I	**Lead aVF**
Normal axis	Positive	Positive
RAD	Negative	Positive
LAD	Positive	Negative
Indeterminate axis	Negative	Negative

PATHOLOGIC LEFT AXIS DEVIATION

As we have stated, a mean QRS axis between −1° and −90° is defined as LAD. But does the presence of a small amount of LAD necessarily imply a disease state?

Actually, many older individuals develop some degree of LAD as a natural part of the aging process. In an attempt to separate such individuals from persons with an underlying conduction system defect, we favor of the term **"pathologic" LAD,** which we define as an axis *more negative than −30°.*

Using this definition, determining whether a patient with LAD has "pathologic" LAD is easy. It may be done at a glance from inspection of just one lead!

Up till now, we have limited our discussion of axis determination to the use of two leads (leads I and aVF). When LAD is present, use of a third lead—lead II—may prove invaluable for assessing the degree of LAD.

Figure 7-14 illustrates the **hexaxial lead system.** The six leads included in the hexaxial lead system are the *standard limb leads* (I, II, and III) and the *augmented limb leads* (**aVR, aVL,** and **aVF**).

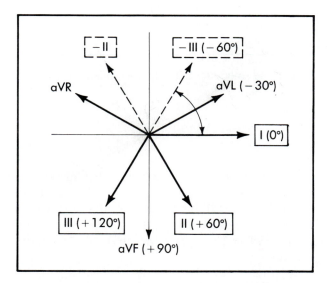

Figure 7-14.   The hexaxial lead system. The **standard limb leads** (I, II, and III) are separated by 60°.

The three **augmented leads** are aVR, aVL, and aVF. Lead aVF is at +90°. Lead aVL bisects leads I and −III, and is at −30°. Lead aVR lies in "no-man's land." *Neither lead aVR nor lead aVL is essential to estimation of axis.*

The **standard limb leads** are separated from each other by 60°. If we start from lead I at 0°, this means lead II lies at +60° and lead III at +120°. Negative lead III (i.e., −III) is 60° away from lead I in the negative direction (at −60°).

The three **augmented leads** are each separated by 120°. Lead aVF lies at +90°. Lead aVL lies 120° away (at −30°) and bisects leads I and −III. Lead aVR lies in "no-man's land." It should again be emphasized that examination of leads aVL and aVR is not essential to axis estimation.

Focus for a moment on lead II at +60°. How far away would the mean QRS axis be if the QRS complex in lead II was isoelectric (Figure 7-15)?

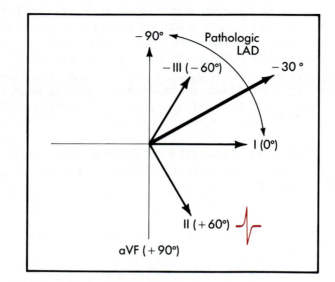

Figure 7-15.   What is the axis if the QRS complex in lead II is isoelectric?

Answer to Figure 7-15

Since we know the mean QRS axis lies perpendicular (90° away) from a lead in which the QRS complex is equiphasic, the axis will be 90° away from lead II in Figure 7-15. Since lead II is at +60° (and assuming the QRS complex in lead I has a net positive deflection as it almost always does), this means the axis will lie exactly at −30°. This is precisely at the point that divides a nonpathologic LAD from one we define as pathologic.

We emphasize that if the net QRS deflection in lead II is more negative than positive, the axis must lie *more than 90° away* from this lead. ***A negative net QRS deflection in lead II therefore means that there must be pathologic LAD.*** Table 7-2 *(which also appears on p. 21 in the pocket reference)* summarizes this information.

Table 7-2
Determination of Pathologic LAD

1. If the net deflection in lead I is positive and lead aVF is negative, there is LAD (see Table 7-1).
2. To determine if this is pathologic LAD, look at QRS morphology in lead II:

Lead II	Axis	Pathologic LAD?
	Less negative than −30°	No
	−30°	Borderline
	More negative than −30°	Yes

HEMIBLOCKS

The subject of hemiblocks is complex. Even in cardiology circles, no consensus exists on what the optimal criteria are for diagnosing the hemiblocks. We simplify this otherwise extensive topic as follows.

There are three major divisions to the ventricular conduction system: the right bundle branch and the two hemifascicles of the left bundle branch. A **hemiblock** is a block (defect) in conduction of the electrical impulse along one of the two major fascicles of the left bundle branch (Figure 7-16).

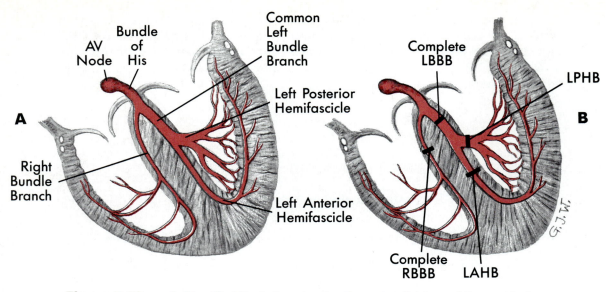

Figure 7-16.   **A,** Simplified illustration showing the major divisions of the ventricular conduction system. After passing through the AV node and the bundle of His, the electrical impulse is carried to the right and common left bundle branches. The latter structure divides into the left anterior and posterior hemifascicles. **B,** Possible sites of block and the conduction defects that may be produced.

We covered the ECG manifestations and clinical implications of complete RBBB and complete LBBB in Chapter 5. As can be seen from Figure 7-16, *B,* complete LBBB may occur as a result of a *proximal* block (i.e., in the common left bundle branch). More distal block (in either the left anterior hemifascicle or the left posterior hemifascicle) produces a hemiblock (LAHB or LPHB, respectively). Simultaneous block in *both* the anterior and posterior hemifascicles would also produce complete LBBB.

LAHB is far more common than LPHB. This is because the left posterior hemifascicle is much thicker than the anterior hemifascicle (Figure 7-16). It also has a dual blood supply (from the left and right coronary arteries), whereas the anterior hemifascicle does not.

For practical purposes, we equate the ECG diagnosis of LAHB with the finding of pathologic LAD. Thus, one only needs to look at lead II to make this diagnosis. *If the net deflection of lead II is negative, the axis is more negative than −30° and LAHB is present.* Clinically, the isolated finding of LAHB usually has little significance, especially when it occurs in an otherwise asymptomatic individual.

LPHB is distinctly uncommon. Because of the thickness of the left posterior hemifascicle and its dual blood supply, LPHB rarely occurs as an isolated finding. Instead, it is most often seen in association with complete RBBB. Although LPHB is often hard to diagnose with certainty, we suspect LPHB *in addition to* RBBB when the S wave in lead I is dramatically deepened. Clinically, LPHB is potentially a much more serious disorder than LAHB (because a much more diffuse conduction disturbance is required in order to produce LPHB).

With a pure hemiblock, the QRS complex is usually not prolonged. In contrast, when a hemiblock occurs in association with RBBB (i.e., when there is *bifascicular* block), the QRS will be prolonged. Clinical implications of bifascicular block are more severe than those of unifascicular block (i.e., isolated RBBB). This is because of the likelihood of a more diffuse conduction disturbance with bifascicular block. However, as we discussed in Chapter 5, on bundle branch block, the key factor determining the significance of a bifascicular block is the clinical setting in which it occurs. The chance that an asymptomatic individual with bifascicular block discovered incidentally on routine ECG will develop complete AV block is small. Neither treatment with drugs nor prophylactic pacemaker insertion is needed in such cases. In contrast, acute development of bifascicular block in association with acute myocardial infarction is definite cause for concern, and is viewed by most cardiologists as an indication for pacemaker insertion.

Check yourself on these concepts by indicating whether a hemiblock and/or bundle branch block is present in the following schematic tracings (Figures 7-17 to 7-21).

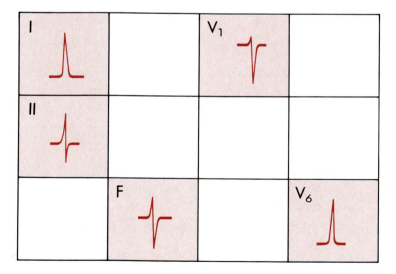

Figure 7-17.   The QRS is of normal duration.

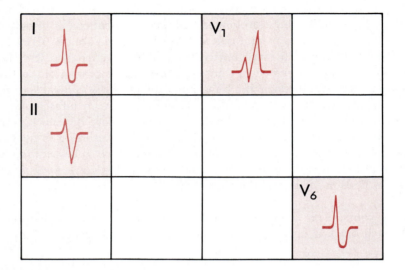

Figure 7-18.   The QRS is prolonged.

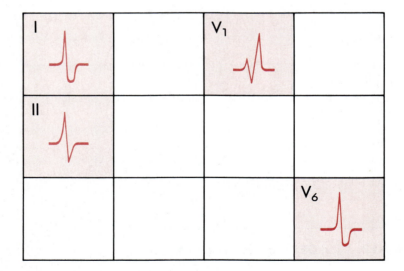

Figure 7-19.   The QRS is prolonged.

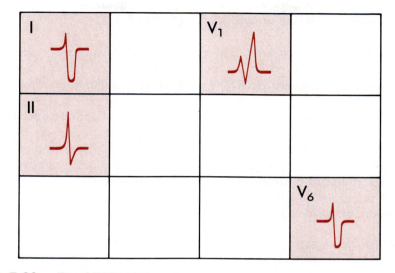

Figure 7-20.   The QRS is prolonged.

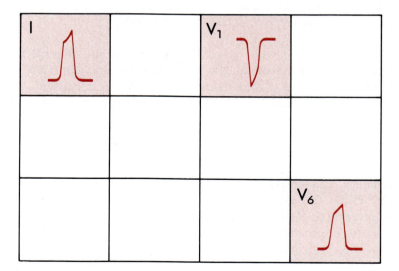

Figure 7-21.   The QRS is prolonged.

Answers

Figure 7-17: The QRS is of normal duration. LAD is present, since the QRS is positive in lead I but has a net negative deflection in lead aVF. However, because the net QRS deflection in lead II is not negative; the axis is *less* than −30°. Thus, there is no LAHB. *Note that one can tell at a glance that LAHB is not present simply by looking at lead II!* (See Table 7-2.)

Figure 7-18: The QRS is wide. The rSR′ in lead V_1 suggests complete RBBB. This diagnosis is supported by the terminal wide S wave in leads I and V_6. *Note that diagnosis of complete RBBB is made from inspection of these three leads alone!*

Axis is often difficult to determine in the presence of complete RBBB, because one never knows how much of the wide terminal S wave in lead I is due to the RBBB and how much is due to an axis shift. Practically speaking, with complete RBBB one really only cares if the axis is normal, markedly rightward (and suggestive of LPHB), or pathologically leftward (and suggestive of LAHB). A glance at lead II in Figure 7-18 tells us that there is LAHB (since the net QRS deflection in this lead is negative). Thus, there is bifascicular block (i.e., RBBB *and* LAHB).

Figure 7-19: The QRS is wide. Inspection of the three key leads (I, V_1, and V_6) tells us that there is complete RBBB. There is no LPHB, since the S wave in lead I is not markedly deepened. There is no LAHB, since the net QRS deflection in lead II is positive.

Figure 7-20: The QRS is wide. Once again inspection of the three key leads confirms the presence of complete RBBB. Note how much deeper the S wave in lead I is here as compared with Figure 7-19. This suggests that LPHB is also present. Thus, there is bifascicular block (RBBB *and* LPHB).

Figure 7-21: The QRS is wide. Lead V_1 clearly indicates that QRS widening is not the result of RBBB. Instead, the monophasic R wave in leads I and V_6, together with the negative (QS) deflection in lead V_1, is consistent with complete LBBB. Since complete LBBB implies the lack of conduction down *both* fascicles of the left bundle branch, complete LBBB may also be viewed as a form of bifascicular block.

• • •

In summary, axis determination is admittedly not essential to the interpretation of many ECGs. Nevertheless, it can often provide information that will be of use to the interpreter. Attention to the basic principles suggested in this chapter greatly facilitates approximation of axis.

Review

Crystallize the concepts we have discussed so far. Examine the following four tracings (Figures 8-1, 8-2, 8-3, and 8-4). Systematically analyze each of them for rate, rhythm, and axis. Be sure to evaluate the three key intervals immediately after determining the rhythm. If the QRS is wide, indicate why. *Feel free to refer to the pocket reference as needed.*

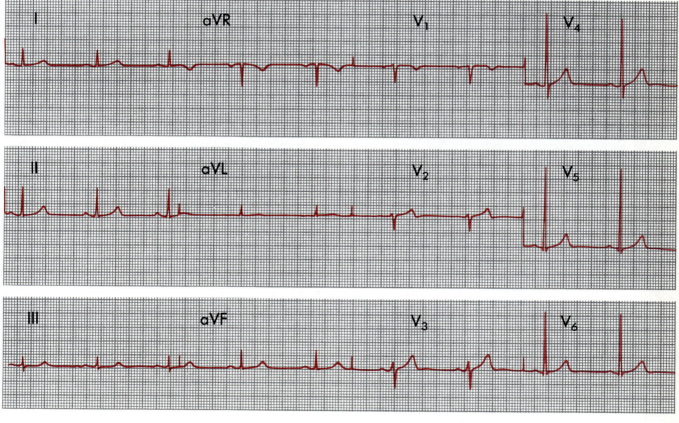

Figure 8-1

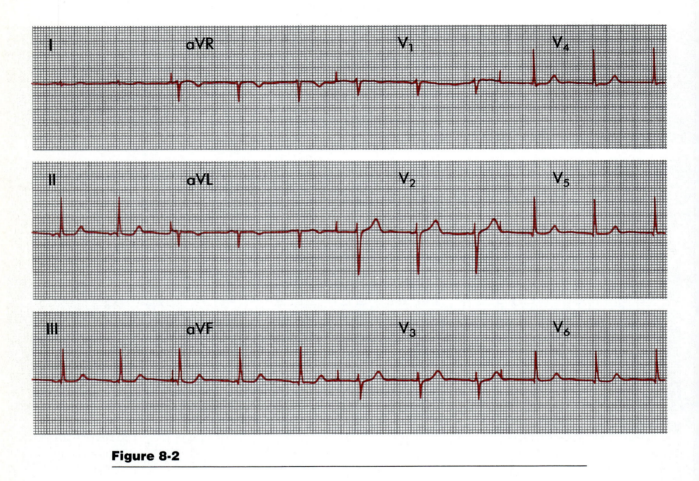

Figure 8-2

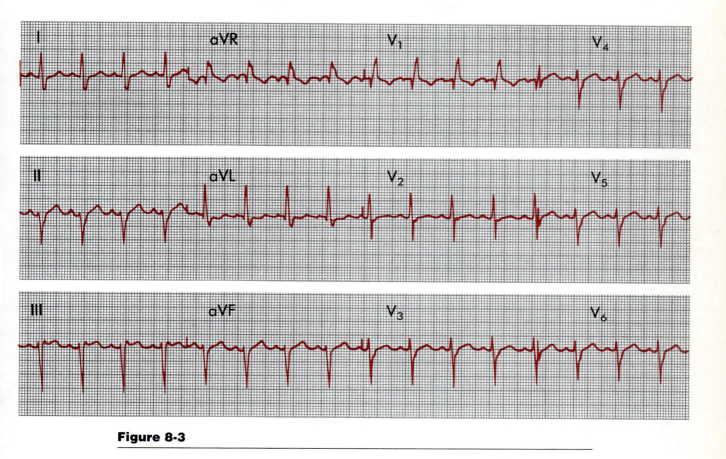

Figure 8-3

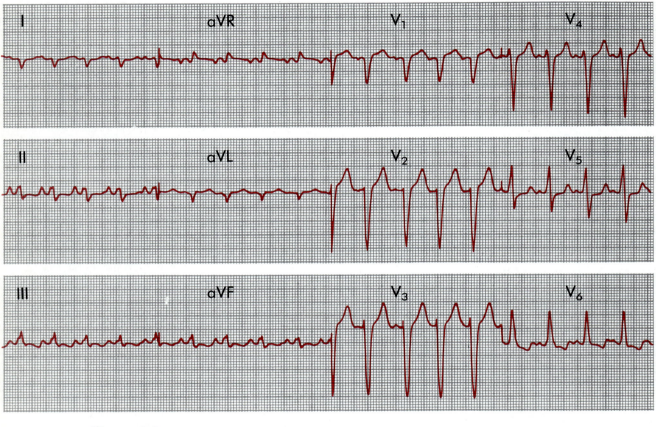

Figure 8-4

Answers

Figure 8-1: The rhythm is fairly regular, at a rate of 55 to 60 beats/minute (since the R-R interval is just over five large boxes). The mechanism is sinus (since the P wave is upright in lead II). Thus, this is sinus bradycardia.

All intervals are normal; that is, the PR interval is less than a large box, the QRS does not exceed half of a large box, and the QT is clearly less than half the R-R interval.

The axis is obviously normal (since the QRS is upright in both leads I and aVF), and approximately $+45°$ to $+50°$ (since the net QRS deflection is ever so slightly greater in lead aVF than in lead I).

Figure 8-2: The rhythm is regular, at a rate of $\approx$70 beats/minute. However, the mechanism is *not* sinus, since the P wave is not upright in lead II. Instead, the P wave is negative in this lead, suggesting that the rhythm is either a low atrial rhythm or a slightly accelerated junctional rhythm.

In the absence of sinus mechanism, the usual lower and upper limits of normal for the PR interval no longer hold true. The QRS complex is normal, and the QT interval is not prolonged.

The axis is normal—but barely so. If the QRS complex was equiphasic in lead I, the axis would be $+90°$. Since the net QRS deflection is ever so slightly positive in this lead, the axis must be ever so slightly less than 90° away, or at about $+80°$ to $+85°$.

Figure 8-3: The rhythm is regular, at a rate of 100 to 105 beats/minute (since the R-R interval is just less than three large boxes). The mechanism is sinus (since the P wave is upright in lead II). Because the rate exceeds 100 beats/minute, this is sinus tachycardia.

The PR interval is normal. However, the QRS is wide (and measures at least 0.13 second). Complete RBBB is suggested by the rSR' in lead V_1. This interpretation is supported by the terminal wide S waves in both leads I and V_6 *(see Figure 5-8 in pocket reference, p. 14)*. Normal secondary ST-T wave changes of RBBB are present, since the T wave is upright in leads I and V_6, and the ST segment is negative in lead V_1 *(see Figure 5-9 in pocket reference, p. 15)*.

In addition, the markedly negative net QRS deflection in lead II suggests LAHB *(see Table 7-2 in pocket reference, p. 21)*. Thus, there is bifascicular block (complete RBBB and LAHB).

The QT interval is more than half the R-R interval, but this may be due to the rate (which exceeds 100 beats/minute) and/or the bundle branch block.

Figure 8-4: The rhythm is almost regular, at 115 to 125 beats/minute. The upright P wave in lead II confirms that this is sinus tachycardia.

The PR interval is normal, but the QRS is obviously widened. Typical RBBB is ruled out by the appearance of the QRS complex in lead V_1. Although QRS morphology in leads V_1 and V_6 would be consistent with complete LBBB, the predominantly negative QRS complex in lead I argues against this diagnosis. Thus, the reason for QRS widening is IVCD—in this case, with RAD *(see Figure 5-8 in pocket reference, p. 14)*.

Once again, QT prolongation is explained by the tachycardia and/or intraventricular conduction defect.

9

Chamber Enlargement

The ECG has long been used as a noninvasive modality for detecting chamber enlargement. Diagnostic criteria abound for this purpose. However, the sad reality is that the ECG is not an extremely accurate diagnostic tool for determining chamber enlargement. Even in the best of hands, *sensitivity* for detecting LVH (left ventricular hypertrophy) does not exceed 60% (although *specificity* may approach 90% to 95%).* Diagnostic accuracy for determining RVH (right ventricular hypertrophy) and atrial enlargement in adults is far less.

Despite these drawbacks, ECG detection of chamber enlargement can still be helpful clinically. In particular, ECG diagnosis of RVH or LVH with "strain" (repolarization abnormalities) may provide important diagnostic and/or prognostic information for patients with disorders such as hypertension, heart failure, valvular disease, or chronic obstructive pulmonary disease (COPD).

SYSTEMATIC APPROACH TO THE ECG DIAGNOSIS OF CHAMBER ENLARGEMENT

Our suggested approach for systematically analyzing the ECG for evidence of chamber enlargement is easy. There are only four cardiac chambers. For each tracing you interpret, look to see whether criteria are met to diagnose:

1. Right atrial abnormality (RAA)
2. Left atrial abnormality (LAA)
3. Left ventricular hypertrophy (LVH)
4. Right ventricular hypertrophy (RVH)

---

*The **sensitivity** of a test is the percentage of abnormal results obtained in a population in which *all* individuals have the condition being searched for. An ideal test would be 100% sensitive, which means that it would be abnormal in *all* individuals with the condition being searched for. Unfortunately, sensitivity for detecting LVH by ECG criteria is poor, and does not exceed 60%. *This means that even the best of electrocardiographers will not be able to detect LVH 40% of the time by looking at an ECG.*

The **specificity** of a test is the percentage of normal results among individuals who *do not* have the condition being searched for. Again, an ideal test would be 100% specific, which means that *all* abnormal tests in a population indicate the presence of the condition being searched for. Despite a poor sensitivity (of no more than 60%) for detecting LVH by ECG criteria, specificity may be quite good (up to 90% to 95%). *This means that when ECG criteria for LVH are met, they indicate true chamber enlargement 90% to 95% of the time.*

ATRIAL ABNORMALITY: GENERAL CONCEPTS

The accuracy of the ECG in detecting atrial chamber enlargement is disappointing for a number of reasons. First, many cases are simply not picked up. *Echocardiography is a far more sensitive tool for this purpose.* Even when ECG criteria for left or right atrial enlargement are present, the reliability (specificity) of these criteria (that they truly reflect enlargement of the respective atrial chamber) is subject to significant error. Finally, one must appreciate that certain conditions other than actual atrial chamber enlargement may also cause alterations in P wave morphology on the ECG. Examples include tachycardia, slender body habitus, and hypokalemia (which may all produce tall, peaked P waves in the inferior leads suggestive of RAE [right atrial enlargement]) and intraatrial conduction abnormalities (which may prolong and distort P wave morphology by altering the path of impulse conduction through the atria).

Because of these shortcomings, we prefer the term atrial ***abnormality*** to atrial ***enlargement.*** This serves as a reminder that conditions other than atrial chamber enlargement may be the cause of the change in P wave morphology. Given the less than optimal reliability of ECG criteria for atrial enlargement, we also favor *underdiagnosing* atrial abnormality. Finally, we tend to avoid the term "borderline" LAA or RAA, especially in the absence of ECG evidence of LVH or RVH, because we don't feel a *borderline* designation for atrial abnormality holds much clinical significance in this setting.

As we discussed in Chapter 3, the best lead to look for P waves in is lead II. By definition, the P wave should *always* be upright in lead II (unless there is lead misplacement or dextrocardia). Next to lead II, lead V_1 is the best lead to look for P waves. These are the two leads we concentrate on to diagnose atrial abnormality.

Figure 9-1 shows the appearance of normal P waves in these two leads with sinus rhythm. Note that the P wave is upright in lead II. Note also that there may be one or two components to the P wave in lead V_1, and that the P wave may *normally* be *negative* or *biphasic* in this lead.

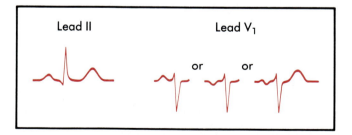

Figure 9-1. Appearance of the P wave in leads II and V_1 with sinus rhythm. With sinus rhythm, the P wave should always be upright in lead II. In lead V_1, the P wave may normally be positive, negative, or biphasic.

Question

When the P wave is biphasic in lead V_1, which component (initial positive deflection, or the terminal negative deflection) represents left atrial depolarization?

Answer

The answer relates back to the basic principle illustrated in Chapter 1 (Figure 1-1). Because the SA node is located in the right atrium, this atrial chamber depolarizes first. As a result, the initial positive deflection in lead V_1 represents right atrial depolarization, and the terminal negative deflection left atrial depolarization.

We raise this point because many clinicians automatically equate the finding of a negative P wave component in lead V_1 with LAA. The left atrial (i.e., the negative) component of the P wave in lead V_1 suggests atrial abnormality *only* when it is abnormally deepened or widened!

ATRIAL ABNORMALITY: SPECIFIC CRITERIA FOR DIAGNOSIS

We use two mnemonics to simplify recall of the basic criteria for atrial abnormality: P pulmonale (for RAA) and P mitrale (for LAA). We illustrate the principal findings for each in Figure 9-2 (*which also appears in the pocket reference, p. 24*).

Condition	P Wave Appearance		Mnemonic Features
	Lead II	Lead V_1	
Normal Sinus Rhythm (NSR)	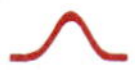	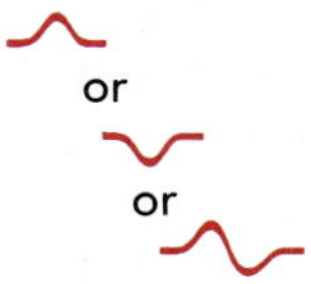 or / or	The P should be upright in lead II if there is sinus rhythm. The P wave may be upright, negative, or biphasic in lead V_1 with sinus rhythm
RAA (= **P P**ulmonale)	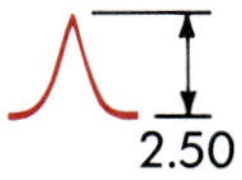 2.50		**P**rominent (≥ 2.5 mm tall) **p**eaked P waves in the **p**ulmonary leads (II, III, and aVF)
LAA (= P **M**itrale)	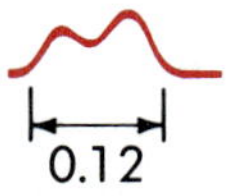 0.12	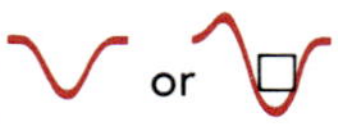 or	**M**-shaped, widened (≥ 0.12 second) P waves in one or more of the **m**itral leads (I, II, or aVL) Deep, negative component to the P wave in lead V_1

Figure 9-2. ECG criteria for diagnosis of RAA and LAA.

P-Pulmonale (Our Mnemonic for RAA)

The P of **p**ulmonale should recall that P waves are **p**rominent (i.e., tall) and **p**eaked in the **p**ulmonary leads with RAA. Patients with COPD often have low-lying diaphragms. As a result, they frequently have a vertically oriented QRS axis.

Leads II, III, and aVF are vertically oriented, which is why we call them the "pulmonary" leads. To satisfy criteria for RAA, P wave amplitude should equal or exceed 2½ little boxes in either lead II or one of the other pulmonary leads. In general, *if P waves are uncomfortable to sit on, think RAA!*

For practical purposes, lead V_1 does not contribute much to the ECG diagnosis of RAA.

P-Mitrale (Our Mnemonic for LAA)

The M of **m**itrale should recall the notched (i.e., **m**-shaped) appearance of P waves in one or more of the mitral leads with LAA. The mitral valve is a left-sided valve (controlling filling of the *left* ventricle from the *left* atrium). We loosely designate left-sided leads I and aVL as well as lead II as "mitral" (left-sided) leads. Since left atrial depolarization occurs later than right atrial depolarization, overall P wave duration may be prolonged.

An even better criterion for the ECG diagnosis of LAA is deepening and/or widening of the negative P wave component in lead V_1. Criteria for LAA are met if one can clearly fit a little box in the negative component of the P wave in this lead.

ECG DIAGNOSIS OF LVH

More than 40 criteria exist for the ECG diagnosis of LVH. Whenever an issue generates this many opinions, the obvious implication is that *none* of the criteria are optimal. We simplify this otherwise complex topic by offering three suggestions:

1. If you remember only one number for the ECG diagnosis of LVH, choose to remember the number **35.**
2. If you are able (and willing) to remember two numbers, also remember the number **12.**
3. If you'd like to remember more than two numbers, read on.

If two numbers are enough for you, skip the next section. Refer to Table 9-1 *(which also appears in the pocket reference, p. 22).* Applying the numbers 35 and 12 to the criteria suggested in Table 9-1 will enable you to diagnose LVH in almost all cases when this diagnosis is possible on ECG.

Table 9-1
Simplified Criteria for the ECG Diagnosis of LVH
1. Deepest S wave in lead V_1 *or* V_2, *plus* tallest R wave in lead V_5 *or* $V_6 \geq 35$ 2. R in lead aVL ≥ 12 3. Patient ≥ 35 years old 4. "Strain"

If You'd Like to Remember More than Two Numbers

About 10% of the time, diagnosis of LVH by ECG will be missed if the only voltage criteria used are the two that are shown in Table 9-1. Additional voltage criteria that may be helpful in such cases are listed in Table 9-2 *(which also appears in the pocket reference, p. 22)*. To recall these additional voltage criteria, remember the numbers **20** and **25.**

Table 9-2
Additional Voltage Criteria for the ECG Diagnosis of LVH
1. An R wave $\geq$20 in any of the inferior leads (II, III, or aVF) 2. Deep S waves ($\geq$20-25) in lead V_1 or V_2 3. An R wave $\geq$25 in lead V_5 4. An R wave $\geq$20 in lead V_6

Voltage criteria for LVH generally reflect the fact that when the left ventricle enlarges, left-sided leads (V₅, V₆ and/or aVL) see a greater amount of electrical activity *approach* this chamber. As a result, the amplitude of the R wave in these leads tends to increase. Similarly, right-sided leads (V₁ and V₂) will see a greater amount of electrical activity moving *away* from the right. The amplitude of the S wave in right-sided leads may therefore deepen (Figure 9-3).

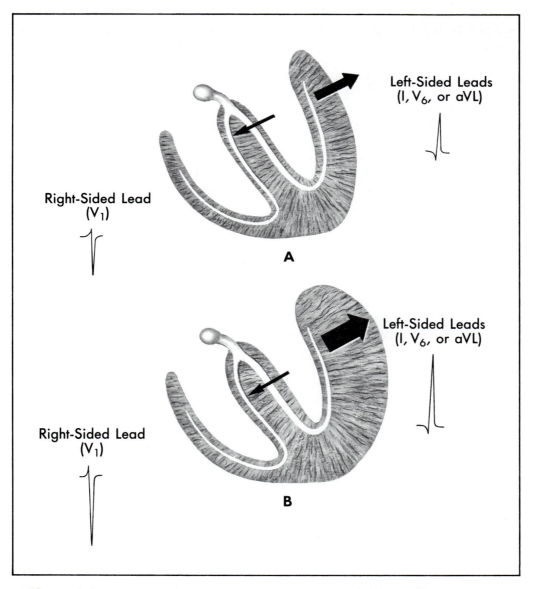

Figure 9-3.   Rationale for voltage criteria changes with LVH. **A,** Schematic representation of normal ventricular activation. **B,** Because of the increase in size of the left ventricle with LVH, more electrical activity is directed *toward* left-sided leads (V₅, V₆, and/or aVL) and *away* from right-sided leads (V₁ and V₂). As a result, the R wave tends to become taller in left-sided leads and the S wave deeper in right-sided leads.

Explanation of the Criteria for LVH

The most important voltage criterion for LVH is the one based on the number **35.** One takes the *deepest* S wave in either V_1 or V_2—*ADDS* it to the *tallest* R wave in either V_5 or V_6—and if the *SUM* equals or exceeds 35, the voltage criteria for LVH are satisfied *IF the patient is **35 years of age** or older.*

Individuals less than 35 often demonstrate increased voltage in many leads. For them, voltage criteria for LVH should not be considered as satisfied unless the sum of the deepest S wave in V_1 or V_2 plus the tallest R wave in lead V_5 or V_6 exceeds **53** mm *(with 53 conveniently being reversal of the number 35!).* Thus, the number 35 serves a dual function. It recalls the major voltage criterion for LVH, and also reminds us that voltage criteria should only be applied to individuals at least 35 years old.

Lead aVL is a high lateral lead that looks down at the heart from the left shoulder. The voltage criterion of an R wave ≥**12** in this lead is especially useful in patients with LVH and a leftward (superior) axis, in whom the lower lying lateral precordial leads (V_5 and V_6) may not demonstrate sufficient voltage to make the diagnosis.

The specificity (accuracy) of an ECG diagnosis of LVH is greatly limited when voltage criteria are satisfied in the absence of "strain." Specificity may increase to 90% or more when a definite strain pattern is present (Figure 9-4, *which also appears on p. 23 in the pocket reference*). We show the characteristic ECG appearance of "strain" in Figure 9-4, *B*. As opposed to the normal ST segment and T wave (Figure 9-4, *A*), development of strain causes *asymmetric* ST segment depression and T wave inversion.

Sometimes, instead of the typical "strain pattern," a lesser degree of ST-T wave change may be noted—that is, the ST segment may be flat or only slightly depressed, and the T wave decreased in amplitude (Figure 9-4, *C*). When such a change is seen in a patient over 35 who fulfils voltage criteria for LVH, we call it a "strain equivalent." While not as helpful as "typical strain" in solidifying the ECG diagnosis of true chamber enlargement, the presence of a "strain equivalent" does make LVH more likely.

The leads most likely to demonstrate strain are the leads that look at the left ventricle (i.e., leads I, aVL, V_5, and V_6).

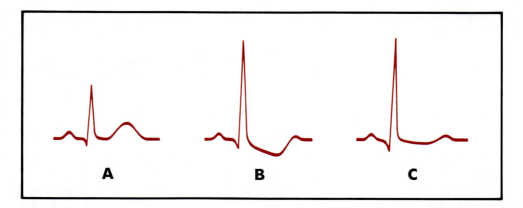

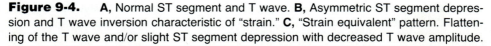

Figure 9-4.   **A,** Normal ST segment and T wave. **B,** Asymmetric ST segment depression and T wave inversion characteristic of "strain." **C,** "Strain equivalent" pattern. Flattening of the T wave and/or slight ST segment depression with decreased T wave amplitude.

It is important to emphasize that only one voltage criterion needs to be satisfied to fulfil the ECG diagnosis of LVH. However, the greater the voltage, and the more voltage criteria that are satisfied, the greater the likelihood that true chamber enlargement is present.

PRACTICE

Apply what we've covered so far. Examine the tracing shown in Figure 9-5. Are criteria for enlargement of any of the cardiac chambers satisfied? If so, how reliable are these criteria for indicating true chamber enlargement?

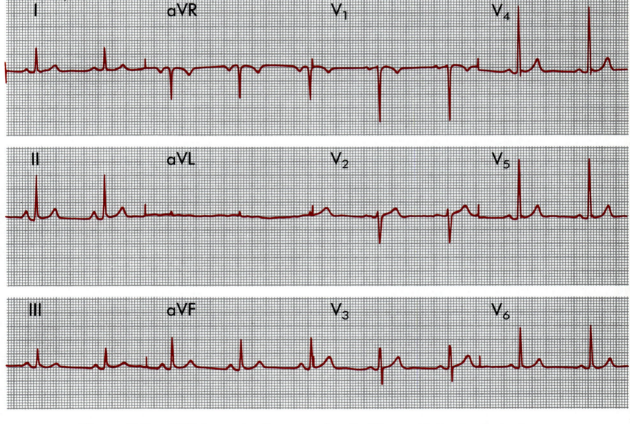

Figure 9-5.   ECG from a healthy, asymptomatic 25-year-old woman. A chest x-ray and a physical exam of this patient are normal (i.e., there is no heart murmur).

Answer to Figure 9-5

Systematic consideration of the criteria for chamber enlargement suggests the following:

RAA? Yes. The P wave is prominent and peaked *(and uncomfortable to sit on)* in the pulmonary (inferior) leads. The height of the P wave attains 2.5 mm in lead II. Even though ECG criteria for **RAA** are satisfied, true right atrial chamber enlargement (i.e., **RAE**) is unlikely in an otherwise healthy 25-year-old woman without a heart murmur.

LAA? No. The P wave is not notched in the mitral leads. The negative component of the P wave in lead V_1 is not at all deepened or widened.

LVH? The two most important numbers to recall are 35 and 12. The R wave in lead aVL is nowhere near 12.

The S wave is deeper in lead V_1 than it is in lead V_2. It measures 20 mm in lead V_1. The R wave is taller in lead V_5 than it is in lead V_6. It measures 21 mm in lead V_5. Therefore, the sum of the *deepest* S wave in lead V_1 or V_2 (20 mm) and the *tallest* R wave in lead V_5 or V_6 (21 mm) exceeds 35. Despite this, voltage criteria for LVH are *not* met, because the patient is under 35 years old. Even if this patient were 35 years old, a diagnosis of true chamber enlargement would be doubtful because of the absence of strain.

Now examine the tracing shown in Figure 9-6. Are criteria for enlargement of any of the cardiac chambers satisfied? If so, how reliable are these criteria for indicating true chamber enlargement?

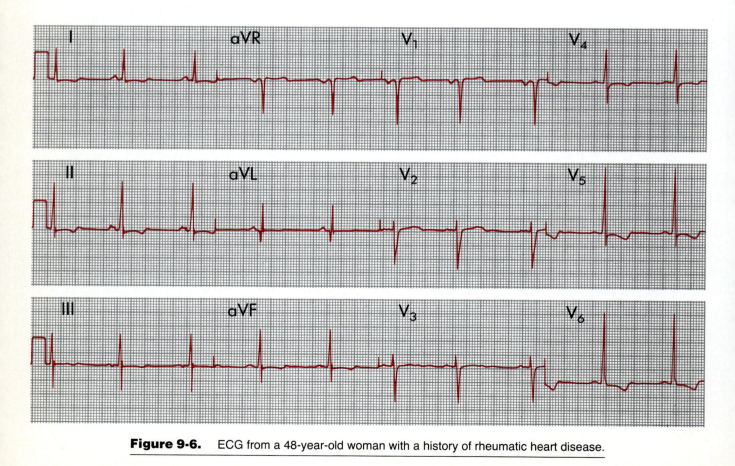

Figure 9-6.   ECG from a 48-year-old woman with a history of rheumatic heart disease.

Answer to Figure 9-6

RAA? No. P waves are neither tall nor peaked in the pulmonary leads.

LAA? Although not significantly widened, m-shaped notching is definitely present in lead II. In addition, a deep, negative component to the P wave is evident in lead V_1. In an adult with a history of rheumatic heart disease, it is likely that these findings reflect true left atrial enlargement.

LVH? The R wave in lead aVL does not quite measure 12. However, the sum of the S wave in lead V_1 (which measures 15 mm) and the R wave in lead V_6 (which measures 26 mm) exceeds 35. In addition, the asymmetric ST segment depression in leads V_5 and V_6 (and to a lesser extent in lead I) is characteristic of "strain" and strongly suggests that true chamber enlargement is present.

ECG DIAGNOSIS OF RVH

We have intentionally saved our discussion of RVH for last. This is because detection of right ventricular enlargement in adults by ECG criteria is often exceedingly difficult. The left ventricle is normally so much larger and thicker than the right ventricle in adults that it masks even moderate increases in right ventricular chamber size.

We look at the ECG diagnosis of RVH as a "detective" diagnosis. Rarely is there any one finding that clinches the diagnosis. Instead, the determination of RVH is usually suggested by a combination of findings.

We list the findings we feel most helpful in suggesting the ECG diagnosis of RVH in adults in Table 9-3 *(which also appears in the pocket reference, p. 25)*.

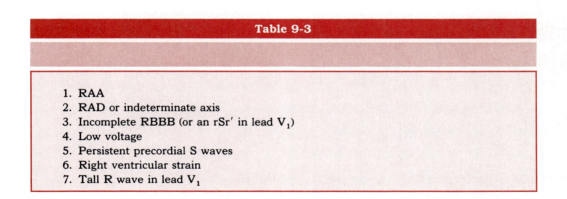

Table 9-3

1. RAA
2. RAD or indeterminate axis
3. Incomplete RBBB (or an rSr′ in lead V_1)
4. Low voltage
5. Persistent precordial S waves
6. Right ventricular strain
7. Tall R wave in lead V_1

Explanation of the Criteria for RVH in Adults

None of the criteria listed in Table 9-3 by itself is enough to make the diagnosis of RVH. However, the presence of several of these criteria, especially in a patient likely to have RVH (such as a patient with COPD, right-sided heart failure, pulmonary hypertension, or pulmonary stenosis) may be strongly suggestive.

The finding of RAA provides strong indirect evidence for RVH. Clinically, true right atrial enlargement is almost never seen without accompanying right ventricular enlargement.

True right ventricular chamber enlargement often produces a right axis shift. Sometimes patients with COPD develop an indeterminate axis instead, because of the shift in their electrical axis. As a result of a rightward and posterior shift in electrical axis, such patients often demonstrate persistent S waves across the precordial leads. Enlargement of the right ventricular outflow tract may give rise to a terminal rightward force in lead V_1 (producing an rSr' or incomplete RBBB pattern in this lead). A huge barrel chest may reduce QRS amplitude in many leads and produce low voltage.

The remaining two findings—right ventricular "strain" and a tall R wave in lead V_1—are usually not seen in adults unless (until) RVH is severe or the disease state is end-stage. With RVH, ST-T wave changes of "strain" appear in leads that look at the right ventricle. Thus, right ventricular strain may be seen either in the inferior leads (II, III, or aVF) or the anterior leads (V_1, V_2, or V_3).

Practice

Examine the ECG shown in Figure 9-7. Is there evidence for atrial enlargement? Is it likely that RVH is present?

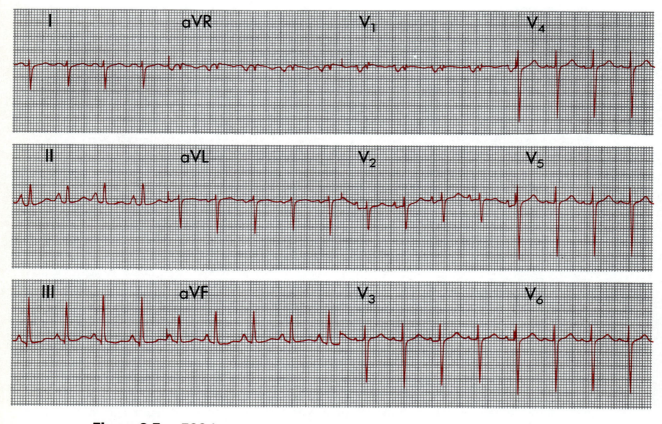

Figure 9-7.   ECG from a 53-year-old woman with long-term and severe COPD.

Answer to Figure 9-7

RAA? Yes. The typical pattern of P-pulmonale is present.

LAA? Yes. The terminal negative component of the P wave in lead V_1 is markedly deepened and widened.

LVH? No. None of the ECG criteria for LVH are met.

RVH? Four of the findings listed in Table 9-3 *(pocket reference, p. 25)* are present. There is RAA. The axis is rightward (negative QRS deflection in lead I; positive QRS deflection in lead aVF). There is an rSr′ (incomplete RBBB) pattern in lead V_1. Transition* never occurs and S waves persist across the precordium. The combination of these findings, especially in an adult with a long-term history of COPD, strongly suggests that RVH may be present.

The ECG Pattern of Pulmonary Disease

Although definitive ECG diagnosis of RVH in adults is often exceedingly difficult, suspicion of the presence of pulmonary disease (such as COPD) may be much more readily apparent. Table 9-4 *(which also appears in the pocket reference, p. 25)* indicates that, once again, a combination of findings may be needed to arrive at this conclusion:

Table 9-4
Findings Suggestive of Pulmonary Disease in Adults
1. RAA 2. RAD or indeterminate axis 3. Incomplete RBBB (or an rSr′ in lead V_1) 4. Low voltage 5. Persistent precordial S waves

Note that, with the exception of the last two findings in Table 9-3 (right ventricular strain, tall R wave in lead V_1), Table 9-4 is identical to Table 9-3. Thus, even though one could not definitively diagnose RVH in Figure 9-7 by ECG criteria, one could at least state that an ECG pattern of ***"pulmonary disease"*** was present.

---

*The precordial zone of **transition** is the place where the QRS complex changes from being predominantly negative to being predominantly positive. Normally this occurs between leads V_2 and V_4. (We discuss the zone of transition more in Chapter 10).

10

QRST Changes

The "heart" of ECG interpretation resides in assessing the tracing for **QRST changes.** The purpose of the mnemonic **Q-R-S-T** is to ensure a systematic approach so that nothing is left out. The most common mistake when a systematic approach is not used is to allow more dramatic ST segment and T wave changes to consume one's attention while subtler but equally important findings (such as a dominant R in V_1 or poor R wave progression) go unnoticed. Forcing oneself to routinely follow a systematic approach not only prevents important findings from being overlooked, but ends up *saving time* in the long run.

For practical purposes, lead aVR can be ignored in your systematic approach. This lead views the heart from afar (looking down from the right shoulder), and rarely contributes useful information to the interpretation.

Our suggested approach to systematic assessment of QRST segment changes is shown in Table 10-1.

Table 10-1
Suggested Approach to Systematically Assessing QRST Changes

1. Ignore lead aVR
2. Scan each of the other 11 leads for **Q waves.** Note the leads in which you find them.
3. Check for **R wave progression:**
    Does transition occur in the usual place?
    Tall R wave in lead V_1?
    rSr' pattern in lead V_1?
4. Look at all leads (except aVR) for **ST segment** and **T wave** changes.

PATTERNS OF LEADS

In Chapter 1 we introduced the basic lead groups and the areas of the heart they represent. Table 10-2 *(which also appears in the pocket reference, p. 27)* reviews this information.

Table 10-2
Basic Lead Groups

Inferior leads: II, III, aVF
Septal leads: V_1, V_2
Anterior leads: V_2 to V_4
Lateral leads:
   Lateral precordial leads: V_4 to V_6
   High lateral leads: I, aVL

Note that there is a lot of overlap within these general lead groups. Thus, the two septal leads are V_1 and **V_2**; the anterior leads are **V_2**, V_3, and **V_4**; and the lateral precordial leads are **V_4**, V_5, and V_6.

We suggest that rather than focusing on individual leads, you aim for a more global assessment. Take in simultaneously *patterns of leads* that view a similar area of the heart.

For example, the three inferior leads are II, III, and aVF. With inferior infarction, one would expect to find similar changes in *each* of these leads. If a small q wave or subtle ST segment change is present in only one of these three leads, it is much less likely to be clinically significant than if it were found in all three leads.

To crystallize this point, examine panels *A* and *B* in Figure 10-1. Is the q wave and ST segment elevation in lead III of panel *A* likely to be a real finding? Is it likely to be significant? Or is this small q wave and subtle ST segment elevation more likely to be significant in panel *B?*

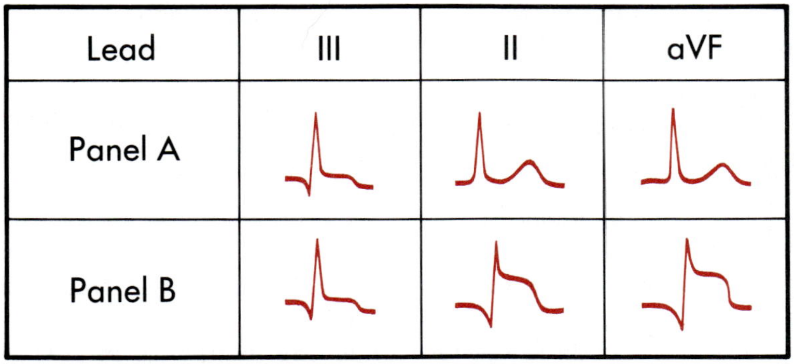

Lead	III	II	aVF
Panel A			
Panel B			

Figure 10-1

Answer to Figure 10-1

The identical complex is shown for lead III in both panel *A* and panel *B*. However, the normal findings in leads II and aVF of *A* make it much less likely that the small q wave and subtle ST segment elevation in lead III represents an acute (and significant) change. On the other hand, the obvious abnormalities in leads II and aVF of *B* leave little doubt that the findings in lead III are real and suggestive of an acute change!

Looking at patterns of leads makes you sound (and think) more like an experienced electrocardiographer, improves your accuracy, and saves time. Try it in Figure 10-2. Is the shallow T wave inversion in lead V_3 of panel *A* likely to be significant? Is it more likely to be significant in panel *B?*

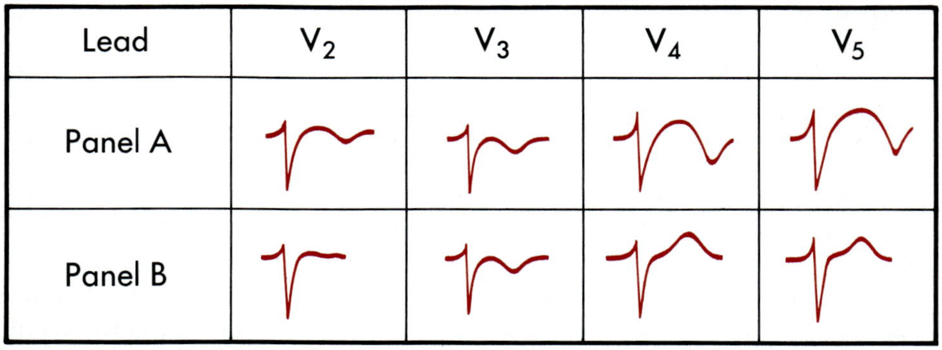

Lead	V_2	V_3	V_4	V_5
Panel A				
Panel B				

Figure 10-2

Answer to Figure 10-2

Once again, the identical QRS complex is shown for lead V_3 in both panel *A* and panel *B*. Once again, neighboring leads provide the answer. ST segment coving and deep T wave inversion in *A* strongly suggest acuity. In contrast, the isolated T wave inversion in lead V_3 of *B* is a relatively nonspecific finding (in the absence of T wave inversion in other leads), and much less likely to reflect acute ischemia. (The isolated T wave inversion in lead V_3 is a particularly unusual finding, considering that the T wave is not inverted in lead V_2 and not inverted in lead V_4.)

ꝗ WAVES

Q waves embody the essence of myocardial infarction. Dead (necrosed) tissue is electrically inert, and accounts for the initial negative deflection away from an infarcted zone. It is this initial negative deflection directed *away* from the monitoring lead that produces a Q wave in the area of infarction.

Reference is often made to the term *significant* with respect to Q waves. According to those using this reference, a Q wave is labeled as "significant" (i.e., indicative of infarction) if it is at least one little box wide and/or at least 25% of the height of the R wave in the lead in question. This is in contrast to the **normal** small ("insignificant") **septal q waves** routinely seen in otherwise healthy individuals in one or more of the lateral leads (i.e., I, aVL, V_4, V_5, or V_6).

We have difficulty with this terminology for several reasons. First, certain leads may normally display moderate- or even large-sized Q waves, making it difficult at times to distinguish between normal and pathologic Q waves on the basis of size alone (Table 10-3, *which also appears in the pocket reference, p. 27).* Moreover, not all infarctions produce "significant" Q waves. Some infarctions don't produce any Q waves at all (so-called non-Q-wave infarctions). Q waves that do reflect prior infarction do not always persist. With time they may diminish in size or completely disappear. Thus, the tiny remnant of a previously large Q wave may still be clinically "significant" (i.e., reflect prior infarction) despite its seemingly insignificant size and otherwise benign electrocardiographic appearance. Finally, many conditions other than infarction may produce Q waves (including IHSS,* dilated cardiomyopathy, axis shifts, COPD, intraventricular conduction defects, technical errors, etc.).

Table 10-3
Leads That May Normally Display Moderate- to Large-Sized Q Waves*
Lead III Lead aVF Lead aVL Lead V$_1$ (and sometimes also lead V$_2$) Lead aVR†

*NOTE: Small and narrow **normal septal q waves** are often seen in one or more of the lateral leads (I, aVL, V$_4$, V$_5$, and/or V$_6$) in asymptomatic individuals without heart disease.
†In general we ignore lead aVR, since it rarely contributes useful information to our interpretation.

For all these reasons, we suggest you *not* concern yourself with the significance of Q waves at this point in the interpretive process. Instead, content yourself with merely identifying and listing those leads that have Q waves. The significance of Q waves will usually become apparent later on when the ECG is interpreted in light of the clinical history, other findings (accompanying ST-T wave changes), and comparison with prior tracings (if available).

THE ZONE OF TRANSITION

Normally, the QRS complex is predominantly negative in lead V$_1$. This is because this right-sided lead for the most part views the heart's electrical activity as moving *away* from the right as the left ventricle is depolarized (Figure 10-3, *which also appears in the pocket reference, p. 30).*

In contrast, the QRS complex in left-sided leads V$_5$ and V$_6$ is usually positive, reflecting the fact that the general direction of left ventricular depolarization is *toward* these leads (i.e., toward the left).

We define the zone of **transition** as the place where the QRS complex changes from being predominantly negative to being predominantly positive. Normally this occurs between leads V$_2$ and V$_4$. If the QRS complex becomes predominantly positive sooner (i.e., between leads V$_1$ and V$_2$), we say there is **early transition.** The extreme case of early transition is when the R wave is entirely positive

---

*IHSS = Idiopathic hypertrophic subaortic stenosis. This type of cardiomyopathy is characterized by marked hypertrophy of the interventricular septum. Septal thickening may produce Q waves that are not due to infarction. A more recent term for the disorder is obstructive hypertrophic cardiomyopathy.

in lead V_1. The most obvious example of this occurs with severe RVH (from pulmonary stenosis, pulmonary hypertension, or end-stage pulmonary disease), because of the tremendous increase in right ventricular forces. In addition to RVH, there are several other entities that may give rise to a ***tall R wave in lead V_1.*** (We defer discussion of these until Chapter 13.)

In contrast to early transition, the R wave may sometimes not become predominant until later (i.e., until after lead V_4). When this is the case, we say there is ***delayed transition.*** Occasionally, transition may *never* occur. This is most commonly seen in patients with COPD, in whom relatively deep S waves tend to persist across the precordial leads. We have already seen an example of this in Figure 9-7.

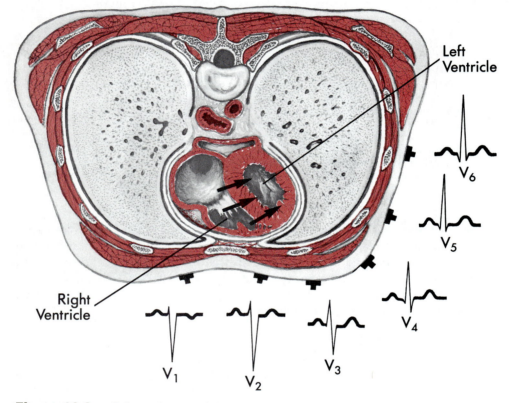

Figure 10-3.   Schematic view of the heart. The arrows depict the general direction of left ventricular depolarization. The QRS complexes in the precordial leads show normal R wave progression.

Question

Between which two leads does transition occur in Figure 10-3? Is this a normal area of transition?

Answer

The QRS complex is predominantly negative in lead V_2. It becomes predominantly positive in lead V_3. Therefore, *transition* occurs between leads V_2 and V_3. This is a normal area for transition to occur.

R WAVE PROGRESSION

R wave progression is normal in Figure 10-3; that is, the R wave gradually increases in amplitude as one moves across the precordial leads.

There are several points to emphasize regarding R wave progression:

1. It is a purely descriptive electrocardiographic finding. It does not by itself imply any organic pathology.

2. The R wave may not necessarily become taller in each successive precordial lead. Thus, the R wave may normally "peak out" in lead V_5, or even in lead V_4 (Figure 10-4).

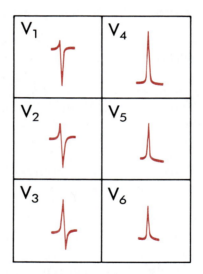

Figure 10-4.   Example of normal R wave progression despite the fact that the amplitude of the R wave in leads V_5 and V_6 is *less* than that in lead V_4. Transition occurs between leads V_2 and V_3. R wave progression is normal because the R wave does "progress" (increase in amplitude) from V_1 to V_4.

3. There are many causes of poor R wave progression (Table 10-4, *which also appears in the pocket reference, p. 31*). One of the most common causes (if not **THE** most common cause) is lead misplacement. We do not include the causes of R wave progression as one of our "Essential Lists" (and therefore do *not* advocate committing Table 10-4 to memory) because other findings on the tracing will usually suggest the cause.

Table 10-4
Common Causes of Poor R Wave Progression
LVH RVH Pulmonary disease (i.e., COPD, long-standing asthma) Anterior or anteroseptal infarction Conduction defects (i.e., LBBB, LAHB, IVCD) Cardiomyopathy Chest wall deformity Normal variant Lead misplacement

4. Despite its common usage (and all that we have said up to now), we feel it important to realize that "R wave progression" is an ambiguous term, and different expert electrocardiographers may perceive an entirely different meaning when using it. Practically speaking, the morphology of the QRS complex in the precordial leads may be more effectively communicated by use of one or more of the following descriptors:

   QS complex in lead(s) V_1; V_1 and V_2; or V_1 to V_3 (as the case may be)

   Loss of R wave in lead V_2, V_3, or V_4 (as the case may be)

   Delayed transition

5. A final condition to be aware of is the finding of an **rSr′ pattern in lead V_1.** As we discussed in Chapter 5, *complete RBBB* is diagnosed when the QRS complex is widened (to ≥0.11 seconds) and there is an rSR′ (or RBBB-equivalent pattern) in lead V_1 and a wide terminal S wave in leads I and V_6. *Incomplete RBBB* is diagnosed if QRS morphology is typical of RBBB, but the QRS complex is not widened.

   Sometimes QRS morphology suggests incomplete RBBB in lead V_1 (i.e., there is an rSr′ in this lead), but lateral S waves are missing. No consensus exists as to whether this pattern represents incomplete RBBB. We therefore acknowledge the finding as an **"rSr′ pattern"** (i.e., rSr′ in V_1, no S waves in I or V_6).

   Incomplete RBBB and the rSr′ pattern are exceedingly common findings that have identical clinical implications. Although they may occur in patients with COPD, RVH, or certain types of congenital heart disease (especially atrial septal defect), they are seen most often as incidental findings (normal variants) in otherwise healthy young adults. *It is easy to pick up the rSr′ pattern if you routinely look for it when inspecting lead V_1 for R wave progression.*

Examine the sets of precordial leads shown in Figures 10-5 through 10-11. Despite the fact that all seven of these sets might be described by an expert as showing "poor R wave progression," the clinical implications of each are quite different. For each example, describe QRS complex morphology in the anteroseptal leads (i.e., V_1 through V_4), indicate whether r wave amplitude increases appropriately or decreases, and note where transition occurs. *Is there an rSr′ pattern in lead V_1?* Finally, choose the clinical cause(s) from Table 10-4 most likely to produce this precordial lead appearance.

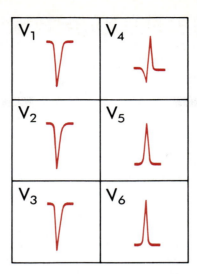

Figure 10-5. Precordial leads of a 75-year-old woman with a history of "angina" for years. The QRS complex is narrow.

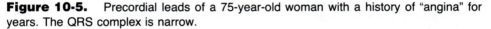

Determine the following for Figure 10-5:

QRS morphology in leads V_1 to V_4 *(Is there an rSr' pattern in lead V_1?)*

Whether the r wave increases appropriately or decreases in amplitude

The zone of transition

The likely cause (from Table 10-4) of the poor R wave progression

Answer to Figure 10-5

There is a QS complex in leads V_1 to V_3 and a QR in V_4. Strictly speaking, there is poor R wave progression (since there is no r wave at all in leads V_1 to V_3), but transition occurs normally between leads V_3 and V_4.

Clinically, this picture suggests anteroseptal infarction, since there are Q waves in leads V_1 to V_4 *(see Table 10-2 in the pocket reference, p. 27).*

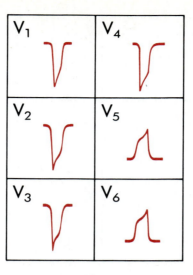

Figure 10-6. Precordial leads of a 70-year-old man with a history of heart failure. The QRS complex is *wide*. Lead I (not shown) looks identical to lead V_6.

> **Determine the following for Figure 10-6:**
> QRS morphology in leads V_1 to V_4 *(Is there an rSr' pattern in lead V_1?)*
> Whether the r wave increases appropriately or decreases in amplitude
> The zone of transition
> The likely cause (from Table 10-4) of the poor R wave progression

Answer to Figure 10-6

There is a QS complex in leads V_1 to V_4. Transition is slightly delayed and occurs between leads V_4 and V_5. *But the most significant finding on this tracing is QRS widening.* Morphology in the three key leads (considering we are told that lead I looks identical to lead V_6) suggests that the patient has complete LBBB.

Clinically, QS complexes are a normal finding in the anterior precordial leads with LBBB. One cannot say anything about the possibility of prior infarction, and the area of transition means little with this conduction defect.

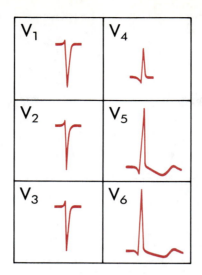

Figure 10-7. Precordial leads of a 50-year-old man with long-standing hypertension. The QRS complex is narrow, and QRS amplitude is markedly increased in leads V_5 and V_6.

Determine the following for Figure 10-7:
  QRS morphology in leads V_1 to V_4 *(Is there an rSr' pattern in lead V_1?)*
  Whether the r wave increases appropriately or decreases in amplitude
  The zone of transition
  The likely cause (from Table 10-4) of the poor R wave progression

Answer to Figure 10-7

There is an rS complex in leads V_1 to V_3, and a qR in V_4. Although technically the small initial r wave in lead V_1 does not "progress" (increase in size) as one moves from V_1 to V_3, this is not necessarily abnormal, since an r wave *IS* present in these leads and transition occurs normally (between leads V_3 and V_4).

Clinically, the markedly increased QRS amplitude in leads V_5 and V_6, together with characteristic ST-T wave changes of strain in these leads, suggests LVH as the reason for poor R wave progression in this example.

Question

Do you think the q waves in leads V_4 to V_6 in Figure 10-7 are "significant" (i.e., do these q waves reflect infarction?). Is there another possible explanation for these q waves?

Answer

The q waves in leads V_4 to V_6 could reflect lateral infarction. However, they are neither deep nor wide, and are more likely to be normal septal q waves that are not indicative of any pathology.

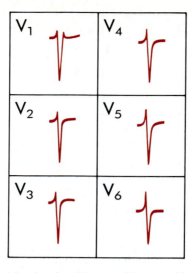

Figure 10-8.   Precordial leads of a 60-year-old man with a long history of smoking. There is diffuse wheezing on examination. The QRS complex is narrow. There is low voltage in the limb leads, RAD, and tall, pointed P waves in the inferior leads suggestive of RAA.

Determine the following for Figure 10-8:
 QRS morphology in leads V_1 to V_4 *(Is there an rSr' pattern in lead V_1?)*
 Whether the r wave increases appropriately or decreases in amplitude
 The zone of transition
 The likely cause (from Table 10-4) of the poor R wave progression

Answer to Figure 10-8

There is an rSr' pattern in lead V_1 and an rS complex in leads V_2 to V_4. R wave amplitude increases only slightly as one moves across the precordial leads, and transition never occurs.

Without knowing if there is an S wave in lead I, it is impossible to tell if the patient has a true incomplete RBBB or just an rSr' pattern in lead V_1. Practically speaking, it doesn't matter, because the clinical significance of these two entities is the same. The combination of low voltage, RAD, RAA, an rSr' pattern in lead V_1, and persistent S waves across the precordium in a 60-year-old man with a history of smoking and wheezing suggests pulmonary disease (and possible RVH) as the cause of the poor R wave progression.

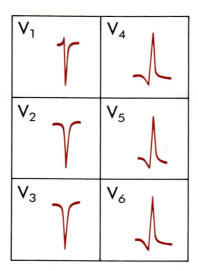

Figure 10-9.   Precordial leads of a 60-year-old woman with coronary artery disease. The QRS complex is narrow.

Determine the following for Figure 10-9:
QRS morphology in leads V_1 to V_4 *(Is there an rSr' pattern in lead V_1?)*
Whether the r wave increases appropriately or decreases in amplitude
The zone of transition
The likely cause (from Table 10-4) of the poor R wave progression

Answer to Figure 10-9

An rS complex is seen in lead V_1. There is then **loss of R wave** in leads V_2 and V_3, and development of a wide Q wave (a QR complex) in V_4 (that persists in leads V_5 and V_6). Despite these Q waves, transition occurs normally between leads V_3 and V_4.

Even though lead misplacement is probably the most common cause of loss of R wave in the precordial leads, this is not the case here. Instead, the deep QS complexes in leads V_2 and V_3, and the wide Q waves in leads V_4, V_5, and V_6, strongly suggest infarction. *Note how much wider and deeper the Q waves are in leads V_4 to V_6 in this example than they were in Figure 10-7.*

Question

Is the infarction suggested in Figure 10-9 anteroseptal, anterior, or anterolateral? (You may wish to refer to Table 10-2 (on *p. 27 of the pocket reference)* before giving your answer.)

Answer

The infarction is not defined as septal because the initial r wave in lead V_1 remains intact. Q waves are seen in the anterior leads (V_2 to V_4) and persist across the lateral precordial leads (V_4 to V_6), making this an *anterolateral* infarction.

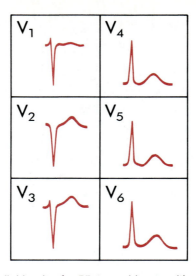

Figure 10-10. Precordial leads of a 55-year-old man with no history of heart disease. The QRS complex is narrow.

Determine the following for Figure 10-10:
QRS morphology in leads V_1 to V_4 *(Is there an rSr′ pattern in lead V_1?)*
Whether the r wave increases appropriately or decreases in amplitude
The zone of transition
The likely cause (from Table 10-4) of the poor R wave progression

Answer to Figure 10-10

An rS complex is seen in lead V_1. There is then *loss of R wave* in lead V_2 (which shows a QS complex) and resumption of a small r wave in lead V_3 (which shows an rS complex). There follows an abrupt change to an upright QRS complex (R wave) in lead V_4. Transition occurs normally between leads V_3 and V_4.

As opposed to Figure 10-9, loss of r wave (and the QS complex in lead V_2) is an isolated finding in this example. Lead V_3 shows resumption of an r wave, and the remaining precordial leads show no evidence of infarction. Thus, although one cannot absolutely rule out infarction, in an otherwise healthy 55-year-old man the isolated QS complex in lead V_2 is much more likely to be due to lead misplacement.

Question

If the loss of R wave and QS complex in lead V_2 of Figure 10-10 was due to infarction, would you label the infarction as septal, anteroseptal, or anterior?

Answer

The infarction would be *anterior,* since the initial r wave in lead V_1 remains intact.

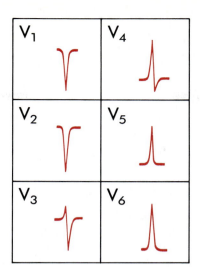

Figure 10-11.   Precordial leads of a 45-year-old woman with no history of heart disease. The QRS complex is narrow.

Determine the following for Figure 10-11:

QRS morphology in leads V_1 to V_4 *(Is there an rSr' pattern in lead V_1?)*

Whether the r wave increases appropriately or decreases in amplitude

The zone of transition

The likely cause (from Table 10-4) of the poor R wave progression

Answer to Figure 10-11

A QS complex is seen in leads V_1 and V_2. An R wave develops by lead V_3 and becomes predominant in lead V_4. Transition occurs normally between leads V_3 and V_4.

Clinically we are faced with a problem similar to the one that confronted us in the previous example. There is simply no way to know for sure whether the QS complexes in leads V_1 and V_2 represent infarction. Statistically, however, in an otherwise healthy 45-year-old woman with no history of heart disease, it is more likely that they do not. Contrast this example with the set of precordial leads shown in Figure 10-5. In that example, a QS complex was seen in leads V_1, V_2, and V_3, **and** a wide Q wave was present in lead V_4. In addition, the patient was older and had a history of angina for years. The combination of these factors argues strongly for infarction.

As stated in Table 10-3 *(pocket reference, p. 27)*, leads V_1 and V_2 may sometimes normally display Q waves (QS complexes). In such cases it may be extremely difficult to exclude the possibility of infarction. However, when a QS complex is seen in leads V_1, V_2, **and** V_3, it becomes much more likely that prior infarction has occurred.

Question

If the QS complex in leads V_1 and V_2 of Figure 10-11 was due to infarction, would you label the infarction as septal, anteroseptal, or anterior?

Answer

The infarction would be either *septal* or *anteroseptal,* since the involved leads (the leads with Q waves) are V_1 and V_2 (see Table 10-2).

ST SEGMENT AND T WAVE CHANGES

Assessment of ST segment and T wave changes holds the key to evaluating much of the information available for the interpretation of any given tracing.

The easiest way to approach this assessment is systematically. Look at all leads (except aVR) and note *(write down)* any ST segment and T wave changes as a part of your descriptive analysis. After you have done so, consider these changes and integrate them into your clinical impression in light of the patient's age, the history, available prior tracings, and other abnormalities on the ECG.

Descriptive analysis of ST segment and T wave changes is easy. Simply look at patterns of leads and describe the findings you see.

The Normal ST Segment and T Wave

Figure 10-12 shows the normal appearance of the ST segment and T wave in a lead with a predominantly upright QRS complex *(A)* as well as in one with a predominantly negative QRS complex *(B).*

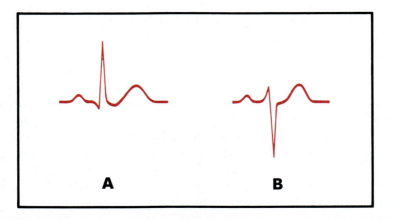

A   **B**

Figure 10-12.   Examples of a normal ST segment and T wave. Note in each case that the ST segment is essentially isoelectric with the baseline (i.e., with the PR segment) and that the T wave is upright. The ST segment itself is smooth, and gradually (and almost imperceptibly) blends with the T wave.

Contrast the normal picture shown in Figure 10-12 with the three variations shown in Figure 10-13. What changes do you see?

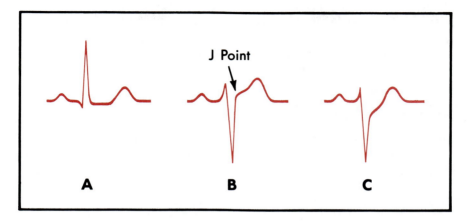

Figure 10-13.   ST segment variations from normal.

Answer to Figure 10-13

Despite the fact that the T wave remains upright for each variation, there are definite changes in the ST segment. In *A,* the ST segment is *flat.* Note how much more abrupt the transition between the end of the ST segment and the onset of the T wave is as compared with the complex in Figure 10-12, *A.*

The ST segment is *elevated* in Figure 10-13, *B*. The **J point** (i.e., the juncture of the end of the S wave of the QRS complex and the beginning of the ST segment) is clearly elevated with respect to the PR segment baseline.

Finally, in Figure 10-13, *C,* the ST segment is depressed (i.e., the J point originates below the PR segment baseline).

ST Segment Elevation

Much more important than the actual amount of ST segment elevation, is the *shape* of the ST segment (Figure 10-14, *which also appears in the pocket reference, p. 31*). While exceptions exist, in general, ST segment elevation with an upward concavity tends to be benign. This is especially true when this type of ST segment elevation occurs in otherwise healthy, asymptomatic adults and is associated with notching of the J point (Figure 10-14, *A* and *B*).

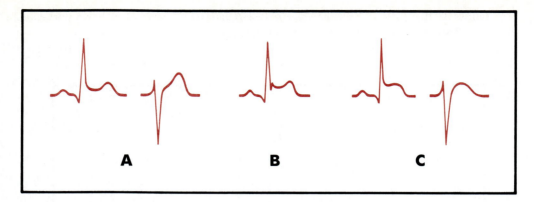

Figure 10-14.   Examples of ST segment elevation. ST segment elevation with an upward concavity **(A)** tends to be benign, especially if there is J point notching **(B)**. ST segment coving **(C)** is much more likely to represent acute injury.

In contrast, ST coving (i.e., with a downward concavity) is much more likely to represent an acute injury current of acute infarction.

To facilitate recall of the usual clinical significance of these two types of ST segment elevation, we like to refer to the upward concavity type as "smiley" ST segment elevation and the coved (downward concavity) type as "frowny" ST segment elevation. A look at Figure 10-15 *(which also appears on p. 28 of the pocket reference)* crystallizes this concept.

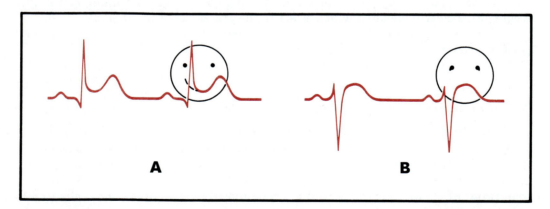

Figure 10-15.   **A,** "Smiley" (upward concavity) ST segment elevation, which is usually benign, especially when it occurs in otherwise healthy, asymptomatic individuals. **B,** "Frowny" (coved) ST segment elevation, which is more often associated with acute injury from acute infarction.

Alterations in T Wave Morphology

T waves may be upright, inverted, or flat. Upright T waves may be tall, pointed, or peaked. Negative T waves may be inverted, either symmetrically or asymmetrically. Negative T waves often blend imperceptibly into a depressed ST segment. Finally, T waves may be biphasic or flat. Examples of these alterations in T wave morphology are shown in Figure 10-16 *(which also appears on p. 29 of the pocket reference)*. Clinical conditions most often suggested by certain morphologic types are also indicated.

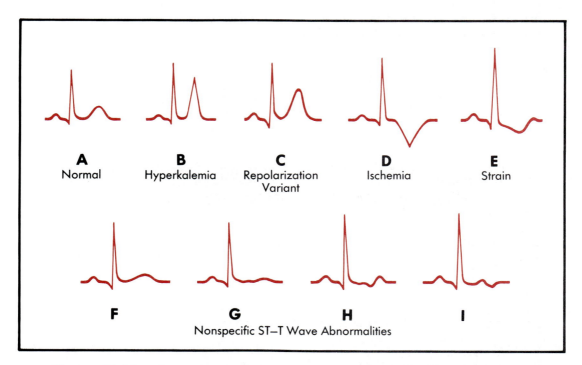

Figure 10-16.   Examples of alterations in T wave morphology. **A,** Normal T wave. **B,** Tall, pointed T wave. **C,** Tall, peaked (but not pointed) T wave. **D,** Symmetrically inverted T wave. **E,** Asymmetrically inverted T wave. **F,** Slightly flattened T wave. **G,** Greater degree of T wave flattening. **H,** Biphasic T wave (initial negative component, terminal positive component). **I,** Biphasic T wave (initial positive component, terminal negative component).

Note from the legend to Figure 10-16 that the descriptions of T wave morphology are merely that—verbal descriptions of T wave appearance. Thus, the T wave in *B* is tall (compared with the normal T wave shown in *A*) and pointed. Tall, peaked (and often pointed) T waves, especially when associated with a narrow base (as is the case here), are characteristic of *hyperkalemia*.

The T wave in *C* is tall and somewhat peaked, but it does not have the same pointed appearance as the one in *B*. Note also that compared with *B*, the base of the T wave is wider and the ascending limb climbs more slowly. This type of T wave is commonly seen as a *normal repolarization* variant.

The T wave in *D* is symmetrically inverted. This appearance suggests *ischemia*, and should be differentiated from the asymmetric T wave inversion seen in *E*. In this latter case, the ST segment only gradually slopes downward and then blends almost imperceptibly into an inverted T wave. The terminal (ascending) limb of the T wave returns to the baseline more rapidly. Asymmetric T wave inversion as seen in *E* is characteristic of *strain*.

The alterations in T wave morphology shown in *F* through *I* are described as nonspecific changes. T wave amplitude is decreased slightly in *F,* and to a greater extent in *G*. In addition to the decrease in amplitude, the T wave becomes biphasic in *H* and *I*. Because the ST segment is relatively isoelectric in each of these four examples, and because it is often difficult to separate the end of the ST segment from the beginning of the T wave, such changes are sometimes referred to as *nonspecific* **ST-T** *wave abnormalities*.

Nonspecific ST-T Wave Abnormalities

It is important to realize that there are many causes of nonspecific ST-T wave abnormalities. We list only a small number of these causes in Table 10-5.

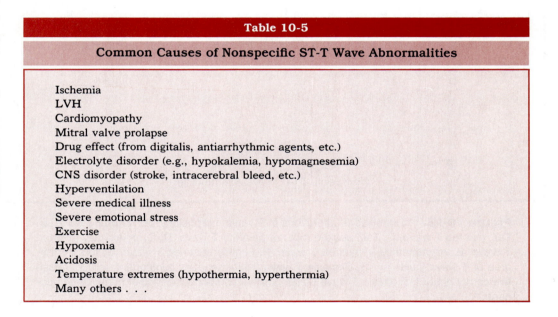

Table 10-5
Common Causes of Nonspecific ST-T Wave Abnormalities
Ischemia LVH Cardiomyopathy Mitral valve prolapse Drug effect (from digitalis, antiarrhythmic agents, etc.) Electrolyte disorder (e.g., hypokalemia, hypomagnesemia) CNS disorder (stroke, intracerebral bleed, etc.) Hyperventilation Severe medical illness Severe emotional stress Exercise Hypoxemia Acidosis Temperature extremes (hypothermia, hyperthermia) Many others . . .

There are two major points to emphasize:

1. Many of the causes of nonspecific ST-T wave abnormalities are completely noncardiac in nature.
2. The appearance of the ST segment and T wave provides no clue to the etiology of the change. This is why such alterations in ST-T wave morphology are termed "nonspecific."

Practice

Check yourself on your ability to characterize the appearance of the ST segment and T wave for the eight patterns shown in Figure 10-17. Indicate the clinical condition suggested by each pattern.

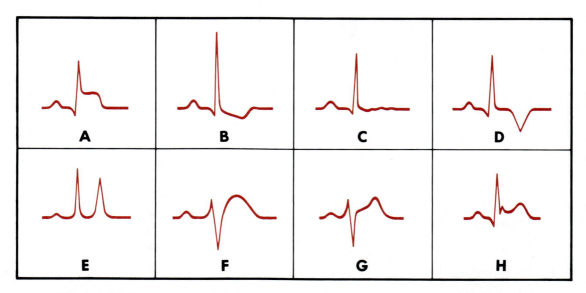

Figure 10-17.   Characterize the ST-T wave changes, and indicate the clinical condition suggested by each pattern.

Our answers appear on the following page (Figure 10-18).

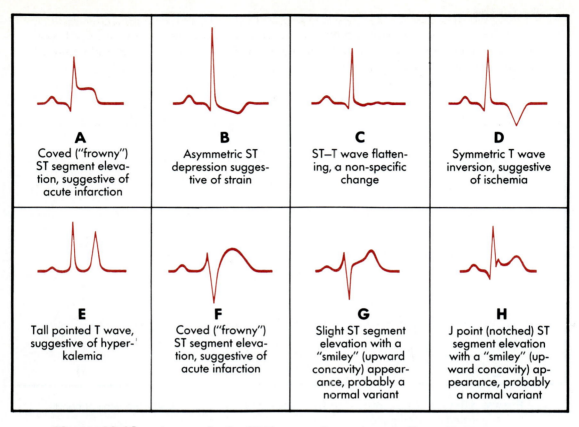

Figure 10-18.   Answers for the ST-T wave patterns shown in Figure 10-17.

Isolated T Wave Inversion

Let us conclude this chapter by introducing a final variant of normal—*isolated* T wave inversion. In certain leads, T wave inversion may be a normal finding and not reflect ischemia (Table 10-6, *which also appears on p. 28 of the pocket reference*). Note that the leads listed in Table 10-6 are conveniently the same leads that may normally display moderate- to large-sized Q waves (Table 10-3, *p. 27 in the pocket reference*)

Table 10-6
Leads That May Normally Display T Wave Inversion
Lead III Lead aVF Lead aVL Lead V$_1$ (and sometimes also lead V$_2$) Lead aVR*

*In general we ignore lead aVR, since it rarely contributes useful information to our interpretation.

As we discussed at the beginning of this chapter, the clinical significance of various electrocardiographic findings often becomes clear when one considers patterns of leads. This is particularly true when one interprets such findings in light of available clinical information. Thus, *isolated* T wave inversion in any of the leads listed in Table 10-6 should be interpreted as a totally normal finding when it occurs in an asymptomatic individual. On the other hand, an identical degree of T wave inversion becomes highly suggestive of ischemia when associated with similar T wave inversion in neighboring leads.

11

Putting It All Together (Writing the Descriptive Analysis)

We are finally ready to put together the concepts we have covered thus far. In this chapter, we present four ECGs. Systematically assess each tracing for the following *(pocket reference, p. 1):*

> **RA**te
> **RH**ythm
>   **I**ntervals (PR/QRS/QT)
>
>   **A**xis
>   **H**ypertrophy
>   **I**nfarct (= **QRST** changes)

The sum of these components represents the **descriptive analysis** portion of your interpretation.

We find it most helpful to *WRITE OUT* all findings noted. Once you have done so, the only step remaining in your interpretation will be to formulate a **clinical impression.** As a challenge, try to formulate a clinical impression for each of the four tracings in this chapter. To do this, consider all findings noted in the descriptive analysis portion of your interpretation in light of the patient's age and clinical history. Feel free to refer to previous chapters and/or the pocket reference as needed for assistance.

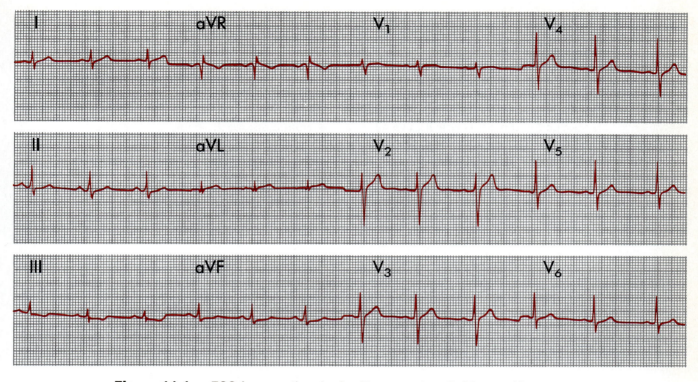

Figure 11-1. ECG from an otherwise healthy, asymptomatic 39-year-old man.

Interpretation of Figure 11-1

Descriptive analysis *(refer to pocket reference, pp. 1 to 4, as needed).* The **rhythm** is slightly irregular, at a **rate** of between 70 and 75 beats/minute. The mechanism is sinus (since the P wave is upright in lead II).

All **intervals** are normal. (That is, the PR interval is less than a large box, the QRS complex less than half a large box, and the QT interval less than half the R-R interval.)

The **axis** is normal (since the net QRS deflection is positive in both leads I and aVF). We estimate the axis to be about +55°, since the net QRS deflection in lead aVF (at +90°) appears to be slightly greater than the net deflection in lead I (at 0°).

Regarding **hypertrophy,** there is no evidence of chamber enlargement. (That is, P waves are not tall and peaked in the pulmonary leads, nor are they notched in the mitral leads, nor is there a deep negative component to the P wave in lead V_1; none of the criteria for LVH are met; and other than persistence of S waves in the precordial leads, there is no suggestion of RVH.)

Assessment of all leads (except aVR) for **infarct** (= QRST) changes reveals a tiny (normal septal) **q** wave in lead aVL, normal **R** wave progression (with transition occurring between leads V_3 and V_4), slight **ST** segment depression in leads III and aVF, and a negative or biphasic **T** wave in lead III.

Clinical impression. Considering this tracing was taken from an otherwise healthy, asymptomatic man, it almost certainly reflects a normal variant. In such an individual, the slight degree of ST segment depression in leads III and aVF should not be cause for alarm. Identical findings in an older individual with chest pain would be much more likely to reflect ischemia.

On normal tracings

Determining what is normal is among the most difficult tasks of the electrocardiographer. Appreciation of the importance of the patient's age and clinical history is invaluable. *In most cases, ECGs obtained from otherwise healthy young adults will not pick up previously unsuspected heart disease.* Electrocardiographic variations from normal are common among such individuals, but considering the context in which they occur, they rarely represent "disease."

Such is the case with Figure 11-1. A systematic approach should have led to the subtle (but definite) finding of ST segment depression in leads III and aVF. Consideration of this finding in light of the clinical context should then suggest that the tracing is probably a normal variant.

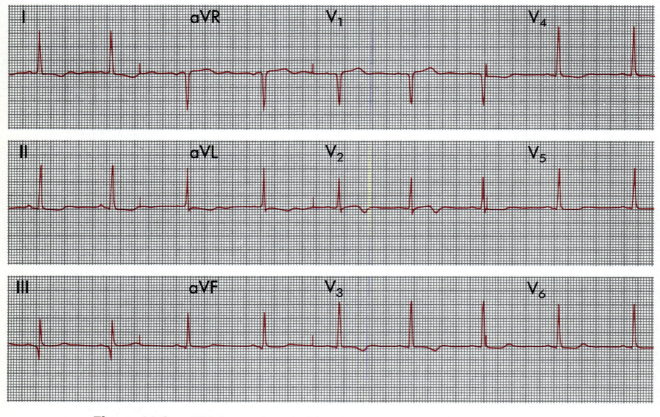

Figure 11-2.   ECG from a 77-year-old woman complaining of chest pain.

Interpretation of Figure 11-2

Descriptive analysis (*refer to pocket reference, pp. 1 to 4, as needed*). The **rhythm** is regular and the mechanism *sinus* (i.e., the P is upright in lead II). Since the R-R interval is just over five large boxes, the heart **rate** must be slightly less than 60 beats/minute ($\approx$58 beats/minute). Thus, the rhythm is *sinus bradycardia*.

All **intervals** are normal. (That is, the PR interval is less than a large box, the QRS complex less than half a large box, and the QT interval less than half the R-R interval.)

The **axis** is normal (since the QRS complex is definitely positive in both leads I and aVF. We estimate the axis to be about $+40°$, since the net QRS deflection of lead I (at $0°$) appears to be slightly greater than the net deflection of lead aVF (at $90°$).

Regarding **hypertrophy,** there is no evidence of atrial abnormality. (That is, P waves are not tall and peaked in the pulmonary leads, nor are they notched in the mitral leads, nor is there a deep negative component to the P wave in lead V_1.)

Regarding LVH, the "35" criterion (deepest S wave in lead V_1 or V_2 plus tallest R wave in lead V_5 or V_6) is not met. However, the "12" criterion *IS* satisfied (since the R wave in lead aVL exceeds 12). There is no evidence of RVH.

Assessment of all leads (except aVR) for **infarct** (= QRST) changes reveals a large, wide Q wave in lead III and small, narrow q waves in the other inferior leads; early transition (with the R wave exceeding the S wave by lead V_2); and generalized changes in the ST segments and T waves. Specifically, the ST segment in lead V_2 is coved and slightly elevated. This is associated with symmetric T wave inversion, which is also seen in lead V_3. Most of the other ST segments and T waves on this tracing demonstrate some degree of flattening compared with what one would expect if the tracing were normal.

Clinical impression. Considering this tracing is from an older woman with chest pain, it is definitely abnormal. LVH is probably present, since voltage criteria are satisfied (in aVL) and ST-T wave changes in leads I, aVL, V_5, and V_6 are at least consistent with a "strain equivalent" (*see Figure 9-4 in the pocket reference, p. 23*).

It is possible that the patient has had a prior inferior infarction, based on the large Q wave in lead III. While q waves are also present in the other two inferior leads (II and aVF), they are much smaller—making it hard to know how much significance to attach to their presence. Although one cannot rule out prior inferior infarction, the lack of ST segment elevation or deep T wave inversion in leads II, III, and aVF makes it unlikely that anything acute is going on.

On the other hand, the coved appearance and slight ST segment elevation in lead V_2, together with symmetric T wave inversion in this lead and V_3, suggest the possibility of ischemia (or even injury) that may be acute (*see Figures 10-15 and 10-16, D, in the pocket reference, pp. 28 and 29*).

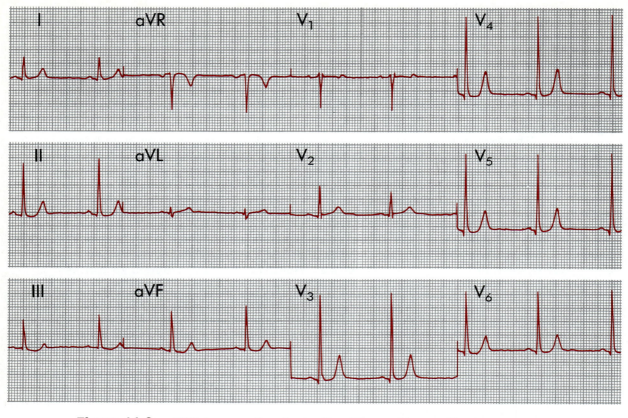

Figure 11-3.   ECG from an otherwise healthy, 55-year-old man without symptoms.

Interpretation of Figure 11-3

Descriptive analysis *(refer to pocket reference, pp. 1 to 4, as needed).* The **rhythm** is regular and the mechanism sinus (since the P wave is upright in lead II). The **rate** is just under 60 beats/minute (since the R-R is just over five large boxes), making this *sinus bradycardia.*

All **intervals** are normal.

The **axis** is normal (since the QRS complex is definitely positive in both leads I and aVF). We estimate the axis to be about +70°, since the net QRS deflection of lead aVF (at 90°) is definitely more positive than the net deflection of lead I (at 0°).

Regarding **hypertrophy,** there is no evidence of either atrial abnormality or RVH. Voltage criteria for LVH are easily met (since the sum of the S wave in lead V_1 plus the R wave in lead V_5 exceeds 35), but there is no evidence of strain.

Assessment of **infarct** (= QRST) changes reveals tiny q waves in multiple leads (I, II, III, aVF, and V_2 to V_6). There is an *rSr′ pattern* in lead V_1. Transition is early (since the QRS complex becomes predominantly positive by lead V_2). T waves are prominent (tall) and pointed (especially in leads V_3 to V_6), and associated with a narrow base. The ST segment is isoelectric.

Clinical impression. In the absence of symptoms and underlying cardiac disease, it is unlikely that the bradycardia, tiny q waves, increased voltage, rSr′ pattern, or early transition carries much clinical significance. Because the appearance of the T waves in this tracing is so typical for hyperkalemia (tall and peaked with a narrow base), the serum potassium level should probably be checked.

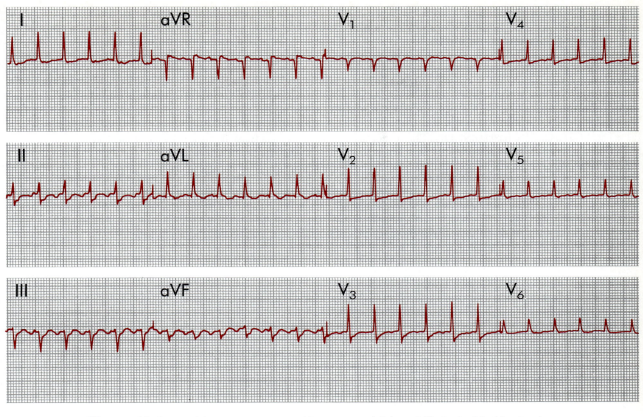

Figure 11-4.   ECG from a 69-year-old man complaining of "fluttering" in his chest.

Interpretation of Figure 11-4

Descriptive analysis *(refer to pocket reference, pp. 1 to 4, as needed).* The **rhythm** is regular, at a **rate** just over 150 beats/minute (since the R-R interval is just under two large boxes). The mechanism is *not* sinus. It can't be, since the P wave is not upright in lead II.

The actual rhythm is *atrial flutter* with 2:1 AV conduction. While the intricacies of this diagnosis extend beyond the scope of this book, three basic concepts should nevertheless be obvious from analysis of this 12-lead tracing:

1. The rhythm is *supraventricular* (since the QRS complex is narrow in *all* 12 leads).
2. The mechanism is *not* sinus (since the P wave is not upright in lead II).
3. The major differential diagnosis is between PSVT and atrial flutter (since the negative P wave in lead II rules out sinus tachycardia, and the regularity of the rhythm rules out atrial fibrillation).

Regarding **intervals,** we have already noted that the QRS complex is narrow (not more than half a large box). In the absence of sinus mechanism, the PR interval loses its meaning (and need not be calculated). Similarly, at rapid heart rates, the QT interval loses its meaning (and need not be calculated).

There is left **axis** deviation (LAD). We know this at a glance because the net QRS deflection of lead aVF is negative while that of lead I is positive. However, *pathologic* LAD (i.e., an axis more negative than $-30°$) is *not* present, because the net QRS deflection of lead II is still positive *(see Table 7-2 in the pocket reference, p. 21).* We estimate the axis to be between $-10°$ and $-20°$.

Regarding **hypertrophy,** we are unable to comment on atrial abnormality in the absence of sinus mechanism. There is no evidence of LVH or RVH.

Assessment of **infarct** (= QRST) changes reveals a tiny q wave in lead aVL, early transition (since the QRS complex becomes predominantly positive by lead V_2), and generalized ST-T wave abnormalities.

Clinical impression. The principal diagnosis is atrial flutter with 2:1 AV conduction (atrial rate $\approx$320 beats/minute; ventricular rate $\approx$160 beats/minute). We interpret the generalized ST-T wave abnormalities as "nonspecific" in nature *(see Figure 10-16, F to I, in the pocket reference, p. 29).* There is definite T wave flattening, but ST segments do not appear to be clearly elevated or depressed. Part of the difficulty in assessment stems from the tachyarrhythmia itself, since flutter waves seem to fall on (and distort) the ST segment and T wave in several leads.

Infarction and Ischemia

One of the most important reasons for obtaining an ECG is evaluation of patients with chest pain and/or possible myocardial infarction. In Table 12-1 *(which also appears in the pocket reference, p. 32)* we summarize the information we hope to learn from an ECG.

Table 12-1
Information Sought from an ECG in Patients with Chest Pain

1. Are there acute changes?
    Is the patient likely to be infarcting? (If so, what area of the heart is likely to
      be involved?)
    Is there ischemia?
    Is there some other condition that might account for the ECG changes?
    Is the patient a candidate for thrombolytic therapy? (an optimal candidate?)
2. Is there evidence of prior infarction?
    If so, is it possible to date such changes?

RECOGNITION OF ACUTE CHANGES ON THE ECG

Our initial priority in evaluating a patient who has chest pain is to determine whether he or she is acutely infarcting. Four principal ECG indicators may assist us with this goal; they are illustrated in Figure 12-1 *(which also appears in the pocket reference, p. 34).*

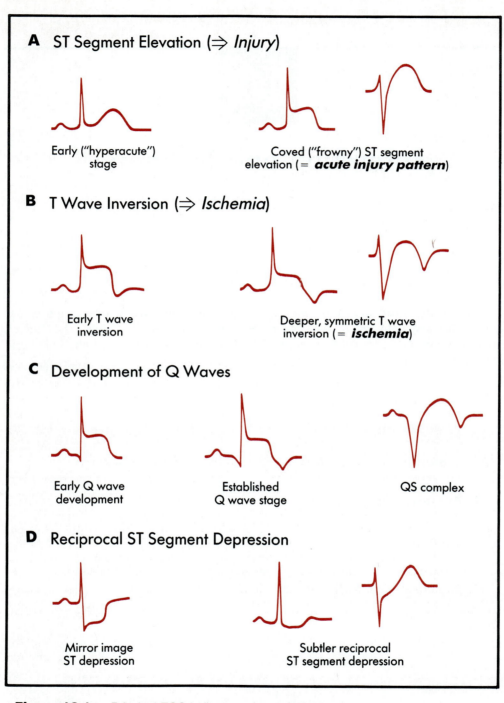

A ST Segment Elevation (⇒ *Injury*)

Early ("hyperacute")
stage

Coved ("frowny") ST segment
elevation (= ***acute injury pattern***)

B T Wave Inversion (⇒ *Ischemia*)

Early T wave
inversion

Deeper, symmetric T wave
inversion (= ***ischemia***)

C Development of Q Waves

Early Q wave
development

Established
Q wave stage

QS complex

D Reciprocal ST Segment Depression

Mirror image
ST depression

Subtler reciprocal
ST segment depression

Figure 12-1.   Principal ECG indicators of acute infarction.

ST Segment Elevation

The hallmark of acute infarction is ST segment elevation. Early on, changes may be quite subtle and represent little more than peaking or widening of the T wave and ever so slight elevation of the J point takeoff ("hyperacute" stage in Figure 12-1, *A*). Definite ST segment elevation with a coved ("frowny") appearance usually follows shortly thereafter. The hyperacute stage is short-lived, and has often already resolved by the time the patient seeks medical attention. *New-onset coved ST segment elevation is known as an* **acute injury pattern,** *and is the most convincing indicator of acute infarction.*

T Wave Inversion

T wave inversion typically follows the stage of ST segment elevation. It almost seems as if the inverted T wave is trying to "pull" the elevated ST segment back to the baseline (Figure 12-1, *B*). T wave inversion is usually *SYMMETRIC,* reflecting the underlying *ischemic* process.

Development of Q Waves

Q waves reflect myocardial necrosis. As discussed in Chapter 10, dead (necrotic) tissue is electrically inert, and accounts for the initial negative (Q wave) deflection *away* from the infarcted zone.

Q waves tend to persist following infarction. However, they don't always remain unchanged. With time they may shrink in size. Sometimes they even disappear.

In the past it was believed that Q waves developed only with transmural (i.e., full-thickness) infarction. We now know this is not always the case. Partial-thickness infarction (i.e., *subendocardial* infarction) may sometimes also produce Q waves. Conversely, infarctions that do involve the entire thickness of the ventricular wall may do so *without* necessarily producing Q waves. As might be expected, such infarctions are often much more difficult to recognize electrocardiographically. History, serial ST segment and T wave changes, and a rise in cardiac enzymes are needed to confirm the diagnosis.

In recognition of the fact that development of Q waves does not uniformly represent transmural infarction, and that transmural infarction may sometimes occur without producing Q waves, simpler terminology has been adopted. Infarctions that produce Q waves are called *"Q wave infarctions";* those that don't are *"non–Q wave infarctions".*

Clinically, non–Q wave infarctions tend to be somewhat smaller and have a better short-term prognosis than Q wave infarctions. However, non–Q wave infarctions also tend to be "incomplete." Recurrence (i.e., "completion" of the infarction) is common, and the long-term prognosis is similar to the prognosis of patients with Q wave infarctions.

Practically speaking, if Q waves do develop in association with ST segment elevation and/or T wave inversion in a patient with new-onset chest pain, one can confidently assume infarction has occurred (Figure 12-1, *C*). If Q waves do not develop, attention to history, serial ST segment and T wave changes, cardiac enzyme results, and/or other diagnostic modalities (such as an echocardiogram or radionuclide myocardial scan) may be needed to confirm the diagnosis.

Reciprocal ST Segment Depression

As we have indicated, new-onset, coved ST segment elevation is the most convincing marker of acute infarction. Noninvolved areas of the heart may also demonstrate changes resulting from acute injury. Instead of ST segment elevation, however, noninvolved areas tend to reflect ongoing infarction by ST segment depression. This is known as a **reciprocal** change. Reciprocal ST segment depression may be the mirror image of ST segment elevation. It may also be a much more subtle change (Figure 12-1, *D*).

Reciprocal changes are most evident at the onset of infarction, and tend to be short-lived. Thus their presence strongly suggests that the infarction is truly acute. Any of the noninvolved areas of the heart may manifest reciprocal changes. Acute inferior infarction (recognized by development of Q waves, ST segment elevation, and T wave inversion in leads II, III, and aVF) may therefore demonstrate anterior and/or lateral reciprocal ST segment depression. Similarly, acute anterior infarction may demonstrate reciprocal ST segment depression in the lateral and/or inferior leads.

It is important to realize that ST segment depression does not always reflect a reciprocal change. It may also reflect ischemia resulting from narrowing of another coronary artery. To illustrate this point, examine the schematic tracing shown in Figure 12-2. Is there evidence of myocardial infarction? If so, is the infarction likely to be acute? What area(s) of the heart is (are) involved?

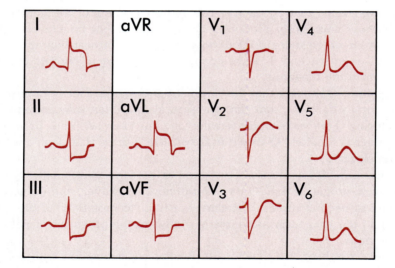

Figure 12-2.   Schematic ECG from a patient with new-onset chest pain.

Answer to Figure 12-2

All four of the principal indicators of acute infarction are present in this tracing. Leads I and aVL each demonstrate q waves, coved ST segment elevation, and beginning T wave inversion. This suggests that the location of infarction is in the high lateral wall of the left ventricle (since leads I and aVL are high lateral leads). Because q waves are small, ST segment elevation is marked, and T wave inversion is only beginning, it is likely that the infarction is still in its early stage. Further support for the acuity of the infarct comes from the presence of reciprocal ST segment depression. Reciprocal ST segment changes are marked in the inferior leads (where they demonstrate a "mirror image" of the ST segment elevation) and somewhat more subtle in the anterior leads.

Acute lateral infarction usually results from acute occlusion of the circumflex branch of the left coronary artery (Figure 12-3, *which also appears in the pocket reference, p. 35*). The inferior and anterior ST segment depression seen in Figure 12-2 may well reflect a reciprocal change of this acute infarction. However, it may also reflect simultaneous inferior and/or anterior ischemia resulting from narrowing of the right coronary artery (RCA) or the left anterior descending (LAD) coronary artery (Figure 12-3).

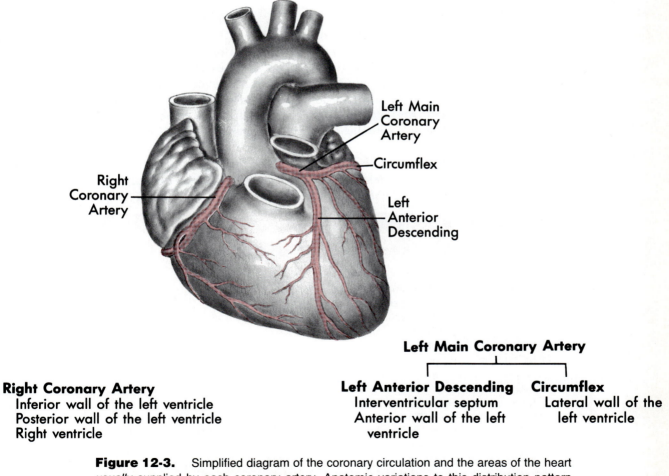

Left Main Coronary Artery

Right Coronary Artery
Inferior wall of the left ventricle
Posterior wall of the left ventricle
Right ventricle

Left Anterior Descending
Interventricular septum
Anterior wall of the left ventricle

Circumflex
Lateral wall of the left ventricle

Figure 12-3. Simplified diagram of the coronary circulation and the areas of the heart *usually* supplied by each coronary artery. Anatomic variations to this distribution pattern exist *(see text).*

As suggested by Figure 12-3, acute inferior, posterior, or right ventricular infarction most often results from occlusion of the right coronary artery. Septal and/or anterior infarction most often results from occlusion of the LAD coronary artery. Lateral infarction most often results from occlusion of the circumflex branch of the left coronary artery.

There are exceptions (anatomic variations) to the simplified diagram of the coronary circulation that we show in Figure 12-3. In about 10% of individuals, the circumflex artery is a much larger vessel (i.e., *"dominant"*) and supplies the inferior and posterior walls of the left ventricle as well as the lateral wall. In such cases, the right coronary artery is a correspondingly smaller and less important vessel. Acute inferior infarction in such patients may result from acute occlusion of the circumflex branch of the left coronary circulation.

Development of collateral vessels is another reason for alterations in the distribution of the coronary circulation. Collateral vessels are most likely to develop in older individuals, especially if they have had angina pectoris for a long period of time. Thus, a patient who has had a prior inferior infarction resulting from total occlusion of the right coronary artery may develop collateral vessels from the left coronary circulation that supply still-viable portions of the inferior wall.

DATING AN INFARCT

Precise dating of infarction is often extremely difficult. This is because all of the electrocardiographic indicators of infarction may overlap in the sequence of their occurrence. Thus, although ST segment elevation is usually the first sign of infarction, it is not always the first sign. Some infarctions never develop ST segment elevation. In such cases, ST segment depression and/or T wave inversion may be the initial ECG change. And although Q waves usually take some time to develop, they may already be well established at the time the initial ECG is recorded.

In acknowledgement of the limitations of the ECG in determining the age of infarction, we prefer to limit our descriptors for dating infarction to the three general terms shown in Table 12-2 *(which also appears in the pocket reference, p. 33).*

Table 12-2
General Descriptors for Dating Infarction

Acute infarction: onset within hours up to a day
    ST segment elevation is hyperacute or coved, and often marked.
    Q waves are small or absent.
    T wave inversion is minimal or absent.
    Reciprocal ST segment depression is often present, and may be marked.
Old infarction: onset over a week ago
    Q waves are present and are often large.
    ST segment elevation is absent.
    T wave inversion is minimal or absent.
    There is no reciprocal ST segment depression.
Recent (i.e., **"subacute"**) **infarction:** onset within a day or so, up to several days to a week
    Q waves are often present; they may be small or large.
    ST segment elevation is minimal or absent.
    T wave inversion is often present and may be marked.
    Reciprocal ST segment depression is minimal or absent.

PRACTICE

For each of the following schematic tracings, indicate whether infarction is likely. If so, what area(s) of the heart is (are) likely to be involved? How would you date the infarction? Which coronary artery(ies) is (are) most likely to be occluded? *(Refer to Table 12-2 [pocket reference, p. 33] and Figure 12-3 [pocket reference, p. 35).*

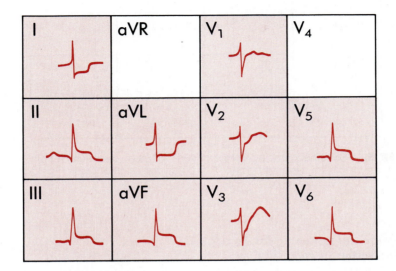

Figure 12-4.   Schematic tracing from a patient with new-onset chest pain.

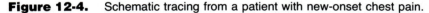

Determine the following for Figure 12-4:
   Is infarction likely?
   If so, what area(s) of the heart is (are) likely to be involved?
   How would you date the infarction?
   What coronary artery(ies) is (are) most likely to be occluded?

Answer to Figure 12-4

Small q waves and coved ST segment elevation are present in the inferior and lateral precordial leads. This suggests *acute inferolateral infarction.* Further support for the acuity of the infarct comes from reciprocal ST segment depression, which is marked in the high lateral leads and subtler in the anterior leads.

Usually, acute inferior infarction results from acute occlusion of the right coronary artery, and acute lateral infarction from occlusion of the circumflex branch of the left coronary artery. However, in patients with a *dominant* circumflex artery, occlusion of this vessel alone may produce acute inferolateral infarction.

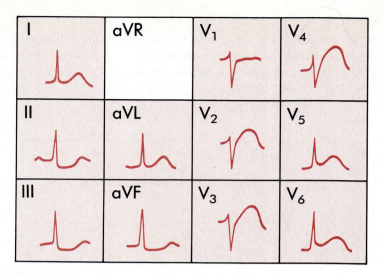

Figure 12-5.   Schematic tracing from a patient with new-onset chest pain.

> *Determine the following for Figure 12-5:*
> **Is infarction likely?**
> **If so, what area(s) of the heart is (are) likely to be involved?**
> **How would you date the infarction?**
> **What coronary artery(ies) is (are) most likely to be occluded?**

Answer to Figure 12-5

Marked, coved ST segment elevation is present in leads V_2 through V_4, and to a lesser extent in leads V_5 and V_6. There are no Q waves and no T wave inversion. These changes suggest acute anterolateral infarction. Reciprocal ST segment depression is seen in the inferior leads.

Acute anterolateral infarction may result from acute occlusion of the LAD and circumflex arteries, or from proximal occlusion of the left main coronary artery.

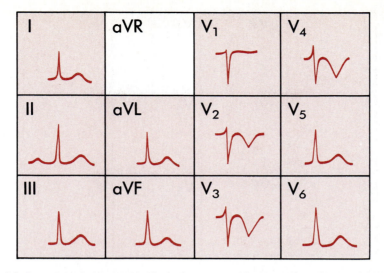

Figure 12-6.   Schematic tracing from a patient with new-onset chest pain.

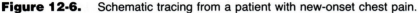

Determine the following for Figure 12-6:
   Is infarction likely?
   If so, what area(s) of the heart is (are) likely to be involved?
   How would you date the infarction?
   What coronary artery(ies) is (are) most likely to be occluded?

Answer to Figure 12-6

Symmetric T wave inversion is seen in leads V_2 through V_4. This suggests anterior ischemia. Otherwise, there is no evidence of infarction (i.e., there are no Q waves and no ST segment elevation or reciprocal ST segment depression).

The schematic tracing shown in Figure 12-6 could be consistent with a non–Q wave infarction if the patient went on to develop elevation of cardiac isoenzymes and evolutionary ST-T wave changes *without* formation of Q waves. T wave inversion in leads V_2 through V_4 is most consistent with involvement of the LAD coronary artery.

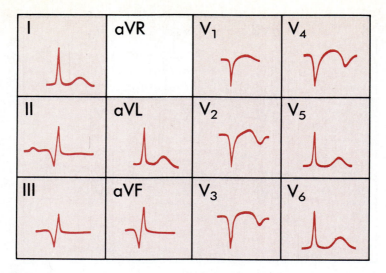

Figure 12-7.   Schematic tracing from a patient with new-onset chest pain.

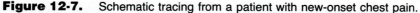

Determine the following for Figure 12-7:
  Is infarction likely?
  If so, what area(s) of the heart is (are) likely to be involved?
  How would you date the infarction?
  What coronary artery(ies) is (are) likely to be occluded?

Answer to Figure 12-7

Deep, wide Q waves are present in the inferior leads, indicating prior infarction. Since the ST segments and T waves in these leads are flat, it is likely that the inferior infarction is *old*.

ST segment coving suggestive of an injury current is seen in leads V_1 through V_4. Deep, established Q waves (actually QS complexes) indicative of infarction are seen in these leads. Symmetric T wave inversion suggestive of ischemia is also seen. Because the degree of ST segment elevation is only slight, it is hard to be sure of the age of the infarct. We would interpret the findings as indicative of anteroseptal infarction of unknown age, possibly quite recent (or even acute).

The old inferior infarction is likely to be due to prior occlusion of the right coronary artery. Anteroseptal infarction is most likely to be due to occlusion of the LAD branch of the left coronary artery. We can speculate that multivessel involvement over time in this patient may have stimulated development of collateral vessels (although cardiac catheterization, if indicated, would be the only way to know this for sure).

WHICH PATIENTS ARE LIKELY TO BENEFIT MOST FROM THROMBOLYTIC THERAPY?

The cause of acute infarction is almost always an occluding thrombus in the involved coronary artery. Reperfusion of the acutely occluded artery can sometimes limit the extent of infarction, and even reverse some of the damage that has already occurred. At the present time, intravenous thrombolytic therapy is the most frequently used method for attempting reperfusion.

Thrombolytic therapy does not always work. Moreover, only a minority of patients with acute infarction are potential candidates for thrombolytic therapy. Although protocols for treatment of acute myocardial infarction are constantly changing and vary greatly from one institution to the next, several generalities can be stated regarding the usual criteria used to select patients for thrombolytic therapy (Table 12-3, *which also appears in the pocket reference, p. 35).*

Table 12-3
Criteria for Considering Thrombolytic Therapy
Age <75 years old History of new-onset ischemic chest pain within the "window of opportunity" (i.e., within 6 hours) Definite ECG evidence of acute infarction No contraindications to thrombolytic therapy

Most institutions prefer not to administer thrombolytic therapy to patients over 75 years of age. This is because benefits seem to be less and complications significantly more in older individuals. The major complication from thrombolytic therapy is bleeding, which may be either local (from catheter insertion) or systemic. As a result, patients at high risk of bleeding are not good candidates to receive this therapy. This includes patients with bleeding disorders or a history of peptic ulcer disease; recent stroke; recent surgery; marked hypertension; trauma victims; or persons who have just received prolonged CPR with external chest compression.

It is essential that patients with dissecting aortic aneurysm or acute pericarditis not be given thrombolytic therapy. This is one of the reasons for requiring definite electrocardiographic evidence of acute infarction. At the time of this writing, *most institutions require at least 1 mm of ST segment elevation in at least two contiguous leads.* Practically speaking, after reviewing the history and initial ECG, the clinician should be comfortable that acute infarction is taking place before deciding to proceed with thrombolytic therapy.

Not all patients with acute infarction benefit from thrombolytic therapy. Assuming that the qualifying criteria in Table 12-3 have been met, two parameters suggest which patients are likely to benefit most from thrombolytic therapy (Table 12-4, *which also appears on p. 36 in the pocket reference).*

Table 12-4
Patients Likely to Benefit Most from Thrombolytic Therapy

Patients treated early
Patients with ECG evidence of large, potentially reversible infarctions:
    Anterior location
    Marked ST segment elevation
    Reciprocal ST segment depression in many leads
    Small or absent q waves

Time is the most important variable. Regarding infarction, *"time is muscle."* At present, most institutions set the upper limit of their "window of opportunity" at 6 hours. That is, symptom onset (i.e., chest pain) must have begun less than 6 hours ago for a patient to qualify as a potential candidate for thrombolytic therapy. Simply stated, *the sooner the thrombolytic therapy is started, the greater the chance that the patient will benefit*. This is especially true if thrombolytic therapy is begun within 3 hours of symptom onset.

The second major variable determining the likely benefit from thrombolytic therapy is the extent of the infarct. *The larger the infarct, the greater the potential benefit*. The ECG initially recorded at the time the patient presents can be extremely helpful in predicting the relative size of the infarct. In general, anterior infarcts are larger than inferior infarcts. The more leads that demonstrate ST segment elevation, and the greater the degree of that ST segment elevation, the larger the infarct is likely to be. This is especially true when *in addition* to ST segment elevation there is also marked reciprocal ST segment depression in multiple leads. Although Q waves do not exclude potential benefit from the thrombolytic therapy, the presence of large new Q waves makes it much less likely that myocardial damage will be reversible. Optimally, Q waves will be either absent or small at the time the patient presents.

Review: Who Should Benefit Most from Thrombolytic Therapy?

Go back to Figures 12-4 through 12-7. Assume that each of these patients is under 75 and presents within 6 hours complaining of ischemic-like chest pain. If there are no contraindications, who among them is (are) likely to benefit most from thrombolytic therapy? *(Refer to Table 12-4 [pocket reference, p. 36] as needed.)*

Answers

Figure 12-4: This patient is an excellent candidate for thrombolytic therapy. Even though the infarct is not anterior, the ECG suggests extensive involvement (of the inferior and lateral walls), with only small q waves and diffuse reciprocal changes.

Figure 12-5: This patient is also an excellent candidate for thrombolytic therapy. Infarction is anterior, Q waves are absent, and there are inferior reciprocal changes.

Figure 12-6: This patient is not a candidate for thrombolytic therapy because there is no ST segment elevation. At the time of this writing, ischemic T wave inversion (even if acute) is not an indication for thrombolytic therapy in most institutions.

Figure 12-7: At best, this patient is only a fair candidate for thrombolytic therapy. The inferior infarction is old. Large Q waves are already present anteriorly, and ST segment elevation in these leads is minimal. It is much less likely that these changes will be reversible.

SILENT INFARCTION

It is important to realize that *at least 25% of all infarctions are clinically silent*. That is, infarction occurs in the complete absence of chest pain. About half of these patients are entirely asymptomatic. In them, prior infarction is only discovered as an incidental finding when an ECG is obtained for some other reason. In the other half, nonspecific symptoms other than chest pain may be present. These include "flu-like" symptoms such as malaise or myalgias, fatigue, abdominal discomfort, shortness of breath, or a change in mental status.

Persons most likely to suffer silent infarction are the elderly, diabetics, and persons with impaired pain sensation or a high pain threshold. Examples of potentially confusing clinical scenarios include peptic ulcer or cholecystitis symptoms (which are common in patients with inferior infarction), acute confusion (without any chest pain) in an elderly patient, and cocaine overdose (which has probably become the most common cause of acute infarction in young, previously healthy adults). *We suggest maintaining a high index of suspicion and having a low threshold for obtaining an ECG on patients presenting with any of the conditions listed in Table 12-5.*

Table 12-5
Clues Suggesting Possible Silent Infarction
New-onset heart failure Acute change in mental status, especially in the elderly Unexplained abdominal pain, especially in older adults or in diabetics Unexplained dyspnea or fatigue, especially in the elderly Cocaine overdose

POSTERIOR AND RIGHT VENTRICULAR INFARCTION

We close this chapter with a few suggestions for diagnosis of acute posterior and right ventricular infarction. There are two reasons why it is important to be aware of these special types of infarction:

1. Overall prognosis from any infarction depends most on the size of the infarct. *The larger the infarct, the poorer the prognosis.* Thus, an infarction that involves the posterior *and* inferior wall of the left ventricle is likely to be larger and associated with a poorer overall prognosis than an isolated inferior infarction.

2. In the case of *right ventricular infarction,* management differs greatly from management of left ventricular infarction. Treatment of right ventricular infarction often entails *fluid infusion* to optimize contractility. Fluid infusion is contraindicated (and likely to aggravate or precipitate heart failure) in most patients with left ventricular infarction. Invasive (Swan-Ganz) monitoring is often needed with right ventricular infarction to ensure optimal hemodynamics, whereas it is not needed in uncomplicated left ventricular infarction.

Clinically, it is impossible to tell at the bedside which area of the left ventricle (anterior, lateral, inferior, and/or posterior walls) is infarcting. In contrast, bedside examination can be very helpful in suggesting acute right ventricular infarction. Such patients often present with signs of isolated right heart failure (i.e., peripheral edema, increased jugular venous distension, and/or hepatomegally with hepatojugular reflux) in the absence of pulmonary congestion. This differs greatly from the clinical presentation of acute left heart failure, in which pulmonary congestion (i.e., rales) is often the most prominent feature.

The ECG can be extremely helpful in suggesting posterior and right ventricular infarction. The problem is that none of the standard leads used on a 12-lead ECG are optimal for viewing either of these "hard-to-get-at" areas of the heart. As a result, special leads or considerations are needed for ECG diagnosis (Figure 12-8).

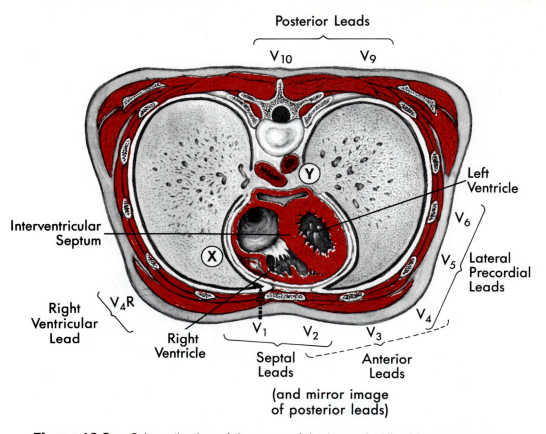

Figure 12-8.   Schematic view of the areas of the heart visualized by the precordial leads (similar to the view we first showed in Figure 1-15). Special leads or considerations are needed to optimally visualize the right ventricular wall *(X)* and the posterior wall of the left ventricle *(Y)*.

As shown in Figure 12-8, leads V_9 and V_{10} (on the back near the spine) provide the optimal view of the posterior wall of the left ventricle. However, application of recording electrodes to the patient in order to obtain these leads would require turning the patient face down (prone) in bed—a position we usually try to avoid. Thus, instead of using posterior leads, we diagnose **posterior infarction** by using anteroseptal leads (V_1, V_2, and V_3) to provide a *mirror image* of the posterior wall of the left ventricle. (Use of the **mirror test** to diagnose acute posterior infarction will be discussed in detail in Chapter 13.)

Right ventricular infarction is diagnosed by observing the typical changes of acute infarction (Q wave, ST segment elevation, and/or T wave inversion) in *lead V_4R.* This special lead looks directly at the right ventricular wall (*X* in Figure 12-8). It is easily recorded by having the ECG technician position the electrode in the anatomic area designated for lead V_4 (i.e., in the midclavicular line in the fifth interspace) on the *right* side of the chest (Figure 12-9).

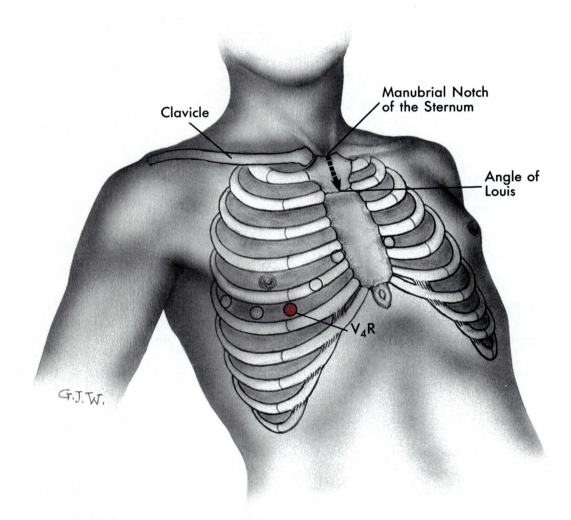

Figure 12-9. Anatomic placement of specialized lead V_4R (in the midclavicular line in the fifth interspace on the *right* side of the chest) for diagnosis of right ventricular infarction.

Problem

There are two clues to look for in the diagnosis of right ventricular infarction. Both are present in Figure 12-10. Can you tell what they are?

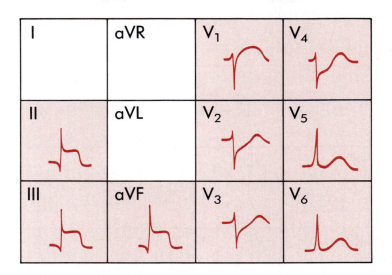

I	aVR	V$_1$	V$_4$
II	aVL	V$_2$	V$_5$
III	aVF	V$_3$	V$_6$

Figure 12-10.   Schematic ECG from a patient with new-onset chest pain. What are the two clues to acute right ventricular infarction in this tracing?

Hint #1: Which coronary artery would you expect to find acutely occluded with acute right ventricular infarction? (See Figure 12-3 [pocket reference, p. 35].)

Hint #2: Is there evidence of acute anterior infarction in Figure 12-10?

Answer

As indicated in Figure 12-3, the right coronary artery usually supplies the inferior and posterior walls of the left ventricle as well as the right ventricular wall. Thus, with acute right ventricular infarction, this is the coronary vessel we would expect to find acutely occluded. Because this same vessel also supplies the inferior wall of the left ventricle, patients with acute right ventricular infarction will almost always also have evidence of acute inferior infarction (as is the case in Figure 12-10). *This is the same reason why patients with acute posterior infarction also almost always have associated acute inferior infarction.*

The other clue to acute right ventricular infarction in Figure 12-10 is found in lead V$_1$. At first glance, the ST segment elevation in this lead may make it appear that the patient is having an acute anterior or anteroseptal infarction. However, none of the other anterior leads demonstrate ST segment elevation. As can be seen from Figure 12-8, V$_1$ is the one standard precordial lead that catches a glimpse of the right ventricle *(broken arrow in this figure)*. This explains why V_1 may show ST segment elevation while none of the other precordial leads do. Thus, *whenever you see ST segment elevation only in lead V_1 in the setting of acute inferior infarction, consider the possibility of associated acute right ventricular infarction.* It is easy to confirm this suspicion by obtaining a right-sided V_4 lead (V_4R), which should show definite ST segment elevation (Figure 12-11).

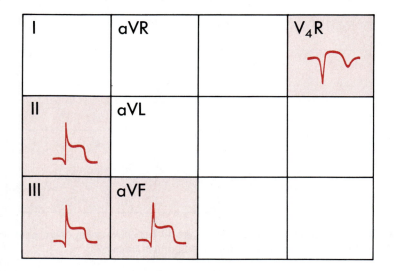

Figure 12-11.   Addition of a V_4R lead to the patient with new-onset chest pain whose 12-lead tracing was seen in Figure 12-10. The limb leads are recorded in the usual fashion, and again show acute inferior infarction. The Q wave, ST segment elevation, and beginning T wave inversion in lead V_4R confirm that acute right ventricular infarction is also present.

Although it is estimated that right ventricular involvement occurs in as many as 25% of all inferior infarctions, symptoms of left ventricular infarction predominate most of the time. The point we wish to emphasize is that in patients with acute inferior infarction who are not optimally responding to treatment, consider the possibility of associated significant right ventricular involvement (infarction), especially if there are clinical signs suggesting right heart failure. In such cases, have a low threshold for recording a V_4R lead.

13

The Five Essential Lists

We advocate recall of five essential lists in electrocardiography (Table 13-1). We define a "list" as a series of conditions to consider in the differential diagnosis of a certain electrocardiographic finding. As soon as you recognize the finding, a "light bulb" should go off, prompting you to run through the entities in the list to see if any might be present. The purpose of making a list is simply to prevent you from overlooking a potentially important ECG diagnosis.

Table 13-1
The Five Essential Lists
1. Causes of a regular, wide-complex tachycardia 2. Common causes of QT prolongation 3. Common causes of ST segment depression 4. Common causes of a tall R wave in lead V_1 5. Causes of anterior ST segment depression in the setting of acute inferior infarction

We devote this chapter to explanation and illustration of our five lists. By limiting the number of lists to five, the amount of material to memorize is also limited. Some of the material is already known to you. The rest builds logically on the basic concepts we have covered thus far. (*For easy reference, we reproduce the Five Lists on p. 4 of the pocket reference.*)

CAUSES OF A REGULAR, WIDE-COMPLEX TACHYCARDIA

Examine the rhythm strip shown in Figure 13-1. What is the rhythm likely to be?

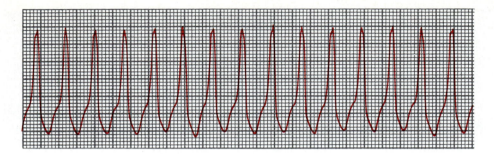

Figure 13-1.   Rhythm strip from a 50-year-old man. The patient is alert and asymptomatic. Blood pressure is 120/80 mm Hg.

Answer to Figure 13-1

The rhythm is regular, at a rate of 185 beats/minute. The QRS complex is wide. Atrial activity is absent. The patient is in a regular, wide-complex tachycardia.

The first (and most important) of our essential lists consists of the five causes of a regular, wide-complex tachycardia (Table 13-2, *which also appears on p. 37 in the pocket reference*). This table was previously presented in Chapter 3 (Table 3-3).

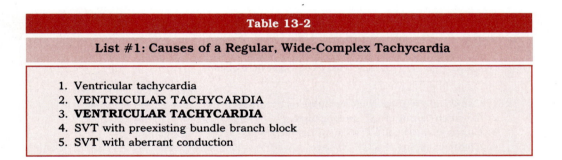

Table 13-2
List #1: Causes of a Regular, Wide-Complex Tachycardia
1. Ventricular tachycardia 2. VENTRICULAR TACHYCARDIA 3. **VENTRICULAR TACHYCARDIA** 4. SVT with preexisting bundle branch block 5. SVT with aberrant conduction

Note that the first, second, and third causes are all the same. *Ventricular tachycardia must always be assumed till proven otherwise.* The fact that the patient is awake, alert, and completely asymptomatic has absolutely no bearing on the likelihood of the entities in this list. Patients may remain asymptomatic and hemodynamically stable despite the persistence of ventricular tachycardia for hours or *even days!*

In Chapter 19 we suggest ways in which a 12-lead tracing may be helpful in determining the cause of a tachycardia. However, when any doubt at all exists, assume a rhythm is "guilty" until proven otherwise:

Assume that the cause of any regular, wide-complex tachycardia in which sinus P waves are absent (or uncertain) is VT until proven otherwise.

CAUSES OF QT PROLONGATION

We have already discussed (in Chapter 6) assessment of the QT interval and how to recognize prolongation of this interval (*Figure 6-2 [pocket reference, p. 18]*). In general:

> *If the heart rate is under 100 beats/minute, the QT interval is probably prolonged if it is greater than HALF of the R-R interval.*

The common causes of QT prolongation make up the second of our lists (Table 13-3, *which also appears in the pocket reference, p. 38*). We have adapted this information from Table 6-2.

Table 13-3
List #2: Common Causes of QT Prolongation

1. **Drugs**
   Type IA antiarrhythmic agents (i.e., quinidine, procainamide, disopyramide)
   Tricyclic antidepressants
   Phenothiazines
2. **"Lytes"**
   Hypokalemia
   Hypomagnesemia
   Hypocalcemia
3. **CNS**
   Stroke
   Intracerebral or brainstem bleeding
   Coma

In addition to the entities indicated in Table 13-3, QT prolongation may also be caused by other conditions such as QRS widening (from bundle branch block or IVCD) or ischemia/infarction. However, the presence of these other conditions will usually be obvious from inspection of the ECG. The point to remember is that *if the QT interval is prolonged in the absence of QRS widening, ischemia or infarction, think "Drugs/Lytes/CNS" as the cause.*

COMMON CAUSES OF ST SEGMENT DEPRESSION

ST segment depression may result from any of the causes shown in Table 13-4 (*which also appears in the pocket reference, p. 39*). Some of these entities may be suggested by associated findings and/or a characteristic appearance of the ST segment and T wave. Thus, strain should be suspected as at least one of the causes of *asymmetric* ST segment depression that occurs in association with increased QRS amplitude (i.e., voltage criteria for LVH). *Symmetric* T wave inversion suggests ischemia. U waves suggest hypokalemia (as we will discuss in Chapter 14).

Table 13-4
List #3: Common Causes of ST Segment Depression
1. Ischemia 2. Strain 3. Digitalis effect 4. Hypokalemia/hypomagnesemia 5. Rate-related changes 6. Any combination of the above

The entities shown in Table 13-4 often overlap in their clinical occurrence. Thus, patients with heart failure are extremely likely to have cardiomegaly (and LVH with *strain*). Such individuals are also likely to be treated with *digoxin* and diuretics. Use of diuretics predisposes to *hypokalemia* (and *hypomagnesemia*). *Ischemia* and/or tachycardia (with its *rate-related changes*) may accompany severe heart failure, especially in patients with concomitant coronary artery disease.

ST segment depression is often nonspecific in its appearance. Thus, *all* of the entities listed in Table 13-4 (either alone or in combination) should be considered as possible causes whenever ST segment depression is present.

It is worthwhile spending a moment on the ST segment changes associated with the use of digitalis (i.e., **digitalis effect**). They may be of three types:
1. Asymmetric ST segment depression identical in appearance to that produced by strain.
2. Scooped ST segment depression
3. Nonspecific ST segment flattening or depression.

ST segment changes associated with digitalis use may appear in multiple leads on the ECG. However, the term "digitalis effect" is a misnomer because the presence of digitalis-induced ST segment changes has virtually nothing to do with the serum digoxin level. Thus a patient may be toxic from digitalis and not manifest any ST segment abnormalities at all. Only about half of those who take the drug develop an ST segment digitalis effect.

Now consider the ECG shown in Figure 13-2. There is a regular, supraventricular tachycardia at a rate of about 230 beats/minute. Note that the ST segments are depressed in multiple leads. What might the diffuse ST segment depression in this example be due to?

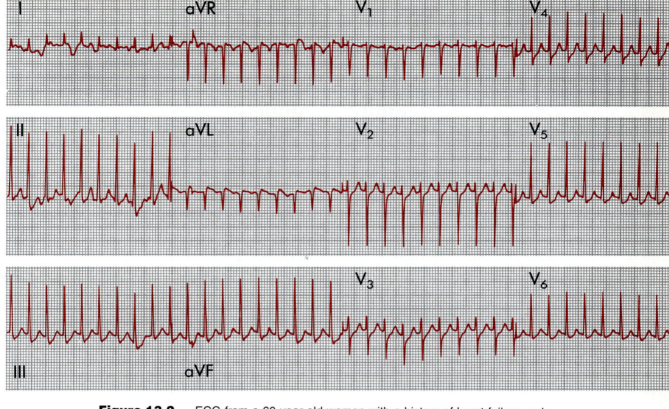

Figure 13-2.   ECG from a 60-year-old woman with a history of heart failure and coronary artery disease. She is taking multiple medications.

Answer to Figure 13-2

The ST segment depression in this example is nonspecific in appearance. It may be due to any of the common causes of ST segment depression that are listed in Table 13-4. The tachycardia is surely fast enough to cause *rate-related changes*. Given the patient's age and medical history, *ischemia* is a definite possibility. Voltage criteria for LVH are satisfied (deep S wave in lead V_2 and tall R wave in lead V_5 >35) in this patient with heart failure, making it likely that some of the ST segment depression is also due to *strain*. *Digitalis* and diuretics are almost certainly among the multiple medications the patient is taking (the latter predisposing to *hypokalemia/hypomagnesemia*). Thus, in this example, *all five* of the causes listed in Table 13-4 may play a role in the ST segment depression.

Question

The QT interval in Figure 13-2 appears to be more than half the R-R interval. Is it fair to say that the QTc (i.e., the *corrected* QT) is prolonged?

Answer

No. As we discussed earlier in this chapter, for the simplified rule to apply (that the QT be less than half the R-R interval), the heart rate should be less than 100 beats/minute. QT interval prolongation is much more difficult to determine at faster heart rates. It is of little clinical significance at the tachycardic rate shown in Figure 13-2.

COMMON CAUSES OF A TALL R WAVE IN LEAD V₁

Normally, the QRS complex in lead V_1 is predominantly negative. This is because this right-sided lead views the heart's electrical activity largely as moving *away* from the right as the left ventricle is depolarized *(see Figure 10-3, on pocket reference p. 30).* The finding of an R wave in lead V_1 that equals or exceeds the S wave in this lead is distinctly unusual. Recognition of this finding should immediately prompt the interpreter to consider one or more of the entities on our fourth list (Table 13-5, *which also appears on p. 39 in the pocket reference)* as the cause.

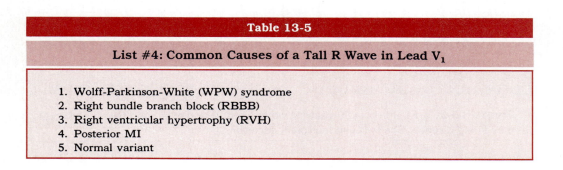

Table 13-5
List #4: Common Causes of a Tall R Wave in Lead V₁
1. Wolff-Parkinson-White (WPW) syndrome 2. Right bundle branch block (RBBB) 3. Right ventricular hypertrophy (RVH) 4. Posterior MI 5. Normal variant

Associated findings on the tracing should provide the clues needed to arrive at the correct diagnosis. We list the clues we find most helpful in Table 13-6 *(which also appears in the pocket reference, p. 40).*

Table 13-6
Helpful Clues for Determining the Cause of a Tall R Wave in Lead V$_1$

1. **WPW:**
    QRS widening
    Short PR interval
    Delta waves (which may be positive or negative)

2. **RBBB:**
    QRS widening ($\geq$0.11 seconds)
    rSR′ (or RBBB equivalent pattern) in lead V$_1$
    Wide, terminal S wave in leads I and V$_6$

3. **RVH:**
    Normal QRS duration
    RAA
    RAD or indeterminate axis
    Low voltage
    Persistent precordial S waves
    Right ventricular strain

4. **Posterior MI:**
    Normal QRS duration
    Evidence of inferior infarction
    Positive "mirror test"

5. **Normal variant:**
    Normal QRS duration
    Diagnosed by exclusion in the *absence* of evidence of WPW, RBBB, RVH, or
        posterior MI
    Often found in an otherwise healthy young adult

Apply the information in Table 13-6 to schematic Figures 13-3 through 13-7. We show only the leads essential for ruling in (or out) the common causes of a tall R wave in lead V$_1$.

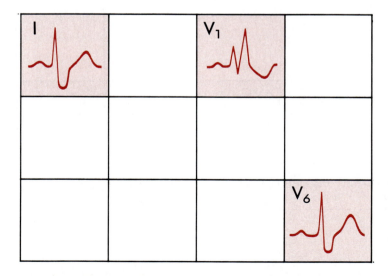

Figure 13-3.   The QRS complex is wide. What is the likely cause of the tall R wave in lead V$_1$?

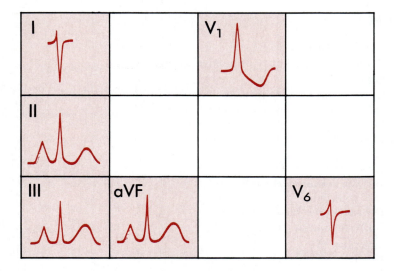

Figure 13-4.   The QRS complex is narrow. What is the likely cause of the tall R wave in lead V₁?

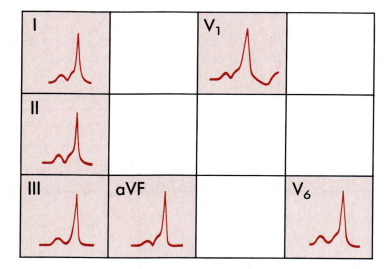

Figure 13-5.   The QRS complex is wide. What is the likely cause of the tall R wave in lead V₁?

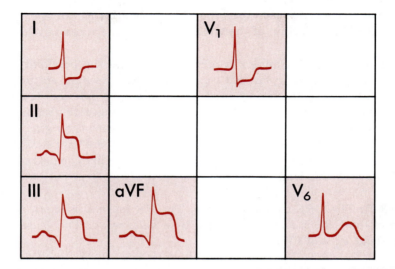

Figure 13-6.   The QRS complex is narrow. What is the likely cause of the tall R wave in lead V$_1$?

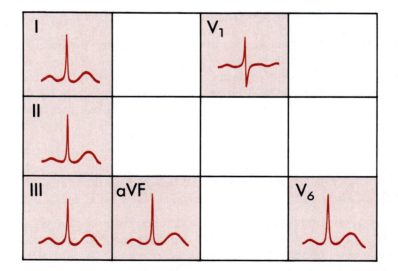

Figure 13-7.   The QRS complex is narrow. The patient is an otherwise healthy, asymptomatic young adult. What is the likely cause of the relatively tall R wave in lead V$_1$?

Answers

Figure 13-3: The QRS complex is wide. An rSR′ is present in lead V_1, and a wide terminal S wave is seen in leads I and V_6. Thus, QRS morphology in the three key leads (I, V_1 and V_6) is typical of complete **RBBB**. Note also that typical ST-T wave changes are seen (i.e., the ST segment and T wave are directed opposite to the last deflection of the QRS complex in the three key leads).

Figure 13-4: The QRS complex is narrow, ruling out the possibility of WPW or RBBB. Marked negativity in lead I indicates RAD. P waves are tall and peaked (and "uncomfortable to sit on") in the pulmonary (= inferior) leads, consistent with RAA. There is also a deep S wave in lead V_6, suggesting significant activity directed *away* from this lateral (leftward) lead, or toward the right. The combination of these findings, in association with the "strain-like" appearance of the ST segment and T wave in lead V_1, suggests **RVH** as the likely cause of the predominant R wave in this lead.

Figure 13-5: The QRS complex is wide. The PR interval is short, and the initial portion of the QRS is marked (slurred) by a *delta* wave. The cause of the tall R wave in lead V_1 is **WPW.**

Figure 13-6: The QRS complex is narrow, ruling out the possibility of WPW and RBBB. Other than the tall R wave in lead V_1, none of the usual findings of RVH are present. Q waves, coved ST segment elevation in leads II, III and aVF, and reciprocal ST segment depression in lead I suggest inferior infarction that is likely to be acute. The finding of a tall R wave in lead V_1 in association with evidence of inferior infarction suggests that **posterior infarction** is present as well. (As we will see momentarily, there is also a positive "mirror test.")

Figure 13-7: The QRS complex is narrow, ruling out the possibility of WPW and RBBB. None of the usual findings of RVH are present. There is no evidence of inferior infarction (making posterior infarction extremely unlikely). Moreover, the patient is an otherwise healthy asymptomatic young adult. All of these factors suggest that the relatively tall R wave in lead V_1 reflects a **normal variant.**

CAUSES OF ANTERIOR ST SEGMENT DEPRESSION IN THE SETTING OF ACUTE INFERIOR INFARCTION

The last of our lists deals with a somewhat less common, but equally important situation. We illustrate it in Figure 13-8. Imagine this schematic ECG was taken from a middle-aged patient complaining of new-onset chest pain. What is going on in the inferior leads?

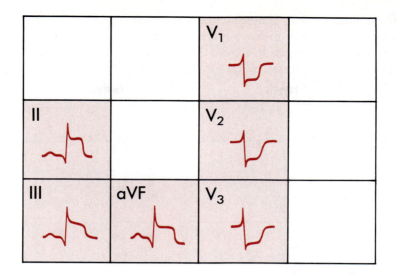

Figure 13-8. Initial schematic ECG from a middle-aged patient with new-onset chest pain.

Answer to Figure 13-8

Each of the three inferior leads (II, III, and aVF) demonstrates Q waves and ST segment elevation. This suggests acute inferior infarction.

ST segment depression is commonly seen in the anterior leads (V_1, V_2, and V_3) *in association with acute inferior infarction.* Note that this is the case in Figure 13-8.

There are three main causes of anterior ST segment depression that occurs in association with acute inferior infarction. Can you think of them?

1.

2.

3.

Hint to Cause #1: As we discussed in Chapter 12, the marker of the acute injury current of acute infarction is ST segment *elevation*. In areas of the heart removed from the infarction, ST segments do not go up. Instead they often go down (become *depressed*). We call such ST segment depression _____ changes.

Hint to Cause #2: Acute infarction is most often caused by sudden, complete occlusion of a coronary artery. In most cases, the acute inferior infarction shown in Figure 13-8 will be due to sudden complete occlusion of the _____ coronary artery *(Figure 12-3, pocket reference p. 35).* But patients with coronary artery disease usually demonstrate involvement (narrowing) of more than one coronary artery. Thus, another possible cause of the ST segment depression in leads V_1, V_2, and V_3 may be anterior _____ resulting from concomitant narrowing of the LAD coronary artery.

Hint to Cause #3: Examine the schematic ECG shown in Figure 13-9. Imagine this is the follow-up tracing for the middle-aged patient with chest pain whose initial ECG was shown in Figure 13-8. Can you now guess the third cause of anterior ST segment depression? (Hint: *Can you explain why the R wave has become so tall in lead V₁?*)

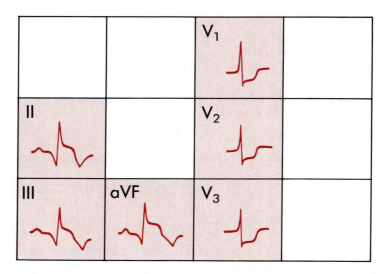

Figure 13-9.   Follow-up (schematic) ECG on the patient whose initial tracing was shown in Figure 13-8. Note that compared with Figure 13-8, there is now a tall R wave in lead V₁. The QRS complex is narrow.

Answer to Figure 13-9

This ECG shows *evolution* of the acute inferior changes first seen in Figure 13-8. That is, Q waves have become deeper in the inferior leads and T wave inversion is beginning as the ST segments are "brought back" to the baseline. **Serial evolutionary changes** of the type shown in Figures 13-8 and 13-9 *confirm* that the patient has had an acute inferior infarction.

Note that the R wave has now become predominant in lead V₁. This should lead you to consider the possibilities in Table 13-5 (*pocket reference, p. 39*) as the cause. We can easily eliminate *WPW* and *RBBB* because the QRS complex is narrow. None of the other findings suggestive of RVH are present—and the ECG in Figure 13-9 is certainly not a *normal variant*. This leaves **posterior infarction** as the remaining possibility, which is supported by associated evidence of acute inferior infarction. *The acute inferior infarction in Figure 13-8 has thus evolved (and/or extended) to now involve the posterior wall.*

Table 13-7 (*which also appears on p. 41 in the pocket reference*) repeats the three main causes of anterior ST segment depression to consider in the setting of acute inferior infarction.

Table 13-7
List #5: Causes of Anterior ST Segment Depression in the Setting of Acute Inferior Infarction
1. Reciprocal changes 2. Concomitant anterior ischemia 3. Posterior infarction 4. Any combination of the above

As is the case in Figure 13-8, you will often not be able to tell which of these three causes is present simply by looking at the tracing. Two, or even all three, of the causes may be present at the same time. ***Thus, whenever a patient presents with evidence of acute inferior infarction and anterior ST segment depression, realize that the ST depression may reflect a reciprocal change, concomitant anterior ischemia, posterior infarction, or any combination of these.***

THE MIRROR TEST

In Chapters 1 and 12, we discussed the areas of the heart that are visualized by the six standard precordial leads. We now repeat this information in Figure 13-10. *Which of the six standard precordial leads directly visualize the posterior wall of the left ventricle?*

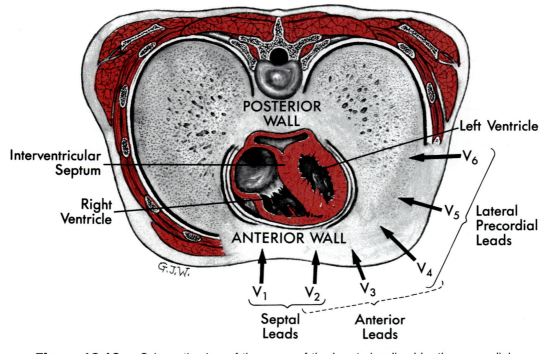

Figure 13-10.   Schematic view of the areas of the heart visualized by the precordial leads.

Answer

None of the standard precordial leads directly views the posterior wall of the left ventricle. Electrocardiographic changes that occur in the posterior wall of the left ventricle must therefore be inferred from *indirect* observation.

One way to do this is with the "mirror test." As can be seen from Figure 13-10, the anterior wall is directly opposite the posterior wall. Thus, one might expect anteroseptal leads (V_1, V_2, and V_3) to demonstrate opposite (i.e., mirror-image) changes with posterior infarction. Examples of what such mirror-image changes might look like are shown in Figure 13-11.

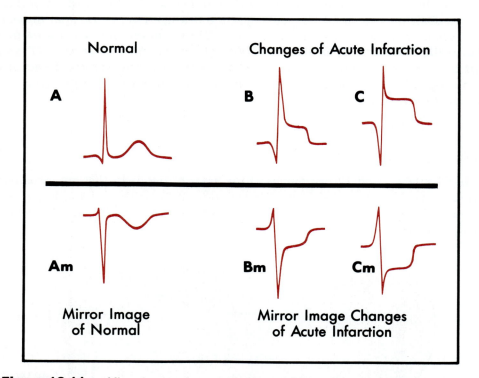

Figure 13-11.   *Mirror image changes.* **A,** Normal QRS complex. **Am,** Mirror-image of normal. **B** and **C,** QRS complex with changes of acute infarction. **Bm** and **Cm,** Mirror-image of the changes of acute infarction.

Figure 13-11, *A,* shows a normal QRS complex. Note that a small (septal) q wave is present, as is often the case. *Am* shows the mirror image of *A.*

B and *C* illustrate changes that may occur with acute infarction. Specifically, a deep Q wave develops and the ST segment becomes coved and elevated. Mirror images of *B* and *C* are shown in *Bm* and *Cm,* respectively. Note that as the Q wave deepens (from *B* to *C*), the respective mirror-image R wave becomes taller (from *Bm* to *Cm*). These are precisely the changes one might expect to see in the anterior leads with posterior infarction.

It is *easy* to apply the mirror test in practice. Simply flip an ECG over, hold it up to the light, and direct your attention to leads V_1, V_2, and V_3 (Figure 13-12, *which also appears on p. 42 in the pocket reference*).

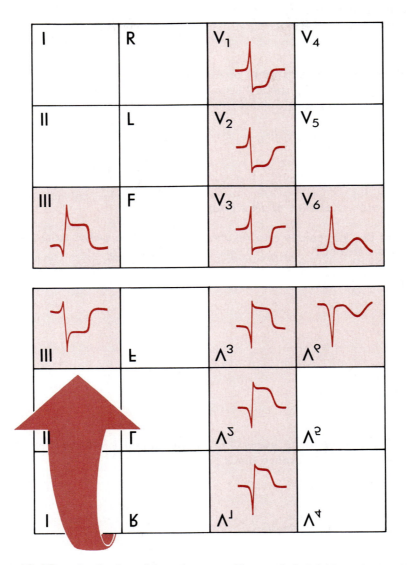

Figure 13-12. Application of the mirror test. The test is helpful in patients with acute inferior infarction when you also suspect posterior infarction. **A,** Schematic 12-lead ECG with changes suggestive of acute inferior infarction in lead III. There is a tall R wave in lead V_1, and ST segment depression in the anterior leads (V_1, V_2, and V_3). **B,** The tracing is flipped over. Looking *through* the paper as it is held up to the light, one would now see Q waves and ST segment elevation in leads V_1, V_2, and V_3. This is a *positive mirror test,* and suggests that the anterior lead changes in **A** reflect associated acute posterior infarction.

Return to Figure 13-6. Do you now see why we said lead V_1 demonstrates a positive mirror test? *(That is, doesn't lead V_1 in Figure 13-6 resemble Figure 13-11, Cm?)*

Finally, return to Figure 13-8. What do you imagine leads V_1, V_2, and V_3 would look like if you applied the mirror test?

Answer

The situation is comparable to of Figure 13-11, *Bm* and *Cm*. Application of the mirror test suggests that the ST segment depression in the anterior leads may be due to posterior infarction.

REVIEW

Check your retention of this chapter.

What are the five causes of a regular, wide-complex tachycardia (in which sinus P waves are absent)?

1.

2.

3.

4.

5.

What are the three main causes of QT prolongation? (Assume there is no ischemia, infarction, or bundle branch block.)

1.

2.

3.

What are five common causes of ST segment depression?

1.

2.

3.

4.

5.

What are five common causes of a tall R wave in lead V_1?

1.

2.

3.

4.

5.

In the setting of acute inferior infarction, what are 3 causes of ST segment depression in the anterior leads?

1.

2.

3.

Answers to these review questions are found in Tables 13-2, 13-3, 13-4, 13-5, and 13-7 *(pocket reference pp. 37 to 41).*

Retention of these five Essential Lists (or ready access to our pocket reference) will go a long way toward narrowing a differential diagnosis, and minimizing the chance that important ECG findings will be overlooked.

14

Electrolyte Disturbances

The ECG is often used to help in evaluation of patients with electrolyte disturbances. Practically speaking, the changes produced are commonly nonspecific and of limited clinical assistance. However, on occasion, the ECG may be the first diagnostic modality to suggest a potentially life-threatening disorder.

The electrolyte disturbances we focus on in this chapter are hyperkalemia and hypokalemia. Other electrolyte abnormalities, such as hyponatremia and hypernatremia, do not produce any characteristic ECG changes. Hypercalcemia may shorten the QT interval—but this is often an extremely subtle and hard-to-recognize change. Hypocalcemia may lengthen the QT interval—but again, this change tends to be subtle and hard to recognize unless the serum calcium concentration is profoundly depressed.

HYPERKALEMIA

The most characteristic finding of hyperkalemia is development of tall, peaked T waves. T wave peaking often begins relatively early in the process (with mild to moderate elevations in serum potassium—between 5.5 and 7.0 mEq/L), and tends to persist with more severe hyperkalemia. As the serum potassium level exceeds 7.0 to 8.0 mEq/L, P wave amplitude decreases and the QRS complex widens. Ultimately (with a serum potassium of 9.0 to 10.0 mEq/L) the electrical waveform takes on a sinusoid pattern. Cardiac arrest usually follows shortly thereafter (Figure 14-1, *which also appears on p. 44 in the pocket reference*).

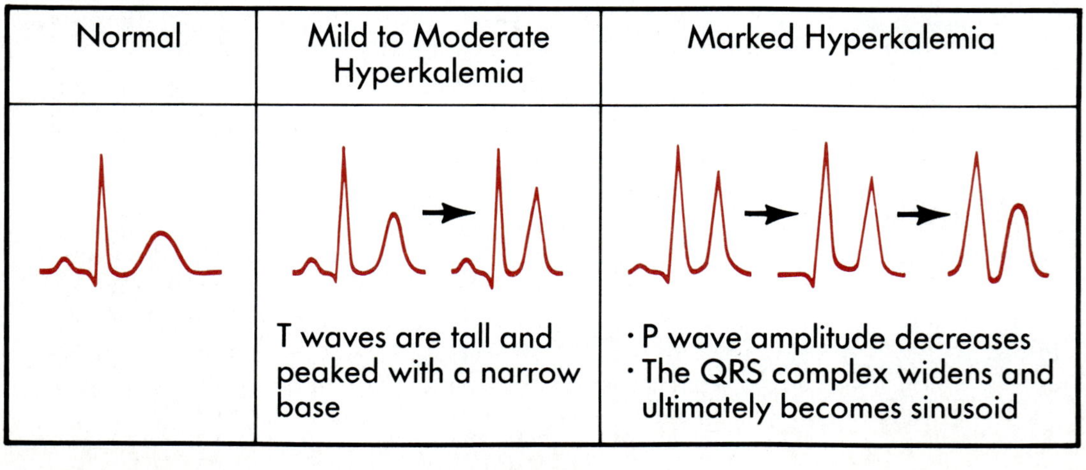

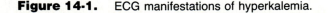

Normal	Mild to Moderate Hyperkalemia	Marked Hyperkalemia
	T waves are tall and peaked with a narrow base	· P wave amplitude decreases · The QRS complex widens and ultimately becomes sinusoid

Figure 14-1. ECG manifestations of hyperkalemia.

Pearls in the ECG Diagnosis of Hyperkalemia

Clinically, the first impulse of many medical providers when told that a patient has an elevated serum potassium level (6 mEq/L or greater) is to validate the reading (and rule out hemolysis) by repeating the blood test. Obtaining a stat ECG may provide the needed information even sooner than the 15 to 40 minutes needed for the laboratory to redraw blood and run stat electrolytes. The finding of tall, peaked T waves is an excellent indicator that the elevated potassium reading is legitimate and merits immediate treatment.

Potential Pitfalls in the ECG Diagnosis of Hyperkalemia

All that produces tall, peaked T waves is NOT necessarily hyperkalemia! T waves are sometimes prominent in certain *normal (repolarization) variants.* When this is the case, the T wave tends to be less pointed and have a broader base *(see Figure 10-16 [pocket reference, p. 29]),* and the ECG is usually from an otherwise healthy and relatively young, asymptomatic adult.

The other possible cause of prominent and often pointed T waves (especially in the anterior leads) is *ischemia.* In this case the tall, pointed T waves reflect a positive mirror test. *(If you flipped the tall, pointed T waves in Figure 14-1 upside down, wouldn't you get deep, symmetric T wave inversion ???).* Suspect ischemia as a possible cause of tall, pointed T waves in leads V_1, V_2, and/or V_3 when there is also evidence on the tracing of inferior ischemia or infarction.

Practically speaking, there are only a handful of clinical situations that commonly produce hyperkalemia (Table 14-1, *which also appears on pocket reference p. 44).* Prominent T waves that occur in an otherwise healthy, asymptomatic young adult taking no medication are much more likely to reflect a normal repolarization variant than hyperkalemia. Thus, before diagnosing hyperkalemia from an ECG, try (if at all possible) to determine if the clinical situation is consistent with this diagnosis.

Table 14-1
Common Clinical Settings Likely to Produce Hyperkalemia
Acute renal failure Chronic renal failure (less common) Acidosis Patients taking potassium-retaining diuretics or angiotensin-converting enzyme (ACE) inhibitors Dehydration

HYPOKALEMIA

The most characteristic ECG sign of hypokalemia is development of U waves. Before this stage, T waves decrease in amplitude and the ST segment may flatten and/or become depressed. Ultimately, U waves may become larger than T waves, or even replace them completely (Figure 14-2, *which also appears on pocket reference p. 45).* This gives the impression of QT prolongation, but in reality is QU prolongation (since growing U waves have replaced the shrinking T waves).

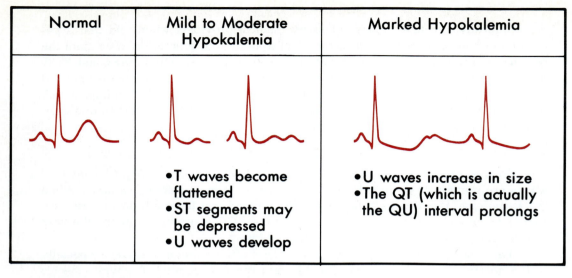

Figure 14-2.   ECG manifestations of hypokalemia.

Pearls in the ECG Diagnosis of Hypokalemia

U waves are recognized as the upright deflection that follows the T wave but precedes the next P wave. When present, they are usually best seen in leads V_2 to V_5, although they may appear in other leads.

Like T waves, U waves may become inverted. This often indicates ischemia and/or severe coronary artery disease. Because of their small amplitude, inverted U waves are usually extremely difficult to recognize. We suggest you *NOT* concern yourself looking for inverted U waves!

Potential Pitfalls in the ECG Diagnosis of Hypokalemia

All that produces U waves is NOT necessarily hypokalemia! U waves may also be seen with bradycardia or LVH.

Although ECG findings of hyperkalemia correlate fairly well with serum potassium values, this is *NOT* the case with hypokalemia. Many patients with low serum potassiums have no ECG changes. Conversely, many patients with ECG abnormalities suggestive of hypokalemia have normal serum potassium values.

ECG changes of hypokalemia are often quite nonspecific (such as diffuse ST-T wave flattening). Maintain a high index of suspicion in patients likely to develop hypokalemia (i.e., those taking diuretics such as furosemide or thiazides, or those on digitalis). Remember that **hypomagnesemia** may produce ECG and clinical manifestations identical to those of hypokalemia. This becomes important clinically because hypokalemia will often be refractory to treatment if undetected hypomagnesemia is present.

Apply the preceding information to the ECG shown in Figure 14-3, taken from an elderly patient in renal failure. Analyze the tracing systematically. Then determine which electrolyte abnormality is likely to be present? How many of the usual findings of this electrolyte abnormality are present?

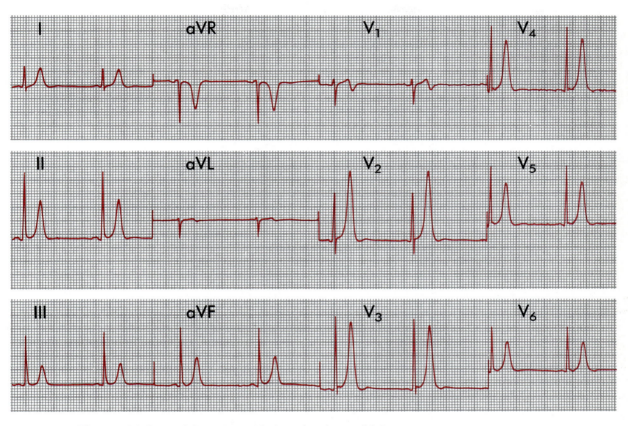

Figure 14-3.   ECG from an elderly patient in renal failure.

Answer to Figure 14-3

The rhythm is regular, at a rate of about 55 beats/minute. The mechanism is sinus, since upright P waves are present in lead II. This is sinus bradycardia.

All intervals (PR, QRS, and QT) are normal.

The mean QRS axis is normal (since the QRS complex is upright in leads I and aVF). It is obviously closer to lead aVF, and we estimate it to be about 70°.

There is no evidence of chamber enlargement.

Tiny septal q waves may be present in the lateral precordial leads. Transition is early (since the R wave exceeds the S wave in lead V_2). But the most remarkable finding on the tracing is the T waves. In addition to being exceedingly tall and peaked in most leads, note the narrow base these T waves have and how symmetric they are. This T wave appearance strongly suggests *hyperkalemia*. Yet despite the tremendous height of the T waves, the QRS complex is of normal duration, and P waves are still present (albeit small)—so the hyperkalemia may not yet have reached a lethal level.

Pericarditis

The easiest way to remember the ECG manifestations of acute pericarditis is to think of them as occurring in four stages:

Stage 1: *everything is UP*
Stage 2:
Stage 3: *everything is DOWN*
Stage 4: normalization

The earliest stage of acute pericarditis is marked by generalized ST segment elevation (*"everything up"* stage) that is seen in virtually all leads except aVR, V_1, and sometimes III (Figure 15-1, *which also appears on pocket reference p. 46*).

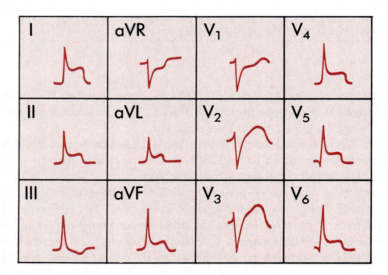

Figure 15-1. Stage 1 of acute pericarditis. There is diffuse ST segment elevation (*"everything up"* stage) in virtually all leads except aVR, V_1, and III.

Stage 1 pericarditis is followed days to weeks later by Stage 3, in which generalized ST segment elevation is replaced by generalized T wave inversion (*"everything down"* stage). ST segments have either returned to baseline or become slightly depressed.

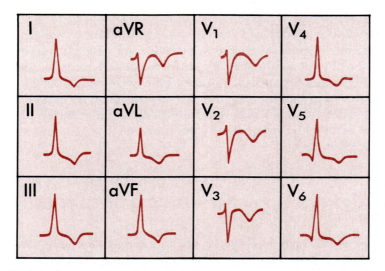

Figure 15-2.   Stage 3 of acute pericarditis. Generalized ST segment elevation has been replaced by generalized T wave inversion (*"everything down"* stage).

Question

If Stage 1 of acute pericarditis is characterized by upright T waves and generalized ST segment elevation (Figure 15-1), and Stage 3 by isoelectric or slightly depressed ST segments and generalized T wave inversion (Figure 15-2, *which also appears on pocket reference p. 47),* what do you think the ST segments and T waves might look like in Stage 2?

Answer

Stages of acute pericarditis:
  Stage 1: *everything UP*
  Stage 2: *transition (= "pseudonormalization")*
  Stage 3: *everything DOWN*
  Stage 4: normalization

Stage 2 pericarditis is therefore a *transitional* stage in which the appearance of the ST segments and T waves may be relatively normal (as elevated ST segments return to baseline before the T waves invert). Stage 2 pericarditis may develop hours, days, or weeks after Stage 1. Thus, if Stage 1 has already passed, it may be extremely difficult to recognize pericarditis electrocardiographically (since Stage 2 may produce a relatively normal ECG)!

Finally, weeks to months following Stage 3, the final stage of pericarditis develops (Stage 4), in which ST segments and T waves gradually normalize.

PEARLS IN THE ECG DIAGNOSIS OF ACUTE PERICARDITIS

Acute pericarditis is not an extremely common disorder in the general population. It is seen much more often following acute infarction or cardiac surgery. Knowledge of the clinical setting may provide a major clue to its recognition. Thus, acute pericarditis should be suspected if chest pain occurs in a young adult without cardiac risk factors, especially if the chest pain is pleuritic in nature. Hearing a pericardial friction rub would clinch the diagnosis. On the other hand, crushing chest pain in an older adult with cardiac risk factors and a history of angina is much more suggestive of acute infarction.

POTENTIAL PITFALLS IN THE ECG DIAGNOSIS OF ACUTE PERICARDITIS

ECG changes of Stage 1 of acute pericarditis may resemble the J point ST segment elevation of early repolarization. Clinical history, the presence of a rub, and comparison with prior tracings (if available) may help make the distinction.

ECG changes of Stage 1 acute pericarditis may also resemble those of acute infarction. Subtle differences may exist. Apply this information to the schematic ECG shown in Figure 15-3, taken from a patient with acute inferior MI. Compare this tracing with Figure 15-1. How do the ECGs differ?

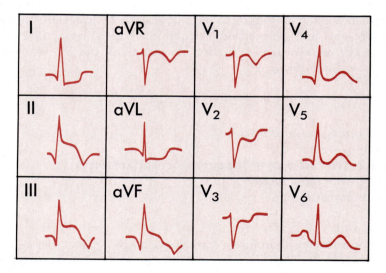

Figure 15-3.   Schematic ECG from a patient with acute inferior infarction.

Answer to Figure 15-3

The schematic ECG of Stage 1 acute pericarditis (Figure 15-1) shows more generalized ST segment elevation. Reciprocal changes are absent. Large Q waves are absent. (The tiny q waves in leads V_5 and V_6 are probably normal septal q waves.)

In contrast, the ST segment elevation in the schematic ECG of acute infarction (Figure 15-3) is localized to the inferior leads. The ST segment is much more coved (i.e., "frowny") than in Figure 15-1. In addition, large inferior Q waves have already formed, and T wave inversion is present. **With acute pericarditis, T waves rarely invert while the ST segment is still elevated.** Finally, reciprocal ST segment depression is seen in the anterior and high lateral leads.

Question

Return to Figure 15-2. Imagine this tracing was obtained from an adult with new-onset chest pain. Could you distinguish between Stage 3 pericarditis and ischemia on the basis of this ECG alone?

Answer

No. ECG manifestations of Stage 3 pericarditis may be identical to those seen with diffuse ischemia. Both may produce generalized, symmetric T wave inversion. History, physical examination, and comparison with prior tracings become all-important in making the distinction.

16

Recognizing Lead Misplacement

Although lead misplacement is not a common problem, it is one that will definitely occur. It is most likely to happen when time is at a premium (i.e., recording a 12-lead ECG during cardiac resuscitation) or when an ECG is obtained by a health care provider not usually assigned to perform the procedure. However, even skilled and experienced ECG technicians eventually make a mistake in ECG recording and at some time fail to correctly apply ECG leads to the proper extremity.

We feel one of the major reasons why lead misplacement is not always picked up is simply that it occurs so infrequently. Because of this, many health care providers are not familiar with its manifestations. This need not be the case. Attention to a few key points is all that is needed to recognize lead misplacement in most instances.

LIMB LEAD MISPLACEMENT

The most common form of lead misplacement results from interchanging the left and right arm electrodes, thus reversing the polarity of the QRS complex in left- and right-sided recording electrodes. Figure 16-1 *(which also appears on pocket reference p. 49)* schematically illustrates the effect this may have on the six standard leads.

Question

Can you identify three clues to lead misplacement in this illustration?

Clue #1:

Clue #2:

Clue #3:

192

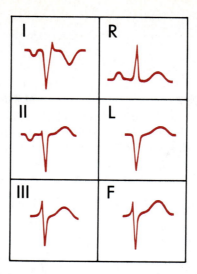

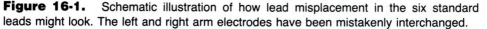

Figure 16-1. Schematic illustration of how lead misplacement in the six standard leads might look. The left and right arm electrodes have been mistakenly interchanged.

Hint to Clue #1: *Is the mechanism of the rhythm sinus?*

Hint to Clue #2: *What should the QRS complex normally look like in lead I?*

Hint to Clue #3: *What should the QRS complex normally look like in lead aVR?*

Answer

The three clues to lead misplacement in Figure 16-1 are:
1. That the P wave in lead II is inverted
2. That there is *"global negativity"* in lead I
3. That the QRS complex is upright in lead aVR.

As we discussed in Chapter 3, the P wave in lead II should be upright if the mechanism of the rhythm is sinus. Although one couldn't rule out a junctional or low atrial rhythm from the appearance of the P wave in lead II in this figure, the finding of a negative P wave in this lead should at least make one consider the possibility of lead reversal as the cause.

Normally the heart lies in the left hemithorax. As a result, electrical activity should travel *toward* the left as the left ventricle is depolarized. Lead I (which is a left-sided lead) should therefore be predominantly positive when leads are placed in their correct positions. Similarly, the QRS complex in a right-sided lead such as aVR should be predominantly negative when leads are placed appropriately.

Question

Will interchanging the left and right arm electrodes affect the appearance of the *precordial* leads?

Answer

No. Only the appearance of the QRS complex in the six standard leads (I, II, III, aVR, aVL, and aVF) is dependent on limb lead placement (i.e., on proper positioning of recording electrodes on the left arm, right arm, left leg, and right leg). Limb lead placement has nothing to do with the appearance of the QRS complex in the precordial leads.

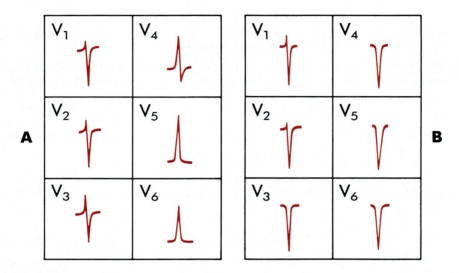

Figure 16-2. **A**, Normal R wave progression in the precordial leads. **B**, *Reverse* R wave progression.

Question

Can you think of an anatomic condition that may produce the identical picture in the six standard leads to that shown in Figure 16-1, but which will also produce "reverse" R wave progression in the precordial leads (Figure 16-2, *B*)? Hint: *On which side in the chest would the heart have to lie to produce a predominantly negative QRS complex in lead I and a predominantly positive QRS complex in lead aVR?*

Answer

If the heart was on the right side (i.e., if there was *dextrocardia*), the QRS complex would be negative in lead I and positive in lead aVR (as seen in Figure 16-1). Dextrocardia would also produce the picture of reverse R wave progression shown in Figure 16-2, *B* (since the heart lies on the right side of the chest in this condition).

Question

Which condition do you think is the more common cause of reversed polarity in the standard leads—lead misplacement or dextrocardia?

Answer

Lead misplacement is *by far* the more common cause of reversed polarity in the standard leads.

Other types of limb lead misplacement are possible. Thus, instead of interchanging the left and right arm electrodes, one of the arm electrodes may be interchanged with a leg electrode. Lead misplacement may still be suspected if any of the findings shown in Table 16-1 *(which also appears in the pocket reference, p. 48)* are present.

Table 16-1
Findings Suggestive of Limb Lead Misplacement
A negative P wave in lead II "Global negativity" (of the P wave, QRS complex, and T wave) in lead I An upright QRS complex in lead aVR

PRECORDIAL LEAD MISPLACEMENT

Lead misplacement may also occur in the precordial leads. One way this may happen is if the angle of Louis is incorrectly identified so that precordial leads are placed one interspace too high. When this occurs, normal R wave progression may be lost (Figure 16-3), giving the impression that anterior infarction is present.

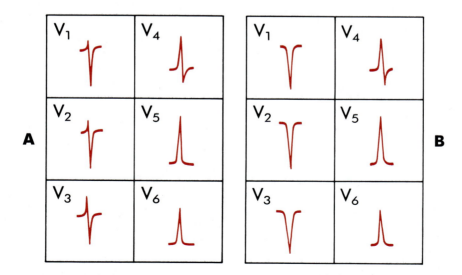

A

B

Figure 16-3.   **A,** Normal R wave progression in the precordial leads. **B,** Loss of R wave progression as may occur if precordial leads are placed one interspace too high.

As you may imagine, it is often extremely difficult to suspect or prove an error in precordial lead placement, and to differentiate between such technical errors and true anterior infarction.

Other types of precordial lead placement errors include misinterpretation of other anatomic landmarks, placing precordial leads on top of the left breast in women (instead of underneath the breast), or mistakenly interchanging two or more of the precordial leads. Errors in identification of anatomic landmarks are especially likely to occur in patients with unusual chest wall configurations, which are often seen in patients with chronic obstructive pulmonary disease or in those with chest wall deformities.

PRACTICE

Examine the following schematic tracings. Would you suspect lead misplacement in any of these examples? If so, why? What other conditions may be present? How could you verify your suspicion?

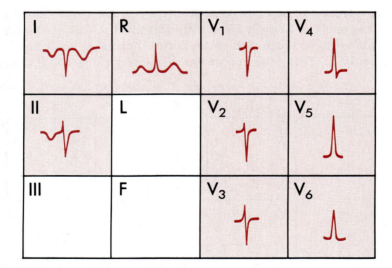

Figure 16-4.   Is lead misplacement likely to be present? If so, why?

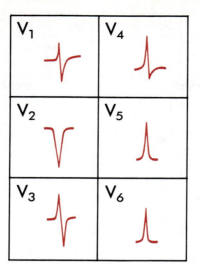

Figure 16-5. Do these precordial leads suggest an error in lead placement? If so, why?

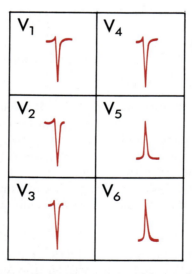

Figure 16-6. Do these precordial leads suggest an error in lead placement? If so, why?

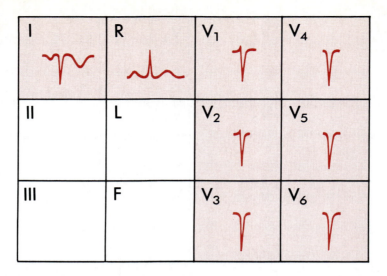

Figure 16-7.   Is lead misplacement likely to be present? Is there another condition that might account for the abnormal finding? If so, how could you verify your suspicion?

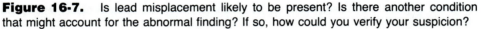

Answers

Figure 16-4: All three of the findings suggestive of limb lead misplacement (listed in Table 16-1) are present in Figure 16-4:

1. A negative P wave in lead II
2. "Global negativity" (of the P wave, QRS complex, and T wave) in lead I
3. An upright QRS complex in lead aVR.

If the only abnormal finding was a negative P wave in lead II, one would suspect a low atrial or junctional rhythm as the cause. However, the associated abnormal appearance of leads I and aVR strongly suggests either limb lead misplacement or dextrocardia. The presence of normal R wave progression in the precordial leads rules against dextrocardia.

Suspicion of limb lead reversal is easy to confirm. Simply repeat the ECG, verifying correct limb lead placement, and the abnormalities seen in Figure 16-4 should disappear.

Figure 16-5: The R wave in lead V_1 is taller than one usually expects. The R wave is then lost in lead V_2, and "regained" in lead V_3. This is an extremely unusual sequence of progression. Although it is possible that the loss of the R wave between leads V_1 and V_2 may be due to an isolated anterior infarction, precordial lead misplacement (i.e., interchanging the lead V_1 and V_2 electrodes) is a much more likely explanation. (Note that this sequence of R wave progression is similar to the sequence we already presented in Figure 10-10).

Again, it should be relatively easy to confirm this suspicion by repeating the ECG, and verifying correct placement of each of the precordial leads.

Figure 16-6: There is "poor R wave progression" in leads V_1 to V_4. Although this may be due to precordial lead misplacement (i.e., mistaken identification of anatomic landmarks and placement of precordial electrodes an interspace too high), it may also simply reflect a normal variant from a patient who has delayed transition. It is also possible that the patient may have had a prior anterior infarction, although the fact that r waves *are* present (albeit small) in *each* of the precordial leads makes this less likely. Suffice it to say that it is much more difficult to distinguish between these possibilities (and the other common causes of poor R wave progression that we listed previously in Table 10-4 [pocket reference p. 31]) than it was in Figure 16-5.

Figure 16-7: At first glance, global negativity in lead I and the upright QRS complex in lead aVR suggest limb lead misplacement as the cause. *Is R wave progression in the precordial leads consistent with this diagnosis?*

No. If the problem was simply the result of interchanging leads I and aVR, R wave progression should be normal. Instead, there is *reverse R wave progression* in the precordial leads. This suggests that the patient has dextrocardia.

You could verify your suspicion of dextrocardia by repeating an ECG with precordial leads positioned on the right side of the chest (Figure 16-8). Doing so should "normalize" R wave progression (Figure 16-9).

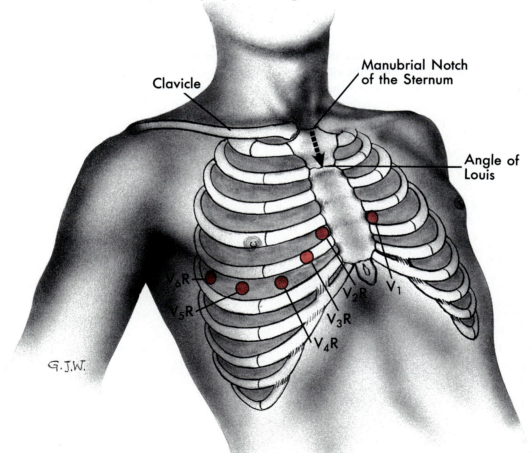

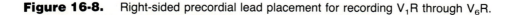

Figure 16-8.   Right-sided precordial lead placement for recording V_1R through V_6R.

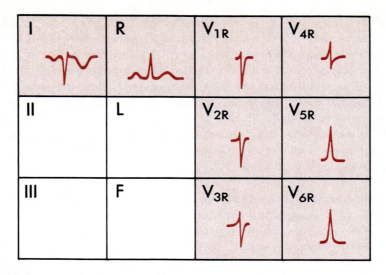

Figure 16-9. Repeat ECG on the patient whose schematic tracing was shown in Figure 16-7, this time with precordial leads placed in a similar anatomic location on the *right* side of the chest. In a patient with dextrocardia, right-sided precordial leads now demonstrate normal R wave progression.

Alternatively, one could verify dextrocardia by obtaining a chest x-ray to see if the heart was on the right side. An even simpler (and more cost-effective) way to verify dextrocardia is to listen for heart sounds on the right side of the chest.

17

When the Patient is a Child

Pediatric electrocardiography is an art unto itself. This is because all of the rules are different. Children's hearts are smaller. They tend to beat faster, and they develop different disease processes than adults' hearts.

Most medical care providers who are not directly involved in the care of children will only rarely be asked to interpret an ECG from a child. As a result, they are usually not familiar with what to expect from a pediatric ECG.

The purpose of this chapter is to review some of the basic differences between pediatric and adult ECGs. Although space constraints prevent us from presenting more than a brief general overview of the topic, our hope is that this will be enough to allow you in most cases to determine whether a pediatric tracing is likely to be normal or not.

PEDIATRIC NORMS

Pediatric norms for rate, rhythm, axis, and intervals differ substantially from those of adults (Tables 17-1 and 17-2, *which also appear in the pocket reference, pp. 50 and 51*). In general, heart rates tend to be faster, especially in younger children. Thus, a sinus rate of 140 beats/minute is still within the normal range for a 2-year-old child, and should not be considered as sinus tachycardia.

Pediatric norms for PR and QRS interval duration are less than for adults. This is simply because the time for conduction is less in a smaller heart. Whereas a PR interval of less than 0.12 second is considered short in adults (see Chapter 4), this is not the case in children, for whom PR intervals of as little as 0.07 second may be normal.

Question

Refer to Table 17-1. Is a PR interval of 0.18 second abnormal for a 3-year-old child? Would it be abnormal for a 12-year-old child? How about a QRS interval of 0.10 second for these age groups?

Table 17-1

Pediatric Norms for Heart Rate and Intervals

Age	Upper normal heart rate limit	Upper normal PR interval limit	Upper normal QRS duration
Newborn to 1 year	180 beats/min	≈0.17 second	≈0.08 second
1-3 years	150 beats/min	≈0.17 second	≈0.08 second
4-10 years	130 beats/min	≈0.17 second	≈0.09 second
>10 years	110 beats/min	≈0.20 second	≈0.09 second
Adults	99 beats/min	≈0.20-0.21 second	≈0.10 second

Answer

As seen from Table 17-1, a PR interval of 0.18 second exceeds the upper limit of normal for a 3-year-old child, and would constitute first-degree AV block in this age group. It would not be abnormal for a 12-year-old child.

A QRS interval of 0.10 second exceeds the upper normal limit for children, and suggests the possibility of an intraventricular conduction defect in the pediatric age group.

Table 17-2 shows normal rhythm and axis findings in children. Sinus arrhythmia is the rule rather than the exception, especially in older children. Sinus arrhythmia commonly demonstrates respiratory variation, with heart rates increasing during inspiration.

Table 17-2

Normal Rhythm and Axis Findings in Children

Rhythm

Sinus arrhythmia is exceedingly common, especially in older children.
Sinus "tachycardia" must be redefined in children (see Table 17-1).

Axis

Pediatric norms for mean QRS axis are often much more *rightward* than for adults:

Age	Approximate normal axis deviation
Up to 30 days	Up to 180°
Up to 1 year	Up to 120°
Up to 16 years	Up to 100°

As can be seen from Table 17-2, a certain degree of right axis deviation is common in the pediatric age group. Thus, a mean QRS axis of 115° should still be considered normal in a 10-month-old child.

PEDIATRIC CHAMBER ENLARGEMENT

The principal reason for obtaining a pediatric ECG in a primary care setting is for assessment of possible chamber enlargement. Most of the time, a heart murmur will have been heard on physical exam. In general, if the child is asymptomatic and the ECG and chest x-ray are both completely normal, the heart murmur is much less likely to be clinically significant.

Pediatric criteria for atrial abnormality/enlargement are similar to adult criteria *(see Figure 9-2 [pocket reference, p. 24])*. In contrast, pediatric criteria for ventricular hypertrophy differ greatly from those in adults. This is because the right ventricle is proportionately much larger in children.

It is important to emphasize that waveforms on an ECG reflect the *net* result after cancellation of electrical forces. This is why combined ventricular hypertrophy (i.e., LVH *and* RVH) is often extremely difficult to detect: increased left ventricular forces are largely balanced (canceled out) by increased right ventricular forces.

In adults, the normal left ventricle is approximately three times the thickness and 10 times the electrical mass of the normal right ventricle. This explains why RVH is so hard to diagnose electrocardiographically in adults. Even if the right ventricle triples or quadruples its electrical mass, its electrical forces will still be overshadowed by normal left ventricular forces.

RVH is much easier to diagnose in children. This is because right ventricular electrical forces are comparable to left ventricular electrical forces at birth, and tend to remain so for the first few years of life. As a result, ***the R wave in lead V_1 may normally remain predominant*** (i.e., *greater than the S wave in lead V_1*) ***for the first 5 years of life.***

In Chapter 9, we referred to RVH as the "detective" diagnosis, since determination of RVH in adults requires a combination of findings. Appreciation of this fact is equally important in diagnosing RVH in children. Insight into application of this principle is evident from Figures 17-1 and 17-2. Imagine that each of these schematic tracings was obtained from a 3-year-old child. Note that each demonstrates a predominant R wave in lead V_1, with associated ST-T wave changes in this lead. Which tracing is likely to reflect RVH? Considering the age of the child, is the other ECG likely to be normal?

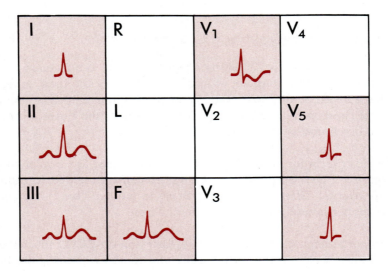

Figure 17-1.   Schematic ECG from a 3-year-old child. Is the predominant R wave in lead V_1 likely to reflect RVH?

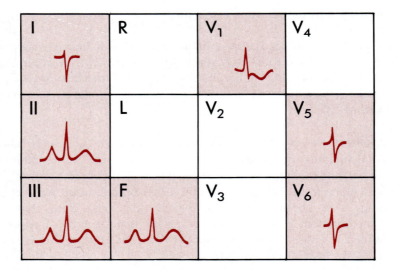

Figure 17-2.   Schematic ECG from a 3-year-old child. Is the predominant R wave in lead V_1 likely to reflect RVH?

Answers

Figure 17-1: Despite the predominant R wave in lead V_1, RVH is unlikely to be present in Figure 17-1. R wave predominance in lead V_1 may normally persist for up to the first 5 years of life. No other evidence for RVH is present: the axis is normal, P waves in the inferior leads are neither prominent nor peaked, and S waves in leads V_5 and V_6 are extremely small. This tracing is likely to be "normal for age."

Figure 17-2: In contrast to Figure 17-1, a number of additional findings support the diagnosis of RVH in Figure 17-2. These include marked RAD, the pattern of P-pulmonale (i.e., RAA), and the presence of deep S waves in the lateral precordial leads *(see Table 9-3 in pocket reference, p. 25).*

Diagnosis of LVH in children is harder to make on clinical grounds. This is because LAD, LAA, and strain are all much less commonly seen in the pediatric age group than they are in adults.

Technically speaking, definitive diagnosis of RVH or LVH in children usually requires confirmation that QRS amplitude has exceeded the normal maximum limit in one or more of the key leads for a particular age group. Comprehensive tables detailing acceptable limits for each lead in each age group are beyond the scope of this book. Suffice it to say that ventricular hypertrophy should be suspected if associated supportive findings are present, or if QRS amplitude exceeds the limits suggested by the *greatly simplified* guidelines we present in Table 17-3 *(which also appears on pocket reference p. 52).*

Table 17-3
Greatly Simplified Voltage Criteria for Diagnosing RVH and LVH in Children

For diagnosis of RVH

Age	Maximum allowable R wave in lead V_1	Maximum allowable S wave in lead V_6
Up to 1 month	30 mm	15 mm
1 month to 16 years	20 mm	6 mm

For diagnosis of LVH

Age	Maximum allowable S wave in lead V_1	Maximum allowable R wave in lead V_5	Maximum allowable R wave in lead V_6
Up to 12 months	20 mm	30 mm	20 mm
1-16 years	30 mm	40 mm	25 mm

Pediatric providers sometimes use additional leads when recording ECGs in children. For example, a V_3R lead may help in the diagnosis of RVH. Similarly, a V_7 lead may help in the diagnosis of LVH. In the interest of simplicity, we have not included voltage criteria for either of these leads in Table 17-3.

Refer to Tables 17-1, 17-2, and 17-3 to answer questions A and B.

Question A

Is RVH likely to be present in a 4-year-old child with a mean QRS axis of +95°, no RAA, an R wave of 12 mm in lead V_1, and an S wave of 4 mm in lead V_6?

Answer to question A

No. The axis, R wave amplitude in lead V_1, and S wave amplitude in lead V_6 are all less than the maximal allowed limits for age.

Question B

Is LVH likely to be present in a 6-year-old child with a mean QRS axis of +20°, no LAA, an S wave of 15 mm in lead V_1, an R wave of 30 mm in lead V_5, and an R wave of 35 mm in lead V_6?

Answer to question B

Maybe. The axis, S wave amplitude in lead V_1, and R wave amplitude in lead V_5 are all within normal limits. However, an R wave of 35 in lead V_6 is more than one would expect for this age group. If the child had a heart murmur, further evaluation (i.e., chest x-ray and possibly echocardiogram and/or referral) might be in order.

JUVENILE T WAVE VARIANT

The final pediatric variant we will present in this chapter is known as the *juvenile T wave variant.*

We emphasized in Chapter 10 that the T wave in adults may normally be inverted in lead V_1 (Table 10-6). Because of enhanced right ventricular electrical forces, T wave inversion may normally be seen in several of the anterior precordial leads throughout the pediatric years. In some individuals (especially women), T wave negativity may even persist into adulthood ("persistent" juvenile pattern).

Examine the schematic ECGs shown in Figures 17-3 and 17-4. What is the likely significance of the anterior precordial T wave inversion seen in each tracing?

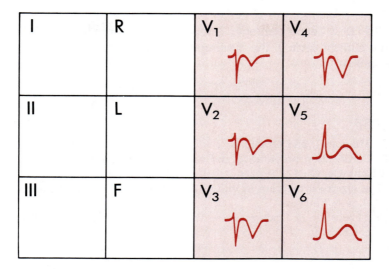

Figure 17-3.   Schematic ECG from a 60-year-old woman with new-onset chest pain. What is the likely significance of the anterior precordial T wave inversion?

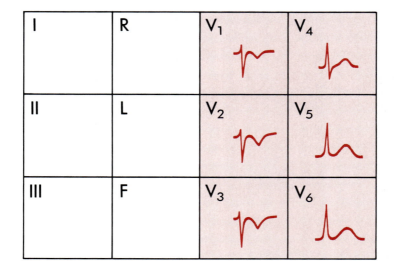

Figure 17-4.   Schematic ECG from a healthy, asymptomatic 8-year-old child. What is the likely significance of the anterior precordial T wave inversion?

Answers

Figure 17-3: Deep symmetric T wave inversion is seen in leads V_1 through V_4. Given the clinical setting, one has to strongly suspect ischemia as the cause of the T wave inversion.

Figure 17-4: Less deep symmetric T wave inversion is seen in leads V_1 through V_3. Given the clinical setting, this finding almost certainly reflects a benign, juvenile T wave pattern.

REFERENCES

Cavallaro D, Hillman J, and Grauer K: Pediatric resuscitation. In Grauer K and Cavallaro D: ACLS: Certification preparation and a comprehensive review, ed 2, St Louis, 1987, The CV Mosby Co, Ch 17.

Garson A: The electrocardiogram in infants and children: a systematic approach, Philadelphia, 1983, Lea & Febiger.

Harris LC and Fernstein E: Understanding ECGs in infants and children, Boston, 1979, Little, Brown & Co.

18

If the Patient Has a Pacemaker

Sophistication of cardiac pacemakers has skyrocketed in recent years. As a result, ECG analysis and interpretation of function of the newer devices now often challenge even cardiologists well versed in their technique. Nevertheless, attention to a few basic points about pacemaker tracings may go a long way toward providing useful information, even when some of the intricacies of the tracing remain unclear.

GENERAL ASPECTS OF PACEMAKER FUNCTION

Discussion of all of the types of cardiac pacemakers is beyond the scope of this book. Even so, one can readily imagine the difficulty that might be posed by a tracing with multiple pacemaker spikes arising from atrial and ventricular pacing at rates that vary according to a patient's activity, and that depend on variable sensing intervals which often remain unknown to all but the programmer of the pacemaker!

Pacemaker function of ventricular demand pacemakers (known as VVI pacemakers) is much easier to assess. These devices used to be the standard pacemaker used. They are less physiologic than the newer, sequential devices because they do not maintain the atrial "kick." Although their use will probably continue to decline in future years, at present they are still among the most common pacemakers found. Understanding the function of VVI pacers is therefore the first step toward understanding pacemaker tracings—and this is our goal for this chapter.

As indicated by the universally accepted classification system, **VVI** pacers PACE *the* **Ventricles,** SENSE *the* **Ventricles,** and are **I**nhibited if a spontaneous beat occurs. They differ from DDD pacemakers, for example, which may pace *either* the atria or the ventricles (**D**ual pacing capability), sense *either* the atria or ventricles (**D**ual sensing capability), and be inhibited *or* triggered by spontaneous beats (capability of being inhibited or triggered also being a **D**ual function).

VVI pacemakers are set at a fixed rate (usually 70 to 72 beats/minute). They are ready to take over pacemaking function whenever (if ever) the patient's underlying rhythm slows *below* the rate at which the pacemaker is set.

Pacemaker function of VVI devices is judged by their ability to **sense** the patient's underlying rhythm, and *pace* (i.e., **capture**) the ventricles when appropriate (i.e., when the patient's inherent rhythm slows down).

209

A pacemaker **spike** indicates that the pacemaker has fired. This is usually seen as a vertical line on the ECG (Figure 18-1, *A*). Pacemaker spikes are most often of small amplitude, although their amplitude may change from one lead to the next, and occasionally from beat to beat in a given lead.

Ventricular **capture** is confirmed when a QRS complex follows a pacemaker spike (Figure 18-1, *B*). Because the origin of the impulse is in the ventricles (since the pacing wire is implanted there), the QRS complex will be wide. Because ventricular depolarization is followed by ventricular repolarization, the QRS complex will be followed by a T wave.

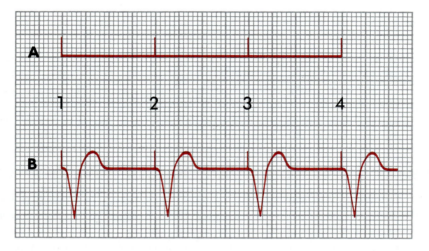

Figure 18-1.   **A,** Four pacemaker spikes are seen at an R-R interval of four large boxes, corresponding to a heart rate of 75 beats/minute (= 300 ÷ 4). There is no ventricular capture. **B,** Each of the four pacemaker spikes successfully captures the ventricles ("100% capture"). Thus, following each spike is a QRS complex (which is wide) and a T wave.

> The easiest way to assess pacemaker function is to imagine yourself as a pacemaker charged with observing the patient's underlying rhythm, and programmed to take over (pace) whenever (if ever) the patient's spontaneous rhythm slows. For example, if you were programmed to pace at a rate of 75 beats/minute, and you didn't see a QRS complex after 0.80 second (i.e., after four large boxes), wouldn't it be time to put out a pacemaker spike?

Apply this principle. Imagine yourself as the pacemaker for the patient whose rhythm is shown in Figure 18-2. Would you have "fired" at point *4* in the tracing? If so, why? Did your pacemaker spike capture the ventricles?

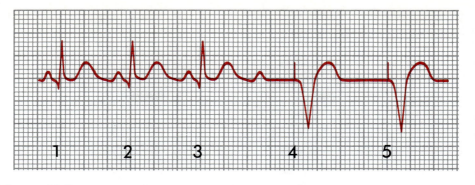

Figure 18-2.   Is the pacemaker functioning appropriately?

Answer to Figure 18-2

The first three beats in this tracing are normal sinus. The fourth P wave fails to conduct. If you were a pacemaker whose sole function in life was to wait four large boxes (= 0.80 second) and then fire if no impulse was forthcoming, you would have put out an impulse at point *4* in this tracing. You would also have put out an impulse four large boxes later (at point *5*), since no spontaneous beat occurred during this interval. Each of these pacemaker spikes successfully captures the ventricles in Figure 18-2, since they are each followed by a wide QRS complex and a T wave. Thus, the pacemaker in this example senses and captures appropriately, and appears to be functioning normally.

Now examine Figure 18-3. There are no pacer spikes at all on this rhythm strip. Does this mean that the pacemaker isn't functioning?

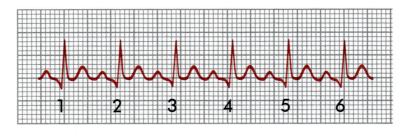

Figure 18-3.   Why hasn't the pacemaker fired?

Answer to Figure 18-3

The rhythm is sinus tachycardia at 125 beats/minute. If you were a pacemaker told to "keep quiet" as long as nothing happened for 0.80 second (= four large boxes), you would not be given an opportunity to speak up in Figure 18-3. This is because the spontaneous rhythm is simply too fast. Thus, it is impossible from Figure 18-3 alone to judge whether the pacemaker is functioning appropriately, since the underlying rhythm never slows below the rate at which the pacemaker is set!

Finally, examine Figure 18-4. If you were the pacemaker in this tracing, would you have acted accordingly?

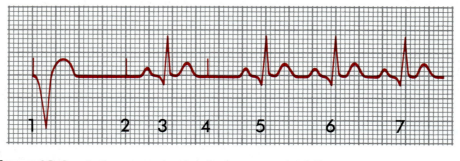

Figure 18-4.   Is the pacemaker functioning appropriately?

Answer to Figure 18-4

Point *1* in the tracing shows a pacemaker spike that successfully captures the ventricles. It is appropriately followed four large boxes (= 0.80 second) later by another pacemaker spike at point *2*. *However, this second pacemaker spike fails to capture the ventricles!* Shortly thereafter follows a spontaneous P wave and sinus-conducted beat at point *3*. This beat is *not* sensed by the pacemaker, which *inappropriately* fires again at point *4*. Not only did the pacemaker fail to sense the spontaneous beat at point *3,* but it also fired early (since the interval between the spike at point *2* and the spike at point *4* is *less* than four large boxes). Spontaneous sinus rhythm at a rate of 100 beats/minute resumes for the last three beats in the tracing. Thus, the rhythm strip shown in Figure 18-4 suggests that the pacemaker is seriously malfunctioning, since it is not reliably sensing and capturing the ventricles.

Several points deserve special mention. First, it is not always possible to determine the precise sensing interval. For example, we are told that the pacemaker in Figures 18-1 through 18-4 has been set to fire at 75 beats/minute. Thus, in the absence of a spontaneous rhythm, a pacemaker spike should appear every four large boxes (as it does in Figure 18-1, *B*). Should the spontaneous rhythm fail (as it does after point *3* in Figure 18-2), one would therefore expect the pacemaker to "kick in" after waiting four large boxes (as it does at point *4* in Figure 18-2). However, the *sensing interval* (i.e., the interval between points *3* and *4* in Figure 18-2) is not always that predictable. This is because it is not always possible to be sure of the exact point in the QRS complex that is being sensed. As a result, it may sometimes appear that the pacemaker is sensing the patient's spontaneous rhythm a little too early or a little too late. As a general rule, if you are in doubt about whether a pacemaker is functioning appropriately, take comfort in knowing that:

> *"Most of the time, the pacemaker is right."*

The accuracy and reliability of these devices are truly amazing. Thus, it is definitely worthwhile to give the pacemaker "the benefit of the doubt," and to look extra hard for a reason that may explain why the pacemaker acted as it did. This is not to say that pacemakers never malfunction. They do. We have already seen one such example in Figure 18-4, when the pacemaker was clearly at fault. However, *most of the time, there's a reason why the pacemaker acted as it did*.

DETECTION OF ISCHEMIA OR INFARCTION IN A PATIENT WITH A PACEMAKER

The task of interpreting a 12-lead ECG in a patient with a pacemaker can be intimidating. Pacemaker spikes may be everywhere! Practically speaking, little useful information is provided by analyzing the morphology of ventricular paced beats. By definition, the electrical impulse from such beats starts in the ventricles (outside of the conduction system), causing the QRS complex to be wide. Because of the unusual (ventricular) origin of these beats, the sequence of repolarization is also altered. As a result, accompanying ST segment and T wave changes of ventricular-paced beats do not reliably reflect underlying infarction or ischemia. *Electrocardiographic diagnosis of acute infarction or ischemia is therefore exceedingly difficult when only a few (or no) spontaneous beats are present!*

Examine the simultaneously recorded 12-lead ECGs in Figures 18-5 and 18-6. Each of these tracings is from an elderly patient complaining of new-onset chest pain. Each patient had a VVI pacemaker implanted years earlier for unknown reasons. Is it possible to diagnose acute infarction or ischemia from either tracing?

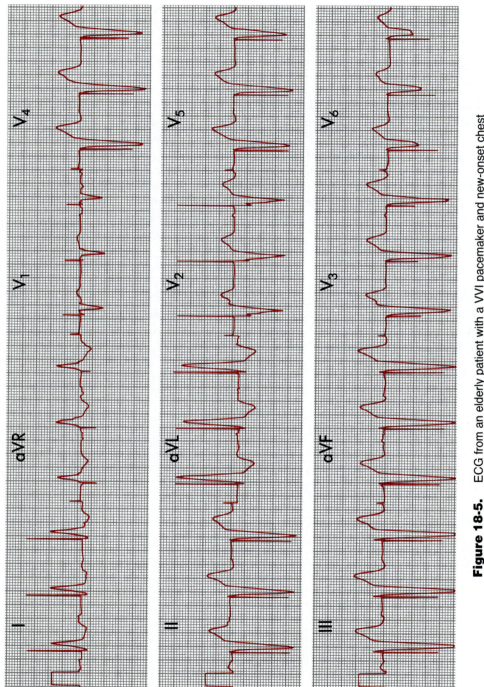
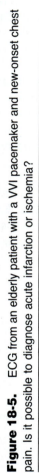

Figure 18-5.   ECG from an elderly patient with a VVI pacemaker and new-onset chest pain. Is it possible to diagnose acute infarction or ischemia?

Answer to Figure 18-5

No. Regular pacemaker spikes appear at a rate of just under 75 beats/minute. There is *100% capture,* since each pacemaker spike is followed by a paced beat (wide QRS complex and T wave). However, since no spontaneous beats occur, it is not possible to assess QRS morphology or the ST segments and T waves for changes suggestive of infarction or ischemia.

Note the different appearance of pacemaker spikes in the different leads. Sometimes spikes are upright; at other times they are directed downward. In this example, spikes are smallest in leads aVR and V_1. Realize that pacemaker spikes may sometimes be so small in certain leads as to pass unnoticed. In such cases, it may only become apparent that the patient has a pacemaker when all leads in a 12-lead tracing are examined.

Finally, note that P waves appear to be present in certain leads in Figure 18-5 (being best seen in simultaneous leads V_1, V_2, and V_3). Occasionally you may even be able to determine a patient's underlying rhythm (and/or the reason the pacemaker was implanted) from assessing spontaneous atrial activity. P waves are not seen well enough to do this in Figure 18-5.

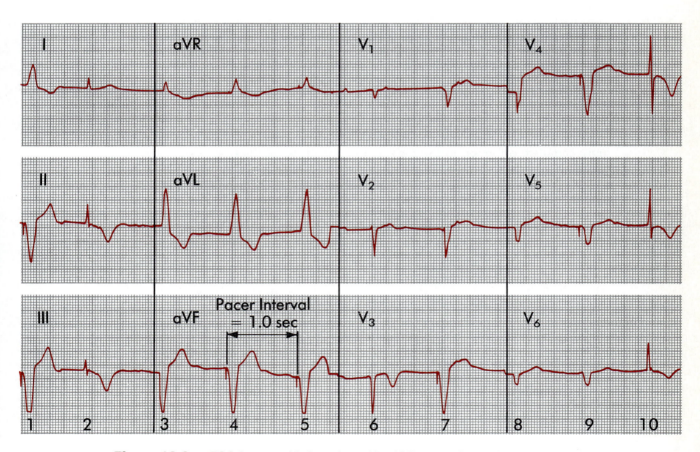

Figure 18-6.   ECG from an elderly patient with a VVI pacemaker and new-onset chest pain. Is it possible to diagnose acute infarction or ischemia?

Answer to Figure 18-6

This ECG is much harder to interpret. Pacemaker spikes are much less numerous. Interpretation of pacemaker function is made more difficult by constant lead changes, so that the only place in the tracing where two pacemaker spikes appear in a row is in lead aVF. It appears from this lead that the pacer interval is five large boxes (= 1.0 second), corresponding to a rate of 60 beats/minute. Clearly, a long rhythm strip would be needed to adequately judge pacemaker function. Nevertheless, several basic points can be stated. All pacemaker spikes seen on the tracing are followed by a QRST complex. This suggests appropriate capture. Note that pacemaker spikes are extremely small in some leads (such as aVR) and not at all evident in others (such as aVL). Knowing that the ECG was simultaneously recorded explains QRS widening in these leads.

Spontaneous beats are seen in several leads. These spontaneous beats appear to occur at an interval of *less* than five large boxes (i.e., less than 1.0 second) from the previous beat. This is consistent with our assumption that the pacemaker is set for a rate of 60 beats/minute and appears to be functioning appropriately (although as already stated, a much longer rhythm strip would be needed to verify this).

However, our main purpose for including this otherwise very complex tracing is to highlight the QRST morphology of the spontaneous beats. *Focus on these spontaneous beats.* They can be identified by the fact that they have a narrow QRS complex and are not preceded by a pacemaker spike. Does the QRST morphology of these spontaneous beats suggest acute infarction or ischemia?

Yes! Note deep, symmetric (and worrisome) T wave inversion in spontaneous beats seen in leads II, III, and V_3 through V_6. This suggests underlying ischemia.

In summary, although the intricacies of pacemaker tracings may be exceedingly complex, attention to the basic principles presented here will surprisingly often allow you to determine the adequacy of pacemaker function, especially for ventricular demand (VVI) pacemakers. Identification and evaluation of QRST morphology of spontaneous beats may also provide insight into the presence of underlying infarction or ischemia.

19

When 12 Leads are Better than One

Use of the 12-lead ECG for dysrhythmia interpretation

Twelve leads are better than one. Yet despite the intuitive logic of this principle, many medical care providers do not seem to regularly apply it in their practice.

The aspect of electrocardiography that we feel is aided most by regular application of the 12-lead principle is dysrhythmia interpretation. All too often, diagnostic and therapeutic decisions are based on information provided from the one lead being monitored by telemetry. Doing so is like playing cards with an incomplete deck. Information is missing. Conclusions may or may not be justified.

For example, would you say a chest x-ray was normal if you didn't get to look at the lateral view? Could you say the x-ray was normal if you saw the lateral, but didn't get to look at the posteroanterior (PA) view? Would you comment on a patient's acid-base status if all you were told was the Pco_2? How then can one be sure that a QRS complex is truly narrow (or that atrial activity is truly absent) by inspection of only one lead?

Medical care providers often work in settings where the patients they are caring for are monitored by telemetry. *Decisions need not be based solely on the one lead being monitored.* The goal of this chapter is to highlight how the use of additional information (from other monitoring leads or from a 12-lead ECG) may tremendously enhance diagnostic skill and improve patient management.

To bring this point home, examine the following seven rhythm strips taken from patients A through G (Figures 19A-1, 19B-1, 19C-1, 19D-1, 19E-1, 19F-1, and 19G-1, respectively). For each tracing, interpret the rhythm to the best of your ability. Considering the clinical scenario given in the legend of each figure (and assuming each patient is hemodynamically stable), imagine what your initial approach to management would be. To help crystallize your impressions, *write your answers down!* Our suggestions follow.

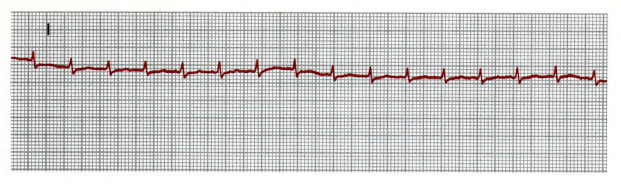

Figure 19A-1. Rhythm strip from **Patient A,** a 60-year-old woman presenting because of a "rapid heart beat." Her blood pressure is 140/90 mm Hg. Patient A is not having chest pain, and is not on any medications. *What could the rhythm be? How would you proceed?*

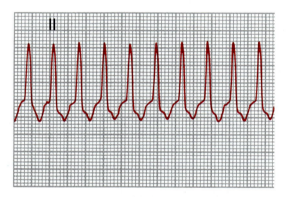

Figure 19B-1. Rhythm strip from **Patient B,** a 50-year-old man with a history of coronary artery disease. His blood pressure is 160/100 mm Hg. Patient B is aware of a rapid heart beat, but is not having chest pain. *What could the rhythm be? How would you proceed?*

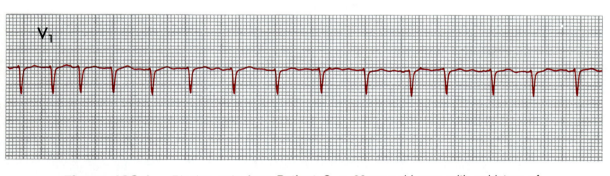

Figure 19C-1. Rhythm strip from **Patient C,** a 60-year-old man with a history of chronic obstructive pulmonary disease. Patient C had been told in the past that he had a "rapid heart beat." He is wheezing at the time this tracing is recorded, and has a blood pressure of 130/80 mm Hg. *What could the rhythm be? How would you proceed?*

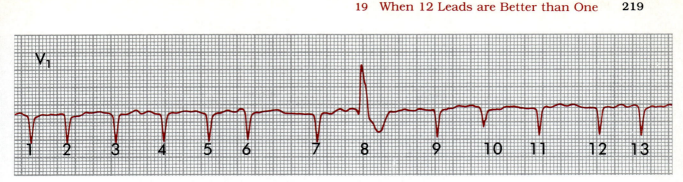

Figure 19D-1.   Rhythm strip from **Patient D,** a 60-year-old man presenting with palpitations. Patient D has a history of coronary artery disease. He is not having chest pain and has a blood pressure of 140/90 mm Hg at the time this tracing is recorded. *What is the underlying rhythm? What is beat #8? Are there any other unusual beats in this tracing?*

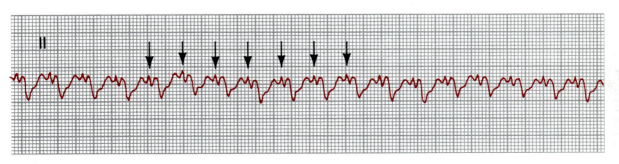

Figure 19E-1.   Rhythm strip from **Patient E,** a 65-year-old woman with a history of prior myocardial infarction. Patient E has a blood pressure of 150/80 mm Hg at the time this tracing is recorded. She is not having chest pain, but is bothered by "palpitations." *Should you treat her sinus tachycardia?*

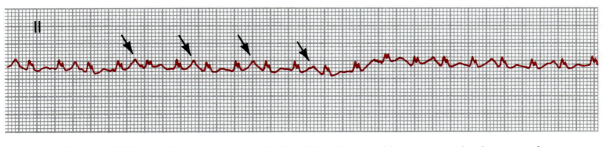
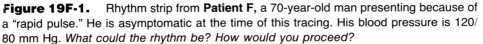

Figure 19F-1.   Rhythm strip from **Patient F,** a 70-year-old man presenting because of a "rapid pulse." He is asymptomatic at the time of this tracing. His blood pressure is 120/80 mm Hg. *What could the rhythm be? How would you proceed?*

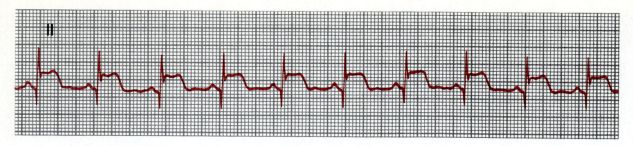

Figure 19G-1.   Rhythm strip from **Patient G,** a 70-year-old woman presenting with a history of new-onset chest pain. The initial 12-lead ECG, obtained 2 hours earlier, was entirely normal. Patient G's chest pain has suddenly increased. Her blood pressure is 140/90 mm Hg. *What is the rhythm? How would you proceed?*

ANSWERS

Figure 19A-1

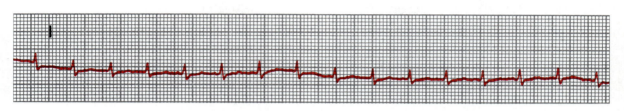

Figure 19A-1.   Rhythm strip from **Patient A,** a 60-year-old woman presenting because of a "rapid heart beat." Her blood pressure is 140/90 mm Hg. The patient is not having chest pain, and is not on any medications. *What could the rhythm recorded be? How would you proceed?*

The rhythm in Figure 19A-1 is fairly regular, at a rate just under 150 beats/ minute (i.e., the R-R interval is just over two large boxes). Although there are slight undulations in the baseline, definite P waves are not evident in the one lead shown. For all the world this appears to be PSVT *(see Chapter 3)*.

The *KEY* lies in the second question: *How would you proceed?* Although one might try a vagal maneuver (in an attempt to slow AV conduction and bring out atrial activity) and/or medication (such as verapamil) to try to convert the rhythm, a more reasonable (and less invasive) first step might be to simply collect more information (Figure 19A-2).

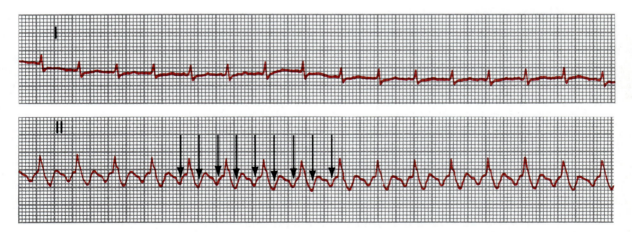

Figure 19A-2.   Simultaneously recorded lead II for Patient A, whose lead I rhythm strip was shown in Figure 19A-1. *Does this facilitate diagnosis of the rhythm?*

The simultaneously recorded lead II in Figure 19A-2 reveals atrial activity (with a sawtooth appearance) at a rate of about 300 beats/minute *(see arrows).* Thus, the rhythm is actually **atrial flutter** with a 2:1 AV response (atrial rate about 300 beats/minute; ventricular rate about 150 beats/minute).

In our experience, atrial flutter is by far the most commonly overlooked arrhythmia. A look at the 12-lead ECG of patient A explains why (Figure 19A-3).

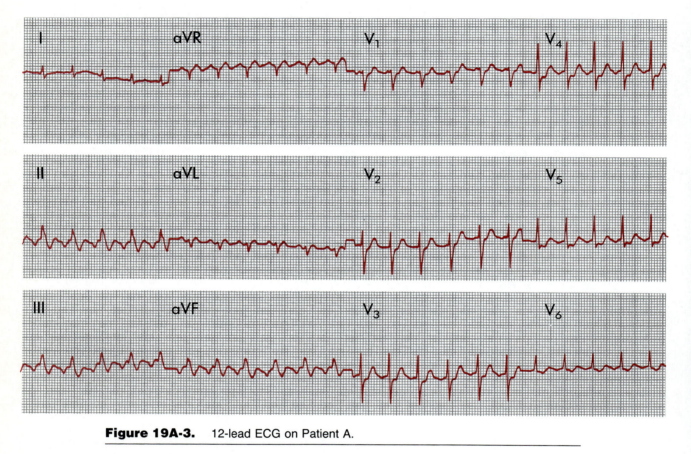

Figure 19A-3.   12-lead ECG on Patient A.

Although flutter activity is evident in each of the three inferior leads (II, III, and aVF), it is not at all obvious from inspection of the remaining nine leads that the rhythm is flutter. One might imagine how easy it could be to overlook this rhythm if flutter waves are not apparent in the lead being monitored. This was the case in Figure 19A-1. As we emphasized in Chapter 3, the key to recognizing atrial flutter is to always maintain a high index of suspicion. In adults, the atrial rate for *untreated* flutter is almost always close to 300 beats/minute (range of 250 to 350). The most common ventricular response is 2:1. Therefore:

> *Whenever you have a regular, supraventricular tachycardia with a ventricular response close to 150 beats/minute, **think flutter till proven otherwise**—especially if normal (upright) P waves are not evident in lead II.*

Again, the process we used to arrive at the diagnosis of flutter is to carefully review all 12 leads of the ECG shown in Figure 19A-3. The rhythm is regular, and the QRS complex is narrow (not greater than half a large box). The negative P wave in lead II rules out sinus tachycardia. Recognizing that the ventricular response is about 150 beats/minute then brings to mind the axiom we just stated: *think flutter till proven otherwise!* Further dissection of the waveform in the inferior leads (as shown by the arrows in Figure 19A-2) confirms atrial activity at the telltale rate of 300 beats/minute.

Figure 19A-4 shows the 12-lead ECG of patient A following conversion to normal sinus rhythm. Note that the P wave is once again upright in lead II. Note also that the negative deflection that seemed to form the terminal portion of the QRS complex in the inferior leads in Figure 19A-3 has disappeared, confirming that these deflections were really flutter waves. Careful (retrospective) *caliper-aided* analysis of other leads in Figure 19A-3 (such as aVR, aVL, and V_4 to V_6) in comparison with the postconversion tracing (Figure 19A-4) now also reveals that exceedingly subtle flutter activity had been present all along.

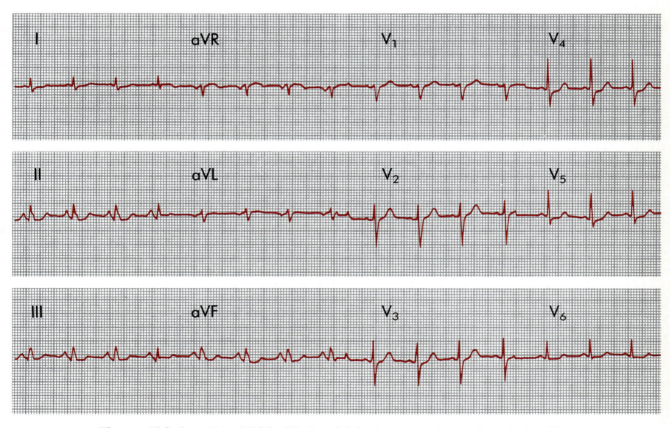

Figure 19A-4.   12-lead ECG of Patient A following conversion to sinus rhythm. Note that the P wave is now upright in lead II. Comparison with Figure 19A-3 *retrospectively* reveals subtle flutter activity during the tachycardia. Note also that much of the ST segment depression that had been present during the tachycardia (in Figure 19A-3) has disappeared now that the rate has slowed.

Routinely obtaining a *12-lead **postconversion ECG*** is an excellent habit to develop. As we have just seen, comparison of preconversion and postconversion tracings may provide invaluable insight into true QRS morphology. Occasionally the postconversion tracing may also suggest the etiology of the arrhythmia (i.e., if delta waves or changes of acute infarction are now seen). Finally, the postconversion ECG helps evaluate the significance of ST-T wave changes that may have been present during the tachycardia. Note in Figure 19A-4 that the ST segment depression seen during the tachycardia (in Figure 19A-3) has largely resolved. This suggests that much of the ST segment depression seen earlier (in Figure 19A-3) was due either to the negative deflections of the flutter waves or to the tachycardia itself (i.e., rate-related ST segment changes), rather than being the direct result of ischemia *(see Table 13-4 in the pocket reference, p. 39, which lists the common causes of ST segment depression)*.

In summary, we admit to being deceptive in providing you with only one lead in Figure 19A-1. Nevertheless, we hope doing so has emphasized the high index of suspicion needed to diagnose many cases of atrial flutter.

Hint: *We become even more deceptive in some of the following tracings.*

Figure 19B-1

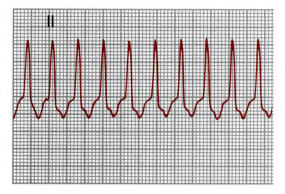

Figure 19B-1.   Rhythm strip from **Patient B,** a 50-year-old man with a history of coronary artery disease. His blood pressure is 160/100 mm Hg. Patient B is aware of a rapid heart beat, but is not having chest pain. *What could the rhythm be? How would you proceed?*

The rhythm is regular, at a rate of 210 beats/minute. Atrial activity is absent, and the QRS complex does not really appear to be wide. Considering that the patient is awake, alert, and normotensive, one's first impulse might be to assume that the rhythm is PSVT. This could be a potentially lethal mistake if one were to treat accordingly.

What do we know about the arrhythmia?

We know the following:
1. The rhythm is rapid and regular.
2. Atrial activity is absent and the QRS does not appear to be wide in the lead being monitored.

Question. Do we know anything about the width of the QRS complex in other leads?

Answer. No.

(See *Figure 19B-2.*)

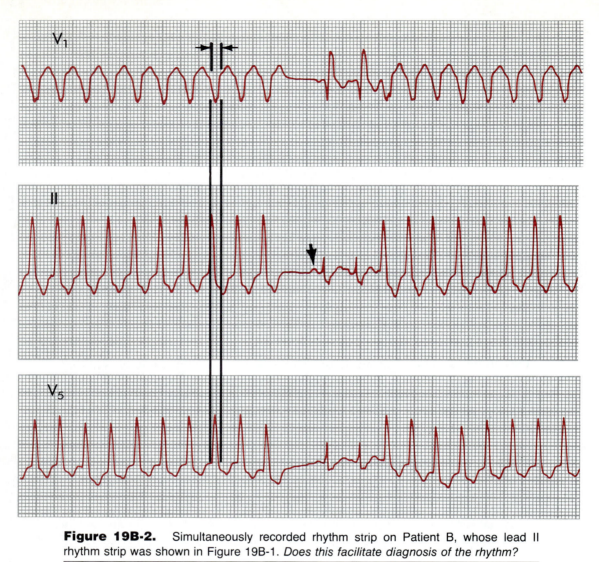

Figure 19B-2. Simultaneously recorded rhythm strip on Patient B, whose lead II rhythm strip was shown in Figure 19B-1. *Does this facilitate diagnosis of the rhythm?*

Although the QRS complex does not appear to be more than 0.10 second in either lead II or lead III, it certainly looks wide ($\geq$0.12 second) in lead V_1. Vertical time lines in the simultaneously recorded rhythm strip in Figure 19B-2 show why: a portion of the QRS complex in leads II and III lies on the baseline.

Before going further, let us interject a word on the **simultaneously recorded rhythm strip** displayed in Figure 19B-2. Simultaneous recording of the three leads shown facilitates comparison of P wave and QRS morphology in different leads at different times. *The three leads most commonly used for this purpose are V$_1$, II, and V$_5$.*

Lead II is selected because it is usually the best lead for visualizing atrial activity. As we have already emphasized, with sinus rhythm the P wave must be upright in this lead. Lead II is also an excellent lead for identifying flutter waves or retrograde P waves (which appear as negative deflections in lead II).

Leads V$_1$ and V$_5$ are the other two leads commonly selected. We emphasized in Chapter 5 that when the QRS complex was wide, the type of bundle branch block could be determined by evaluating QRS morphology in three key leads (I, V$_1$, and V$_6$). Our simultaneously recorded rhythm strip uses only two leads to assess QRS morphology: the right-sided lead V$_1$ and lead V$_5$. For practical purposes, lead V$_5$ provides adequate left-sided morphologic information (and is usually quite similar in appearance to lead V$_6$).

In addition to allowing determination of the type of bundle branch block, assessment of QRS morphology may provide invaluable information for differentiating between ventricular ectopy and aberrantly conducted beats, as we shall see shortly.

Focus for a moment on the beat in the middle of Figure 19B-2 that follows a brief pause, and whose P wave is highlighted by the arrow in the tracing for lead II. This beat appears to be sinus conducted, since it is preceded by an upright P wave with a normal PR interval. It is followed by a second sinus-conducted beat before the tachycardia resumes. (The P wave preceding the second sinus-conducted beat is partially hidden by the preceding T wave.)

In each of the three leads monitored (leads V$_1$, II, and V$_5$), note how different the QRS morphology is for the two sinus-conducted beats compared with the beats during the tachycardia.

QRS morphology for the two sinus-conducted beats is consistent with underlying RBBB: there is a QR complex (which is an *RBBB-equivalent pattern*) in lead V$_1$ *(see Figure 5-13 on pocket reference p. 14),* and a wide terminal S wave in left-sided lead V$_5$.

QRS morphology during the tachycardia is quite different: there is a QS complex in lead V$_1$ and a monophasic R wave in lead V$_5$. Since the two beats with underlying RBBB are sinus conducted, the etiology of the very different-appearing beats in the tachycardia must be ventricular. Thus, the rhythm shown in Figure 19B-1 had to have been **ventricular tachycardia.**

That the patient was in ventricular tachycardia is easier to conceptualize after analysis of the simultaneously recorded rhythm strip shown in Figure 19B-3.

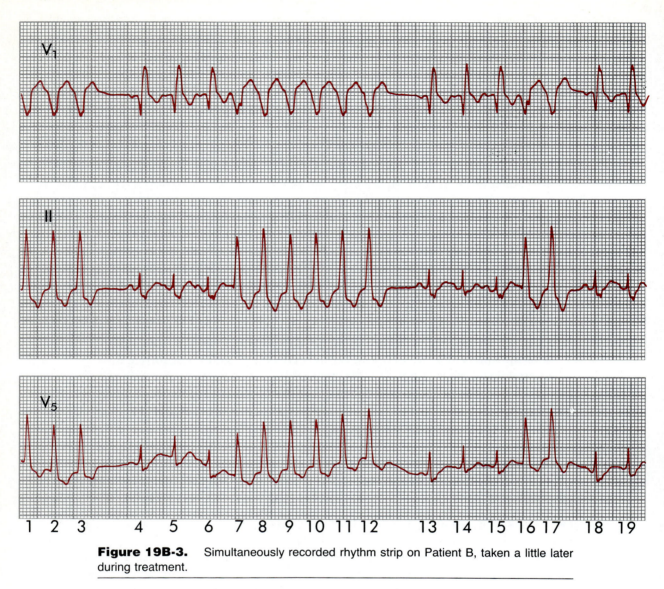

Figure 19B-3.   Simultaneously recorded rhythm strip on Patient B, taken a little later during treatment.

The patient remained awake and alert at the time Figure 19B-3 was recorded. Beats *4, 5,* and *6* are clearly sinus conducted. Sinus rhythm is then interrupted by a run of ventricular tachycardia (beats *7* to *12*). Following a short pause, sinus rhythm resumes with beats *13* to *15*. A ventricular couplet intervenes (beats *16* and *17*), but the last two beats of the rhythm strip are sinus (beats *18* and *19*).

Several points deserve special emphasis:

1. Patients may remain awake, alert, and hemodynamically stable for extended periods of time despite being in ventricular tachycardia. *A normal (or even elevated) blood pressure in no way rules out this diagnosis!*

2. Just because the QRS complex does not appear wide (≥0.12 seconds) in one lead does not necessarily mean that it will not be wide in other leads. *Whenever possible, 12 leads are better than one.* If the patient remains hemodynamically stable, there will usually be enough time to obtain additional leads (and ideally a 12-lead ECG) to help in making a definitive diagnosis.

3. Verapamil should *NEVER* be used for treatment unless one can be relatively certain that the rhythm is not ventricular tachycardia.

Verapamil is an excellent drug. It is a treatment of choice for PSVT. It is also extremely useful in management of atrial flutter and atrial fibrillation. However, if it is mistakenly given to a patient in ventricular tachycardia, there is a high likelihood that the rhythm will deteriorate to ventricular fibrillation. *Verapamil would therefore be contraindicated for treatment of the rhythm shown in Figure 19B-1. This rhythm should not be assumed to be PSVT without first obtaining additional leads.*

4. Analysis of QRS morphology can be exceedingly helpful in differentiating between ventricular ectopy (PVCs, ventricular tachycardia) and supraventricular beats (PACs or SVT with aberration).

Let us expound on this last point. Morphologic characteristics in right- and left-sided monitoring leads may be the best clue to the true etiology of wide beats or of a wide-complex tachycardia. In general, the presence of a typical right or left bundle branch block morphology *(as shown in Figure 5-8, on pocket reference p. 14)* is consistent with a supraventricular etiology. Deviation from the typical pattern either is of no diagnostic help or suggests ventricular ectopy *(Figures 19B-4 and 19B-5, which also appear on pocket reference p. 56).*

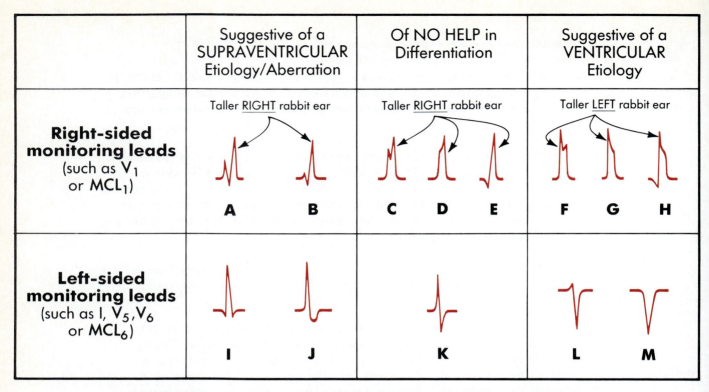

	Suggestive of a SUPRAVENTRICULAR Etiology/Aberration	Of NO HELP in Differentiation	Suggestive of a VENTRICULAR Etiology
Right-sided monitoring leads (such as V_1 or MCL_1)	Taller <u>RIGHT</u> rabbit ear **A** **B**	Taller <u>RIGHT</u> rabbit ear **C** **D** **E**	Taller <u>LEFT</u> rabbit ear **F** **G** **H**
Left-sided monitoring leads (such as I, V_5, V_6 or MCL_6)	**I** **J**	**K**	**L** **M**

Figure 19B-4. Differentiation of wide beats **When the QRS Complex is Upright in V_1.**

	Suggestive of a SUPRAVENTRICULAR Etiology/Aberration	Of NO HELP in Differentiation	Suggestive of a VENTRICULAR Etiology
Right-sided monitoring leads (such as V_1 or MCL_1)	**N** **O**		**P** **Q**
Left-sided monitoring leads (such as I, V_5, V_6 or MCL_6)	**R** **S**		**T** **U** **V**

Figure 19B-5. Differentiation of wide beats **When the QRS Complex is Negative in V_1.**

Thus, ***when the QRS complex is upright in lead V_1,*** an RsR′ or rsR′ pattern (Figure 19B-4, *A* and *B*) in which there is a taller right "rabbit ear" (i.e., in which the R′, or second upright component of the QRS, is taller) is consistent with beats of a supraventricular etiology. This is especially true when the QRS complex has an S wave in the lateral leads (Figure 19B-4, *I* or *J*).

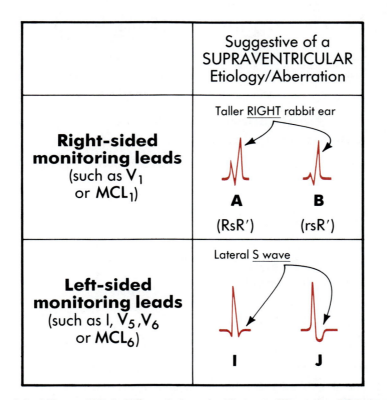

A, B, I, and **J** of Figure 19B-4. Differentiation of wide beats **When the QRS Complex is Upright in V_1.**

In contrast, the presence of a taller left rabbit ear (in which the first upright component of the QRS is taller) strongly suggests ventricular ectopy (Figure 19B-4, *F*, *G*, and *H*). A predominantly negative or totally negative complex in the lateral leads is also strongly suggestive of ventricular ectopy (*L* and *M*).

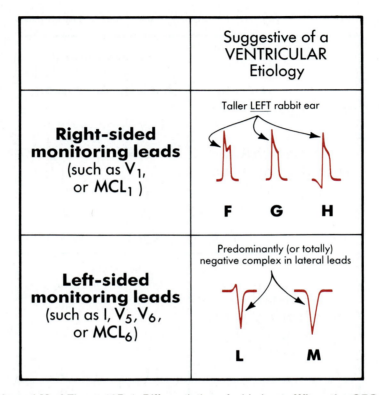

F, G, H, L, and M of Figure 19B-4. Differentiation of wide beats **When the QRS Complex is Upright in V₁.**

QRS morphology is of little help in differentiation for intermediate forms *C*, *D*, and *E* (which do not have a clear rsR′ with an S wave that descends back to the baseline) or *K* (which has neither a predominant R wave nor a predominant S wave).

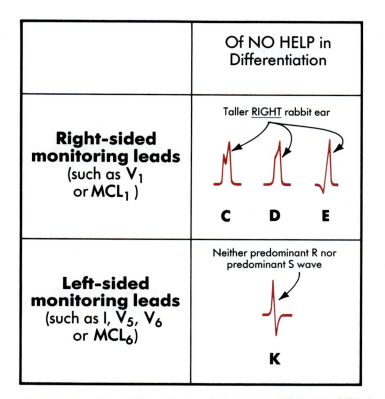

C, D, E, and K of Figure 19B-4. Differentiation of wide beats **When the QRS Complex is Upright in V₁.**

Emphasis for evaluation of QRS morphology changes *when the QRS complex in question is negative in lead V₁* (Figure 19B-5). A supraventricular etiology is suggested by a rapid downslope of the QRS complex in a right-sided lead (*N* and *O*). In contrast, if the initial upward deflection in lead V_1 or MCL_1 is wide (i.e., if the initial r wave is fat, as it is in *P*), or if the downward deflection is slurred or delayed (as it is in *Q*), ventricular ectopy is likely.

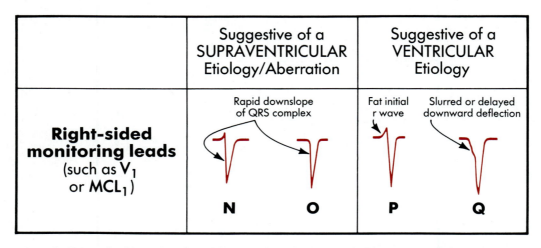

N, O, P, and **Q** of Figure 19B-5. Differentiation of wide beats **When the QRS Complex is Negative in V₁.**

An upright R wave in a left-sided monitoring lead is consistent with supraventricular beats (*R* or *S*), whereas the presence of any Q wave *(T)*, or a predominantly negative *(U)* or totally negative *(V)* complex, in a left-sided lead is strongly suggestive of ventricular ectopy.

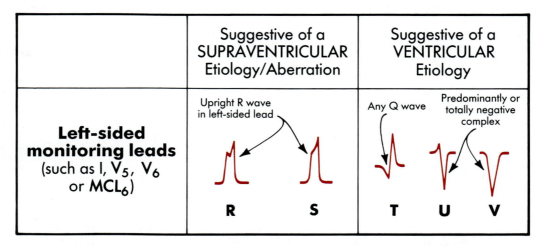

R, S, T, U, and **V** of Figure 19B-5. Differentiation of wide beats **When the QRS Complex is Negative in V₁.**

The information in Figures 19B-4 and 19B-5 can be simplified (for easier recall) as follows:

> **If the QRS is UPRIGHT in lead V₁** (Figure 19B-4):
> A supraventricular etiology is suggested by typical RBBB morphology (rsR′ or RsR′ in lead V₁ or MCL₁ **and** a wide terminal S wave in lateral leads).
> Ventricular ectopy is suggested by a taller left rabbit ear in lead V₁ **or** a totally or predominantly negative complex in lateral leads.
>
> **If the QRS is NEGATIVE in lead V₁** (Figure 19B-5):
> A supraventricular etiology is suggested by typical LBBB morphology.
> Ventricular ectopy is suggested if there is a fat initial r wave **or** slurred/delayed downslope in lead V₁ or MCL₁ **or** a totally or predominantly negative QRS complex in a lateral lead.

Return now to Figure 19B-2. Assess QRS morphology during the tachycardia in leads V₁ and V₅. Use Figure 19B-5 for guidelines, since the QRS complex is negative in lead V₁.

Answer. The QRS complex in lead V₁ is completely negative. Note that the downslope is slurred and delayed (as in Figure 19-B5, *Q*, adding further support to the conclusion that the tachycardia in Figure 19B-2 is of ventricular origin (and not supraventricular with aberration).

Practice

Analyze the fairly regular wide-complex tachycardia shown in Figure 19B-6. Although there are undulations in the baseline in lead II, there are no definite P waves. Is QRS morphology in leads V₁ and V₆ more suggestive of a supraventricular etiology or a ventricular etiology? *(Refer to Figure 19B-4, since the QRS complex is upright in lead V₁).*

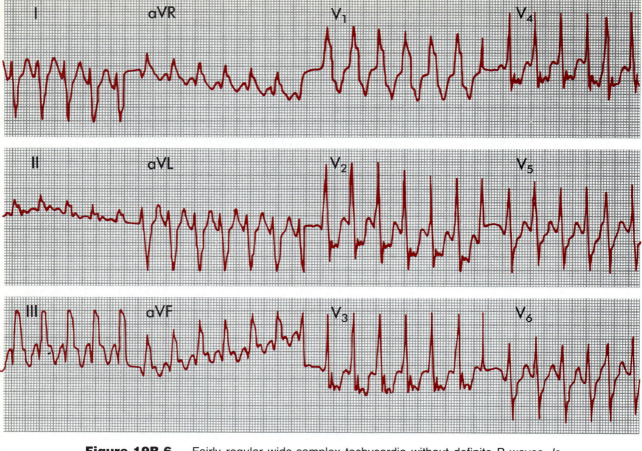

Figure 19B-6. Fairly regular wide-complex tachycardia without definite P waves. *Is QRS morphology in leads V₁ and V₆ more suggestive of a supraventricular etiology or a ventricular etiology?*

Answer to Figure 19B-6

QRS morphology in lead V_6 is not helpful, since neither the R wave nor the S wave is predominant. However, the taller left rabbit ear of the QRS complex in lead V_1 (which resembles Figure 19B-4, *G*), strongly supports our previous assumption that the tachycardia is ventricular in origin.

A final clue to the etiology of this tachyarrhythmia lies with determination of the QRS **axis.** The finding of either marked RAD or marked LAD strongly suggests ventricular tachycardia. This is the case in Figure 19B-6, in which the predominantly negative QRS complex in lead I indicates marked RAD.

Finally, analyze the regular wide-complex tachycardia shown in Figure 19B-7. It is hard to determine if the upright deflection between QRS complexes in lead II represents the terminal portion of the T wave, a P wave, or both. Is QRS morphology in leads V_1 and V_6 more suggestive of a supraventricular etiology or a ventricular etiology? *(Refer again to Figure 19B-4, since the QRS complex is upright in lead V_1).*

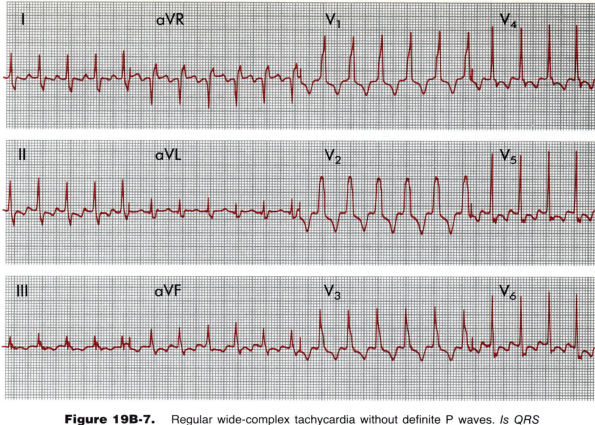

Figure 19B-7. Regular wide-complex tachycardia without definite P waves. *Is QRS morphology in leads V₁ and V₆ more suggestive of a supraventricular etiology or a ventricular etiology?*

Answer to Figure 19B-7

QRS morphology in the key lateral leads (I and V₆) is consistent with a supraventricular etiology, since the R wave is relatively tall and the wide terminal S wave expected with typical RBBB conduction is present. Unfortunately, morphology of the QRS complex in lead V₁ (which resembles Figure 19B-4, *D*) is not helpful in differentiation. Thus, all one can say about the rhythm in the 12-lead ECG in Figure 19B-7 is that there is a regular, wide-complex tachycardia without definite atrial activity. As always, *ventricular tachycardia must be assumed until proven otherwise.* (Fortunately, a prior ECG from the patient was found that demonstrated an identical pattern of QRS widening during sinus rhythm. In the absence of a prior tracing, however, it would be impossible to rule out ventricular tachycardia from the information presented in Figure 19B-7).

Question. Is the QRS axis in Figure 19B-7 normal? Does this favor a supraventricular etiology or a ventricular etiology for the arrhythmia?

Answer. The QRS axis in Figure 19B-7 is normal because the QRS complex is upright in leads I and aVF. Although this is consistent with a supraventricular etiology for the arrhythmia, it does not rule out ventricular tachycardia. *It should be emphasized that determination of QRS axis is helpful in differentiating between supraventricular and ventricular tachycardia ONLY when there is MARKED axis deviation (RAD or LAD).*

Figure 19C-1

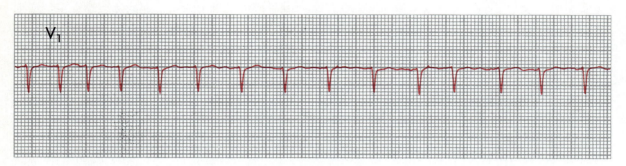

Figure 19C-1.   Rhythm strip from **Patient C,** a 60-year-old man with a history of chronic obstructive pulmonary disease. Patient C had been told in the past that he had a "rapid heart beat." He is wheezing at the time this tracing is recorded, and has a blood pressure of 130/80 mm Hg. *What could the rhythm be? How would you proceed?*

The rhythm is irregularly irregular. The QRS complex appears to be narrow, and there is no definite atrial activity. For all the world, this appears to be atrial fibrillation.

Question. Is there another rhythm that might give the identical appearance of irregular irregularity without atrial activity in a single monitoring lead? (**Hint:** *Patient C has COPD!*)

Answer. Once again the *KEY* lies in the second question we posed above: *How would you proceed?* Whenever doubt exists about the true nature of P waves or the QRS complex in one monitoring lead, *seek additional viewpoints!* Does the simultaneously recorded rhythm strip in Figure 19C-2 provide an answer?

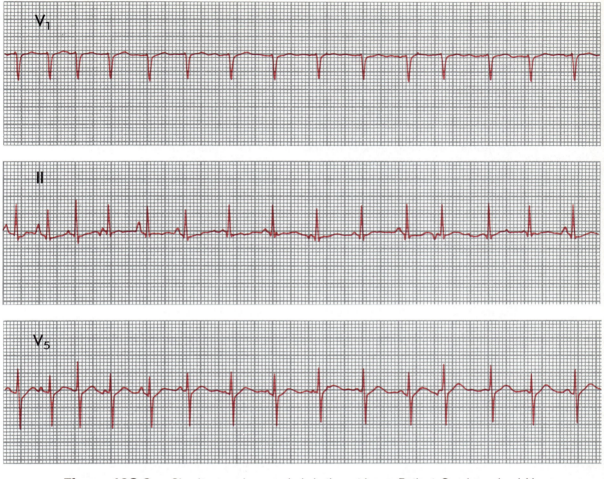

Figure 19C-2.   Simultaneously recorded rhythm strip on Patient C, whose lead V_1 rhythm strip was shown in Figure 19C-1. *Does this facilitate diagnosis of the rhythm?*

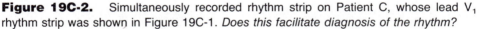

The key lies in lead II. Although the rhythm is again shown to be irregular, definite atrial activity is now evident! The reason why all of the P waves are different in lead II is that the rhythm is ***multifocal atrial tachycardia (MAT).***

MAT is a fairly common rhythm disorder in patients with COPD. It also occurs in sick, intensive care patients with multisystem disease. Clinically, the importance of recognizing MAT is that the rhythm not be misdiagnosed as atrial fibrillation, since management of the two disorders may be vastly different.

Traditionally, digoxin has been the drug most commonly prescribed to slow the ventricular response of rapid atrial fibrillation. In the acute situation, many clinicians tend to give IV increments of the drug until adequate rate control is achieved. Doing the same for MAT is highly likely to result in digitalis toxicity.

The key to treatment of MAT is to recognize and treat the underlying cause. Since in most cases the cause is COPD, optimal treatment often consists of relieving bronchospasm and improving oxygenation. If medication is needed for rate control, however, IV verapamil (rather than digitalis) is the drug of choice.

Figure 19C-3 is the 12-lead ECG of Patient C. How would you interpret this tracing?

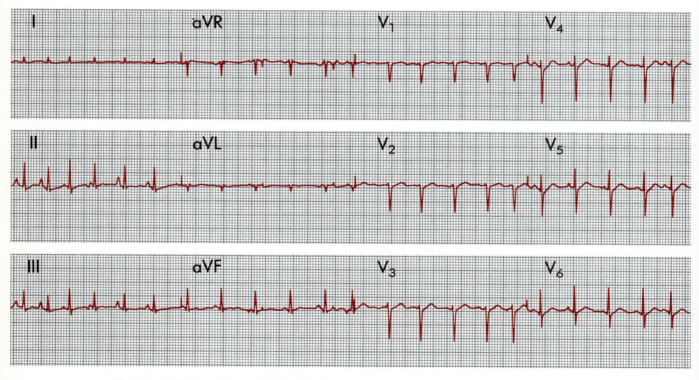

Figure 19C-3.   12-lead ECG of Patient C.

Answer to Figure 19C-3

Descriptive analysis. As already stated, the rhythm is irregularly irregular, and multiple P waveforms are noted in lead II. The rhythm is MAT.

The PR interval varies because of the rhythm. The QRS complex appears to be of normal duration. The relatively rapid rate makes it more difficult to assess the QT interval, but it is probably not prolonged.

The axis is normal. We estimate it to be about +75° (since the net QRS deflection of lead aVF is definitely more positive than the net deflection of lead I).

There is no evidence of LVH.

Small q waves are present in the inferior leads and in lead V_6. There is delayed transition ("poor R wave progression") with persistence of S waves in the lateral precordial leads. There are nonspecific ST segment and T wave abnormalities (flattening) in many leads, but no acute changes.

Clinical impression. Our overall impression of this ECG is that it is consistent with this patient's underlying problem: COPD. Although not meeting strict criteria for low voltage, QRS amplitude is generally decreased. S waves persist across the precordial leads, and there is a relatively vertical QRS axis. And although changing P wave morphology makes it more difficult to assess atrial chamber enlargement, several of the P waves in lead II are prominent and peaked, consistent with RAA. Taken together in the clinical setting, the combination of these findings suggests a *pulmonary disease pattern* (see Table 9-4, on pocket reference p. 25).

In summary, MAT is another rhythm in which a high index of suspicion is often needed in order to make the diagnosis. Atrial activity will *not* always be obvious in every monitoring lead. We therefore suggest the following:

Strongly consider obtaining a 12-lead ECG to verify the cause of an irregularly irregular rhythm, especially in patients with pulmonary disease! *Do not indiscriminately treat with digoxin until you have done so.**

---

*Let us emphasize that digoxin is *not* contraindicated in MAT, and small doses of this drug may be given in an attempt to reduce the ventricular response. However, patients with MAT tend to be extremely susceptible to developing digitalis toxicity, and the drug should not be "pushed" as it sometimes is in treatment of rapid atrial fibrillation. In contrast, IV verapamil effectively slows the ventricular response of both MAT and atrial fibrillation. *We therefore suggest that if you prefer to use large doses of digoxin, be sure the irregularly irregular rhythm is truly atrial fibrillation!*

Figure 19D-1

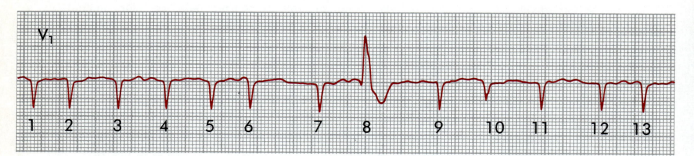

Figure 19D-1. Rhythm strip from **Patient D,** a 60-year-old man presenting with palpitations. Patient D has a history of coronary artery disease. He is not having chest pain and has a blood pressure of 140/90 mm Hg at the time this tracing is recorded. *What is the underlying rhythm? What is beat #8? Are there any other unusual beats in this tracing?*

The rhythm is irregularly irregular. The QRS complex of the underlying rhythm does not appear widened, and P waves are absent. The underlying rhythm is **atrial fibrillation** with a **controlled ventricular response.**

Beat 8 is wider and very different in appearance from the other beats. It has a qR morphology that resembles Figure 19B-4, *H,* and strongly suggests that this beat is a **PVC.**

What about the third question we asked: *Are there any other unusual beats in this tracing?* The simultaneously recorded rhythm strip in Figure 19D-2 answers this question.

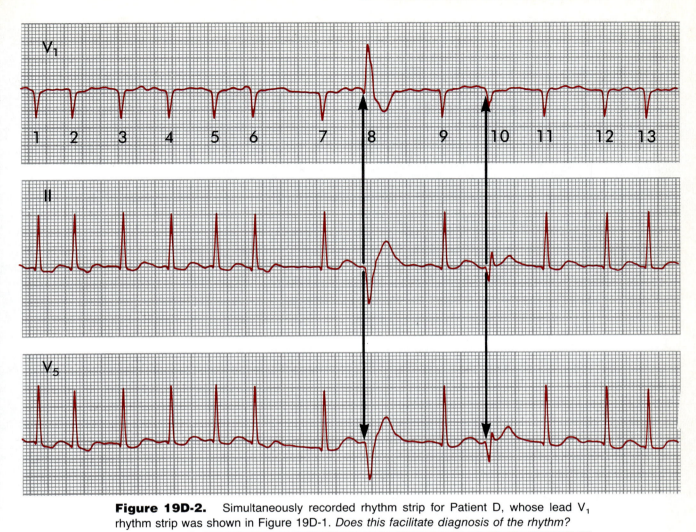

Figure 19D-2. Simultaneously recorded rhythm strip for Patient D, whose lead V$_1$ rhythm strip was shown in Figure 19D-1. *Does this facilitate diagnosis of the rhythm?*

Vertical time lines in Figure 19D-2 show that beat 10 is very different in appearance from the normally conducted beats in leads II and V$_5$. Beat 10 must therefore also be a PVC. Sure, close inspection of beat 10 reveals that it may be slightly wider than the normally conducted beats, and it may begin with a slurring of its downslope, but these are exceedingly subtle changes that might well be due to the normal baseline wander (artifact) of the tracing. *It is virtually impossible (even in retrospect) to tell from lead V$_1$ alone (i.e., from Figure 19D-1) that beat 10 is a PVC.* This is precisely our point! It sometimes is impossible to be certain of the etiology of a beat or a rhythm from only one viewpoint. If accurate interpretation is important clinically, and the patient is hemodynamically stable, **12 leads** (or at the least a second monitoring lead) **will be better than one.**

Figure 19E-1

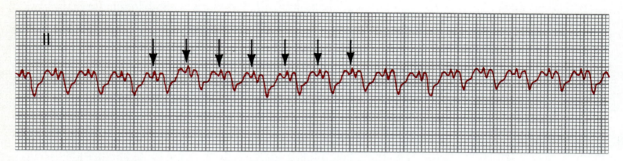

Figure 19E-1.   Rhythm strip from **Patient E,** a 65-year-old woman with a history of prior myocardial infarction. Patient E has a blood pressure of 150/80 mm Hg at the time this tracing is recorded. She is not having chest pain, but is bothered by "palpitations." *Should you treat her sinus tachycardia?*

If by this time you are saying to yourself "help like ours you can do without," you're completely correct. The simultaneously recorded rhythm strip in Figure 19E-2 shows why.

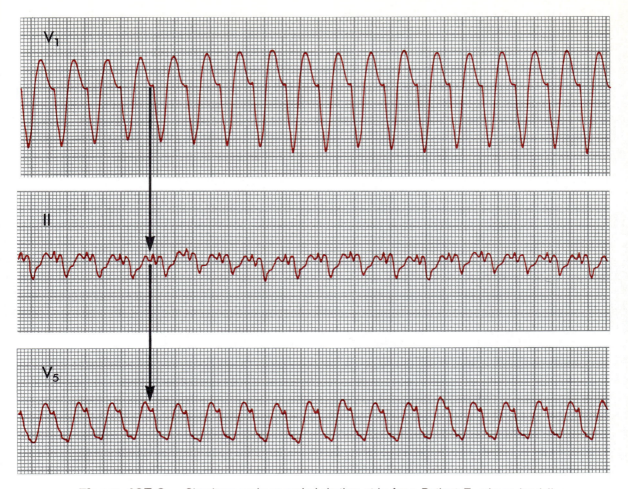

Figure 19E-2.   Simultaneously recorded rhythm strip from Patient E, whose lead II strip was shown in Figure 19E-1. *Does this facilitate diagnosis of the rhythm?*

Despite our "helpful" arrows in Figure 19E-1, this patient is not in sinus tachycardia at all. Vertical time lines show that these "P waves" really form part of the QRS complex. The true QRS complex is markedly widened, and the real rhythm is ***ventricular tachycardia.***

Figure 19E-3 is the 12-lead ECG from Patient E. The diagnosis of ventricular tachycardia is now much more apparent. In particular, QRS morphology in leads V_1 and V_6 strongly suggests a ventricular etiology. The downslope of the QS complex in lead V_1 is definitely delayed (similar to Figure 19B-5, *Q*), and the QRS is predominantly negative in lead V_6 (similar to Figure 19B-5, *U*).

The bizarre QRS morphology makes it difficult to accurately determine the QRS axis in Figure 19E-3. Nevertheless, the QRS complex appears to be predominantly negative in leads aVF and II. This suggests marked LAD and supports the diagnosis of ventricular tachycardia.

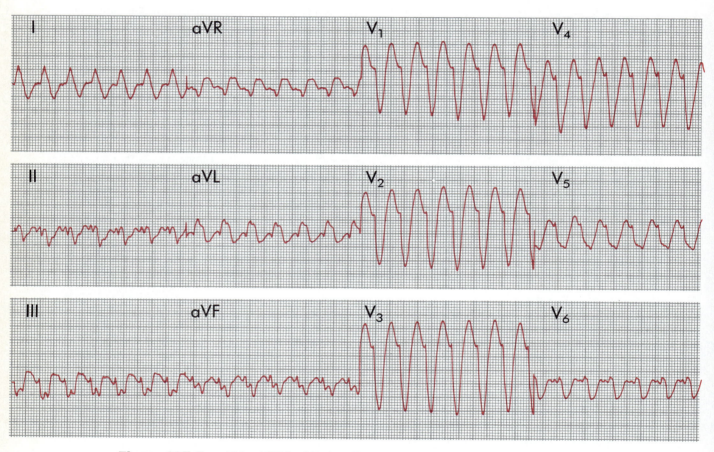

Figure 19E-3.   12-lead ECG of Patient E.

Thus,

all that appears to be "P wave" is not necessarily P wave

and

12 leads are better than one.

Figure 19F-1

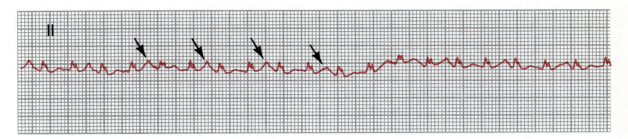

Figure 19F-1.   Rhythm strip from **Patient F,** a 70-year-old man presenting because of a "rapid pulse." He is asymptomatic at the time of this tracing. His blood pressure is 120/80 mm Hg. *What could the rhythm be? How would you proceed?*

The rhythm appears to be regular. Although the QRS complex is somewhat unusual in shape in this lead (it is notched), it does *not* appear to be widened (*greater* than half a large box). Arrows highlight what appear at first glance to be P waves, occurring every other beat.

Once again the key question is: *How would you proceed?* As long as the patient remains stable, obtaining more information (additional leads) should assume high priority. Does the simultaneously recorded rhythm strip shown in Figure 19F-2 help clarify the picture?

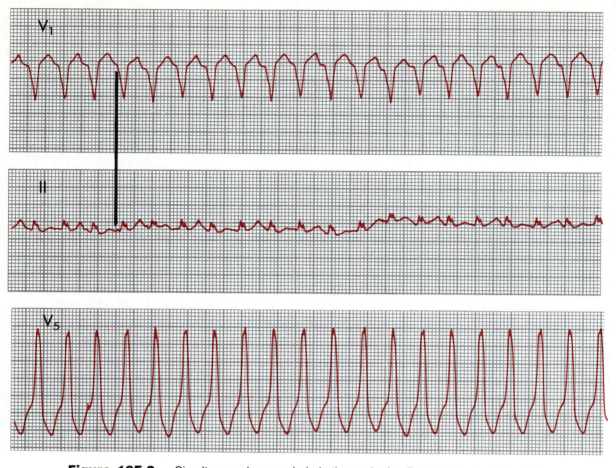

Figure 19F-2. Simultaneously recorded rhythm strip for Patient F, whose lead II rhythm strip was shown in Figure 19F-1. *Does this facilitate diagnosis of the rhythm?*

Although it is still not apparent whether the highlighted upright deflections (marked by arrows) in Figure 19F-1 represent P waves *(or perhaps retrograde atrial activity?)*, what is apparent from the vertical time line is that the QRS complex is really quite wide. This is because a portion of the QRS complex in lead II lies on the baseline. A look at QRS morphology in lead V_1 evokes the picture of Figure 19B-5, *Q,* and strongly suggests that the rhythm is ***ventricular tachycardia.*** This impression is solidified by reviewing the 12-lead ECG of the patient (Figure 19F-3).

Figure 19F-3.   12-lead ECG of Patient F. There is a regular, wide-complex tachycardia. Definite atrial activity is not evident. QRS morphology in lead V_1 strongly suggests ventricular tachycardia.

This example again reinforces the concepts we have tried to demonstrate in this chapter:

12 leads are often a lot better than one.
Evaluation of the rhythm in a single monitoring lead is often not adequate to determine the etiology of a tachycardia.
Upright deflections may for all the world appear to be P waves in one lead, but in reality form part of the QRS complex.
If a portion of the QRS complex lies on the baseline, the QRS may appear deceptively narrow in that monitoring lead.
If the QRS complex is wide (so that you have a wide-complex tachycardia without definite atrial activity), *ventricular tachycardia must be assumed until proven otherwise!*
Hemodynamic status is not a helpful clue to the etiology of a tachycardia.
Assessment of QRS morphology may be an invaluable clue!
Assessment of QRS axis sometimes provides additional information.

Figure 19G-1

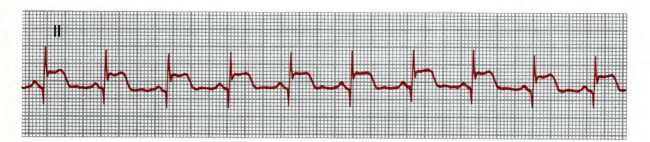

Figure 19G-1.   Rhythm strip from **Patient G,** a 70-year-old woman presenting with a history of new-onset chest pain. The initial 12-lead ECG, obtained 2 hours earlier, was entirely normal. Patient G's chest pain has suddenly increased. Her blood pressure is 140/90 mm Hg. *What is the rhythm? How would you proceed?*

The rhythm is sinus, at a rate of about 85 beats/minute. There is obvious ST segment elevation, as well as a deep (albeit narrow) Q wave. Judging from the above history *(that the initial 12-lead ECG obtained 2 hours earlier was entirely normal),* one would have to be concerned that these findings might be new and reflect development of acute injury/infarction and/or coronary spasm.

Several axioms of telemetry monitoring must be emphasized:

1. Conclusions derived from telemetry monitoring of any one lead about Q wave size, QRS appearance/duration/axis, or ST segment deviations (elevation or depression) *cannot* be relied upon.
2. *Sequential* alterations in Q wave size, QRS appearance/duration/axis, or ST segment deviations in any one lead being *continuously* monitored are more likely to be accurate.
3. The only way to know for sure is to verify the suspicion you have from telemetry monitoring by obtaining a STAT 12-lead ECG!

In the above example, development of ST segment elevation and new Q waves in lead II was real, accompanied by similar changes in the other inferior leads, and reflected acute inferior infarction.

Table 19-1 *(which also appears on pocket reference p. 54)* summarizes the reasons why 12 leads are better than one.

Table 19-1
Reasons Why 12 Leads are Better Than One

Optimizes Evaluation of Atrial Activity

Provides a look at the *KEY LEADS:*
  Lead II
  Lead V_1
  Any of the other 10 leads on the ECG that show P waves

CLINICAL APPLICATION:
  For regular rhythms with a narrow QRS—may allow differentiation between sinus tachycardia, PSVT, and atrial flutter
  For regular rhythms with a wide QRS—may allow differentiation between SVT and ventricular tachycardia
  For irregular rhythms—may allow differentiation between atrial fibrillation, multifocal atrial tachycardia (MAT), and sinus rhythm with multiple PACs

Optimizes Assessment of QRS Morphology

Provides a look at the *KEY LEADS*:*
  Lead V_1 (or MCL_1) and lead V_6 (or MCL_6)

CLINICAL APPLICATION:
  Differentiation of PVCs from aberrantly conducted beats
  Differentiation of ventricular tachycardia from SVT

Allows Determination of QRS Axis

Provides a look at the *KEY LEADS* for axis determination (leads I, II, and aVF)

CLINICAL APPLICATION:
  The finding of either marked RAD or marked LAD strongly suggests ventricular tachycardia.

Allows Verification of Changes Seen in One Lead

CHANGES SEEN/CLINICAL APPLICATION:
  ST segment elevation $\Rightarrow$ Suspect development of acute injury/infarction or coronary spasm
  ST segment depression $\Rightarrow$ Suspect development of ischemia *(silent ischemia?)* or infarction
  A shift in axis $\Rightarrow$ Suspect development of LAHB *(when net QRS deflection in lead II suddenly becomes predominantly negative)*
  A change in QRS morphology $\Rightarrow$ Suspect development of bundle branch block or a change in the site of impulse formation

*Lead II is *not* a useful lead for evaluating QRS morphology!

PRACTICE

Let us conclude this chapter with three final examples illustrating the principle that 12 leads are better than one. Interpret each ECG, paying particular attention to rhythm analysis.

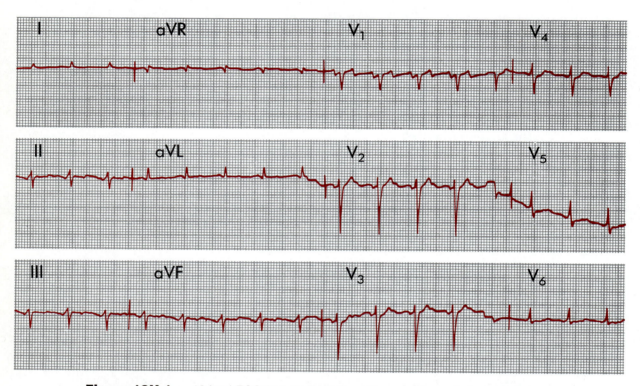

Figure 19H-1.   12-lead ECG from **Patient H,** a 60-year-old man being treated for an arrhythmia with procainamide. *What is the rhythm? Is there anything unusual about the rhythm in this tracing?*

Answer to Figure 19H-1

The rhythm is regular. The ventricular rate is about 110 beats/minute, and the QRS complex appears to be narrow. Normal atrial activity is *not* present, since the P wave is not upright in lead II *(see broken arrow in Figure 19H-2).*

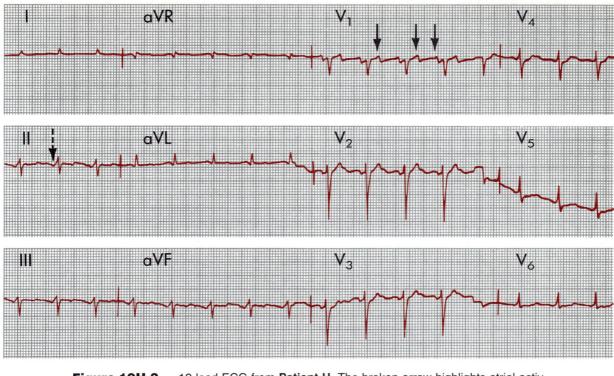

Figure 19H-2. 12-lead ECG from **Patient H.** The broken arrow highlights atrial activity in lead II, while the solid arrow highlights atrial activity in lead V_1.

Close inspection of lead V_1 reveals that there are actually *two* P waves for each QRS complex *(solid arrows in Figure 19H-2)*. Thus, the rhythm is **atrial flutter** with 2:1 AV conduction (atrial rate = 220 beats/minute; ventricular rate = 110 beats/minute). The reason the atrial response is slower than the 250 to 350 beats/minute range one usually expects is that the patient is being treated with procainamide, a type I antiarrhythmic agent with antiarrhythmic properties similar to those of quinidine. Procainamide works by slowing the atrial response of flutter.

Otherwise, the QT interval appears to be normal (at least in lead V_2, which may be the only lead in which one can clearly delineate the end of the T wave). There is LAD (since the net QRS deflection in lead aVF is negative). We estimate the axis to be about $-30°$ because the QRS appears to be isoelectric in lead II. There is no evidence of chamber enlargement (it being exceedingly difficult to evaluate the patient for atrial enlargement, given the rhythm of flutter). There is a small q wave in lead aVL, transition is slightly delayed (occurring between leads V_4 and V_5), and there are nonspecific ST-T wave abnormalities that do not appear acute.

The key to rhythm analysis of this tracing is to recognize that the P wave is not upright in lead II. This rules out a sinus mechanism, and should prompt a search for atrial activity in the remaining leads. It is of interest that flutter waves are apparent in only one lead in this tracing (V_1), emphasizing again how elusive the diagnosis of atrial flutter may sometimes be. The diagnosis is made even more difficult in this particular case because treatment with procainamide decreased the rate of atrial activity below the usual expected range for flutter.

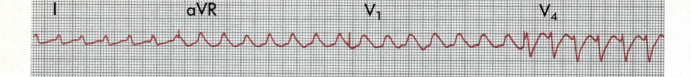

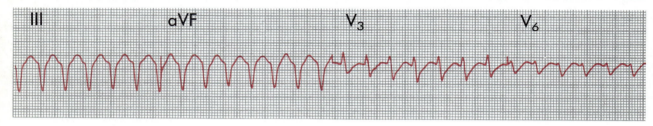

Figure 19I-1.   12-lead ECG from **Patient I,** a 55-year-old man with a history of congestive heart failure. The patient is awake and alert at the time of this tracing. His blood pressure is 150/80 mm Hg. *What is the rhythm? How sure are you of this diagnosis?*

Answer to Figure 19 I-1

The rhythm is regular, at a rate of about 170 beats/minute. The QRS complex is wide. No definite atrial activity is evident. As we have repeatedly emphasized in this chapter *(as in Table 13-2, on pocket reference p. 37),* regardless of the patient's hemodynamic status the differential diagnosis for a regular, wide-complex tachycardia without definite atrial activity should be:

1. Ventricular tachycardia
2. VENTRICULAR TACHYCARDIA
3. **VENTRICULAR TACHYCARDIA**
4. SVT with preexisting bundle branch block
5. SVT with aberrant conduction

Assessment of QRS morphology in lead V_1 is not helpful (since the QRS complex evokes the picture of Figure 19B-4, *D*). However, the predominantly negative QRS complex in lead V_6 (resembling Figure 19B-4, *L*) strongly supports the diagnosis of ventricular tachycardia. This is further supported by the presence of marked LAD (completely negative QRS complex in leads aVF and II).

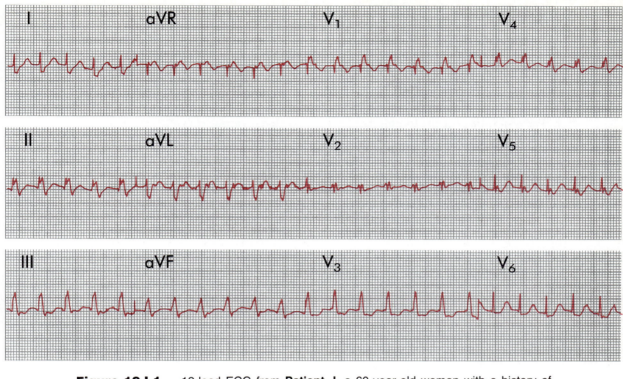

Figure 19J-1.   12-lead ECG from **Patient J,** a 60-year-old woman with a history of renal failure. She is awake and alert at the time of this tracing. Her blood pressure is 130/80 mm Hg. *What is the rhythm? How sure are you of this diagnosis?*

Answer to Figure 19J-1

The rhythm is regular, at a rate just over 150 beats/minute. The QRS complex is wide. Normal atrial activity is absent in lead II, ruling out sinus tachycardia. Thus, we are once again confronted with a regular, wide-complex tachycardia without normal atrial activity. The same differential diagnostic precaution considered in the previous example—*to assume ventricular tachycardia until proven otherwise*—again holds true. However, evaluation of QRS morphology in the key leads (I, V_1, and V_6) suggests that the rhythm may not be ventricular tachycardia. That is, the rSR' in lead V_1 evokes the picture of Figure 19B-4, *A,* and the RS and qRS in leads I and V_6 evoke the picture of Figure 19B-4, *J* and *I.* This suggests a typical RBBB pattern and a supraventricular etiology for the rhythm.

Although accurate determination of the QRS axis is difficult in this example, there does not appear to be either marked RAD or marked LAD. This further supports a supraventricular etiology for the arrhythmia.

In point of fact, the Patient was in PSVT. Subtle notching on the tail end of the QRS complex in lead V_1, and the terminal negative deflection in the inferior leads, represented retrograde atrial activity. Comparison with prior tracings confirmed the long-term presence of complete RBBB. IV verapamil was well tolerated, and rapidly converted the patient to sinus rhythm.

If prior tracings from Patient J were not available, *there would be absolutely NO WAY to be certain from inspection of Figure 19J-1 alone that the rhythm was PSVT with RBBB!!!* All one could say was that the patient was hemodynamically stable and in a regular, wide-complex tachycardia without normal atrial activity, and with morphologic characteristics suggestive of a supraventricular etiology.

We feel it important to emphasize that clinical evaluation of the 12-lead ECG can go only so far. Sometimes, no matter how sophisticated the interpreter, it will NOT be possible to determine the rhythm with certainty. Nevertheless, application of the principles presented in this chapter should greatly narrow the differential diagnosis and minimize the number of times when a solid hunch will not be forthcoming.

20

What Can We Learn From Comparison Tracings?

Imagine a world without comparison. There would be no big or small, no dark or light, no old or new. So it would be with electrocardiography. ECGs would have little (or no) meaning if we couldn't compare. The purpose of this chapter is to emphasize this essential role of comparison in electrocardiography.

Interpret the ECG shown in Figure 20A-1, taken from Patient A, a 52-year-old woman presenting with atypical chest pain of several days' duration. *Are the changes significant? Are they new? Does Patient A need to be admitted to the hospital?*

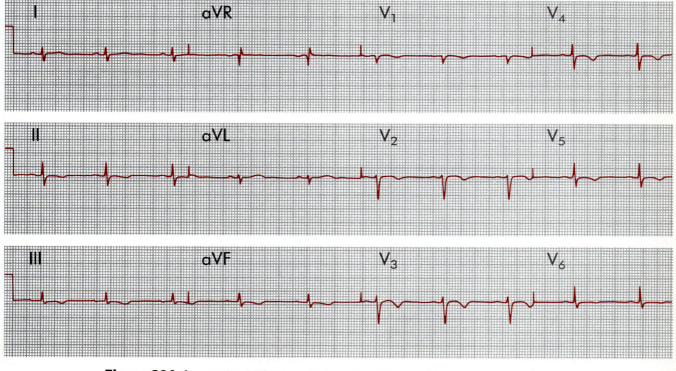

Figure 20A-1.   12-lead ECG from **Patient A,** a 52-year-old woman with atypical chest pain.

Interpretation of Figure 20A-1

Descriptive analysis. There is a regular sinus rhythm, at a rate of about 65 beats/minute. All intervals are normal. The axis is normal and approximately $+90°$ (since the QRS complex appears to be isoelectric in lead I). There is no evidence of chamber enlargement, although several findings consistent with pulmonary disease are present (relatively low voltage, S waves in leads I, II, III, and V_1 through V_6). Q waves are absent, R wave progression is normal (with transition between leads V_3 and V_4), ST segments are ever so slightly coved but not elevated, and T waves are shallow but symmetrically inverted in the inferior and precordial leads.

Clinical impression. The key to the clinical impression lies in answering the questions we posed:

1. *Are the changes significant?*
2. *Are they new?*
3. What should be done clinically? *(i.e., does Patient A need to be admitted to the hospital?)*

The ST segment and T wave changes in Figure 20A-1 definitely could be significant. That is, the shape of the ST segment (particularly in leads III and V_2 to V_5) is coved and could represent a recent injury pattern. Moreover, the T wave inversion is symmetric, and may well represent ischemia. Admittedly, none of these changes are overly impressive; there is no ST segment elevation and the amplitude of the T wave inversion is small. *Nevertheless, they may still reflect acute ischemic heart disease.*

Are the changes new? **How can you tell???** The only way to tell if these electrocardiographic changes are new would be to compare the ECG shown in Figure 20A-1 with a previous tracing. Imagine the following two scenarios:

Scenario # 1: A previous ECG is found and is totally normal.
Scenario # 2: A previous ECG is found and looks identical to the one shown in Figure 20A-1.

If the previous ECG was entirely normal **(Scenario # 1),** the changes seen in Figure 20A-1 would have to be new *(or at least new since the prior ECG was taken).* Despite the minimally impressive history (of atypical chest pain of several days' duration), the wisest course of action would be to admit the patient to the hospital (at least to a telemetry unit) until the clinical picture could be clarified (and infarction ruled out).

On the other hand, one might not necessarily admit Patient A to the hospital if a prior ECG with identical changes was found **(Scenario # 2).** This would imply that the findings in Figure 20A-1 were old. Outpatient management might be appropriate if the physical exam was normal and the history not suggestive of acute ischemic chest pain.

Unfortunately, if no prior (comparison) tracing is available, there would be no way to tell if the ST segment and T wave changes in Figure 20A-1 are new or not. One would have to assume that the changes were new, making it difficult not to admit the patient, even in the absence of a convincing history.

How to Compare ECGs

The technique of ECG comparison is easy. All one does is:

1. Interpret the *earlier* (older) tracing first.
2. Carefully compare each lead in the earlier tracing with the corresponding lead in the newer (more recent) tracing.
3. Comment on any differences.
4. Indicate whether such differences are likely to be clinically significant (or whether they are more likely to be due to positional or lead placement changes).

The technique of comparing newer tracings with older ones is valid regardless of how long ago a prior tracing was obtained. Obviously, the more recent the prior tracing, the better one is able to "date" any changes that are present. Yet the availability of prior tracings may prove invaluable even if they were obtained many years earlier.

The rest this chapter consists of practice in ECG comparison.

•   •   •

The ECG shown in Figure 20B-1 was taken from Patient B, a 69-year-old woman admitted a day earlier for severe pressure sores. The patient developed a syncopal episode at physical therapy. She was alert and hemodynamically stable at the time this ECG was recorded. There was absolutely no history of chest pain. Interpret the ECG.

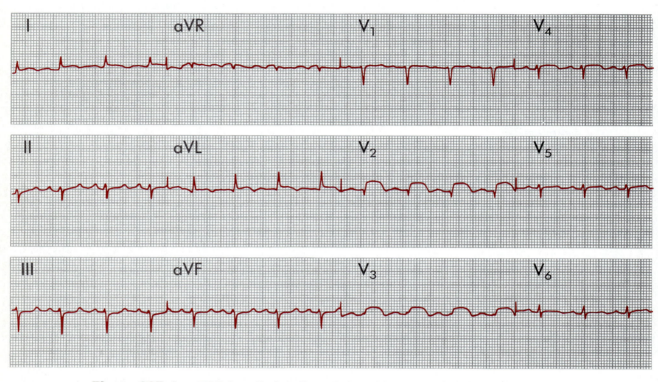

Figure 20B-1.   ECG from **Patient B,** a 69-year-old woman admitted a day earlier for pressure sores. The patient had just experienced a syncopal episode. She was alert, hemodynamically stable, and asymptomatic at the time this tracing was recorded.

Interpretation of Figure 20B-1

Descriptive analysis. The rhythm is sinus, at a rate just under 100 beats/minute. The PR and QRS intervals appear to be normal. Despite the relatively rapid rate (of almost 100 beats/minute), the QT interval looks long (i.e., definitely *more* than half the R-R interval in lead V_2). There is pathologic LAD (LAHB), since the net QRS deflection in lead II is more negative than positive. There is no evidence of chamber enlargement.

However, the most remarkable findings on this tracing reside with QRST analysis. There is a small q wave in lead aVL and a large Q in lead V_2. Transition is delayed (occurring between leads V_5 and V_6), and there is actually loss of the tiny r wave in lead V_1 by lead V_2. Coved ("frowny") ST segment elevation is present in the anterolateral leads, being most marked in leads V_2 and V_3. Beginning T wave inversion is seen in many of these leads.

Clinical impression. Despite the absence of chest pain, this ECG is highly suggestive of *acute anterolateral infarction*. This (and/or an associated arrhythmia) may well be the cause of Patient B's syncopal episode.

•   •   •

Review of patient B's old records reveals that a prior ECG had been obtained approximately 1 year earlier (Figure 20B-2).

Interpret this prior ECG. Compare it with Figure 20B-1. *Does comparison of the two tracings confirm your clinical impression of Figure 20B-1?*

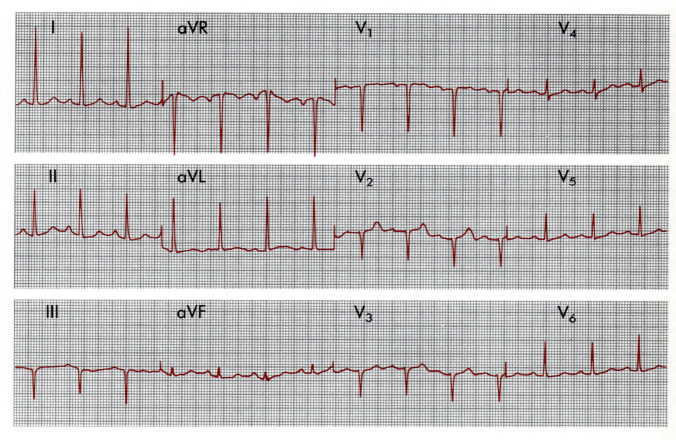

Figure 20B-2.   Prior (comparison) ECG recorded from Patient B one year before the ECG shown in Figure 20B-1.

Interpretation of Figure 20B-2

Descriptive analysis. There is a regular sinus rhythm at a rate of about 85 beats/minute. All intervals are normal. The axis is normal, and probably between $+5°$ and $+20°$ (since the QRS complex in lead I is so much more positive than it is in lead aVF). Voltage criteria for LVH are easily satisfied in lead aVL (where the R wave greatly exceeds 12 mm). There is a QS complex (of unknown significance) in leads III and V_1. A small (but definite) r wave is present in lead V_2, and transition occurs normally between leads V_3 and V_4. There is ST segment flattening and slight ST segment depression in several leads.

Clinical impression: comparison with Figure 20B-1. Considering the patient's age (69 years), the tremendously increased amplitude of the R wave in lead aVL (which measures about 19 mm), and the ST segment and T wave flattening in lateral leads I and aVL (which resembles the "strain equivalent" pattern that we introduced in Figure 9-4, C [on pocket reference p. 23]), it is extremely likely that the patient has LVH.

Otherwise, the ST-T wave changes in Figure 20B-2 are "nonspecific" (i.e., not acute).

Comparison of the two tracings confirms that the coved ST segment elevation and beginning T wave inversion in Figure 20B-1 are acute. But these are *not* the only changes:

What has happened to the axis?
And what has happened to the R wave amplitude in the lateral leads?

Answer: The mean QRS axis in the more recent tracing (Figure 20B-1) has shifted significantly to the left (i.e., LAHB has developed). Note also that R wave amplitude has dramatically decreased in all of the lateral leads (I, aVL, and V_4 to V_6). This may reflect the acute lateral infarction (which causes a loss of lateral forces).

• • •

The ECG shown in Figure 20B-3 was recorded the next day (one day *after* the ECG shown in Figure 20B-1). Interpret Figure 20B-3. *How is it different from Figure 20B-1?*

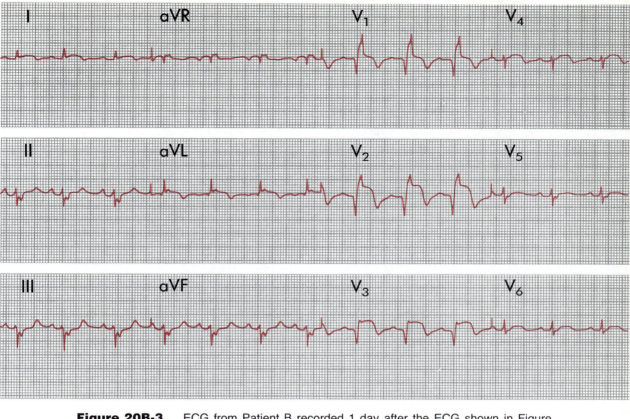

Figure 20B-3. ECG from Patient B recorded 1 day after the ECG shown in Figure 20B-1. The patient remains asymptomatic and hemodynamically stable.

Interpretation of Figure 20B-3/Comparison with Figure 20B-1

Descriptive analysis. Again there is fairly a regular sinus rhythm (at about 75 beats/minute). The QRS complex has now become widened. The QR complex in lead V_1 suggests development of complete RBBB as the cause of QRS widening (although strict criteria for RBBB—wide terminal S waves in leads I and V_6—are lacking). The QT interval is definitely prolonged (in this case as a result of both infarction and the conduction defect). Pathologic LAD (LAHB) is present. There is no evidence of chamber enlargement. Deep, wide Q waves have developed in the anterior leads (V_1 to V_3). The coved ST segment elevation and T wave inversion have become more marked, especially in the anterior precordial leads.

Clinical impression. Interpretation of Figure 20B-3 compared with Figure 20B-1 suggests *ongoing evolution of acute anterolateral infarction*. Bifascicular block may be developing (although, as noted, strict criteria for RBBB are not yet met). In any case, the picture is definitely one of concern, and the patient merits continued close observation in the intensive care unit (despite her absence of symptoms).

The ECG shown in Figure 20C-1 is from Patient C, a 65-year-old woman with a history of coronary artery disease and a known conduction defect. She was having severe chest pain at the time this tracing was taken. How would you interpret Figure 20C-1? *What type of conduction defect does Patient C have? Would you admit her to the hospital?*

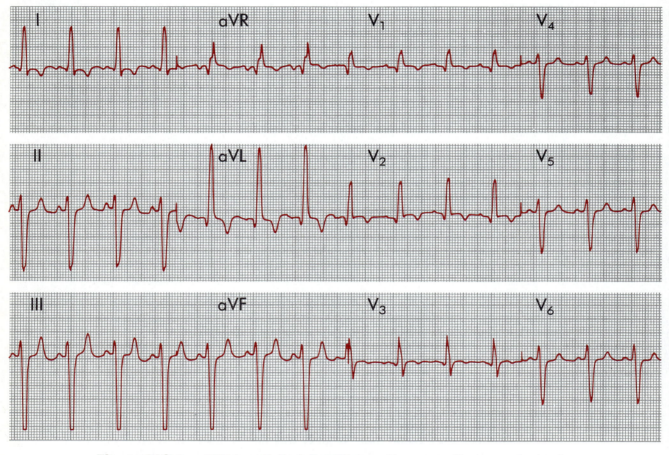

Figure 20C-1.   ECG from **Patient C**, a 65-year-old woman with severe chest pain. What type of conduction defect does she have? Should the patient be admitted to the hospital?

Interpretation of Figure 20C-1

Descriptive analysis. There is a regular sinus rhythm at a rate of about 85 beats/minute. The PR interval is normal. The QRS interval is prolonged.

Examination of the three key leads (I, V_1, and V_6) suggests complete RBBB as the reason for QRS widening—QR (or "RBBB-equivalent") pattern in lead V_1 (*Figure 5-13, on pocket reference p. 14*) and S waves in lateral leads I and V_6 (albeit the S wave in lead I is fairly small and narrow).

Question: Are there *typical* secondary ST segment and T wave changes of RBBB?

Answer: No. As discussed in Figure 5-9 *(on pocket reference p. 15)*, orientation of the ST segment and T wave with typical RBBB or LBBB should be *OPPOSITE* the last QRS deflection in each of the key leads. This is definitely not the case in Figure 20C-1. Although the T wave is upright (as it should be) in lead V_6, it is symmetrically inverted in lead I. The T wave in lead V_1 is inverted (as it should be), but the ST segment appears to be coved and slightly elevated. A look at neighboring leads V_2 and V_3 tells why—each has a Q wave, ST segment coving, and T wave inversion. Thus, in addition to RBBB, there is also evidence of ischemia (anterolateral T wave inversion) and anterior infarction (Q waves in leads V_1 to V_3 with associated ST segment coving) that may be acute.

Now that we've established the reason for QRS widening in Figure 20C-1, we can complete our systematic **Descriptive Analysis:**

The QT interval appears to be prolonged (*greater* than half the R-R interval), but this is probably due to the conduction defect. There is pathologic LAD (LAHB), since the QRS complex is decidedly more negative than positive in lead II. (We estimate the mean QRS axis to be more negative than $-60°$.) Voltage criteria for LVH are easily satisfied in lead aVL, and T wave inversion in this lead probably reflects "strain" and/or ischemia.

Clinical impression. This is *NOT* a simple tracing to interpret! If you recognized that the patient has LVH, LAHB, and a very unusual type of RBBB, you're doing well. If you also suspected ischemia (from the inappropriate T wave inversion in lead I) and possible acute infarction (from the Q waves and ST segment changes in leads V_1 to V_3), you're doing great!!!

What one piece of information would be most helpful in determining whether the potentially worrisome findings in Figure 20C-1 are truly acute?

Answer: A prior ECG.

It turns out that an ECG obtained several months earlier, at the time of Patient C's last hospitalization, shows changes virtually identical to those in Figure 20C-1. What can you conclude?

Answer: The fact that there has not been any interim change means that there is no electrocardiographic evidence of new ischemia or acute infarction.

• • •

Because of Patient C's previous history (of documented coronary artery disease) and the nature of her symptoms (severe chest pain), she is admitted to the hospital. Figure 20C-2 shows a follow-up ECG obtained the next day. What has happened? What is this likely to mean?

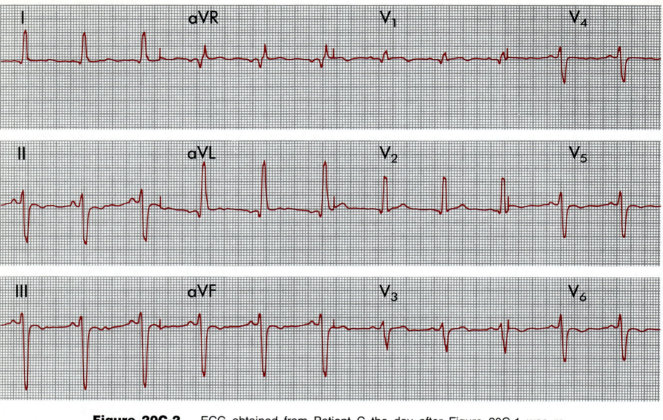

Figure 20C-2.   ECG obtained from Patient C the day after Figure 20C-1 was recorded.

Answer: Lead-to-lead comparison of Figure 20C-2 with 20C-1 reveals the following:

Leads I and aVL: no longer show T wave inversion

Leads II, III, and aVF: now show symmetric (albeit shallow) T wave inversion

Lead V_1: may now show slightly more ST segment elevation

Leads V_2 and V_3: no longer show T wave inversion

Leads V_4, V_5, and V_6: now show either ST segment flattening or T wave inversion (instead of an upright T wave)

Because of this patient's complicated previous history and complex ECG, it would be extremely difficult to interpret the ECG shown in Figure 20C-2 by itself. However, our lead-to-lead comparison shows a marked change from the tracing obtained just 1 day earlier, when the patient was having severe chest pain. In this context, it becomes extremely likely that the changes seen in Figure 20C-2 reflect new ischemia (and/or possible acute infarction)!

We emphasize again that our purpose in presenting Figures 20C-1 and 20C-2 has not been to expound on all of the subtleties contained within these tracings. Instead, our principal goal has been to illustrate how effective lead-to-lead comparison can be in demonstrating that electrocardiographic changes have occurred.

• • •

We conclude this chapter on the role of comparison with a series of ECGs taken from Patient D, a 45-year-old man presenting with new-onset severe chest pain. Symptoms began approximately 4 hours before the ECG shown in Figure 20D-1 was obtained. The patient had previously been completely healthy, and was not on any medications. No prior tracing is available. How would you interpret the ECG shown in Figure 20D-1? Is the patient a candidate for reperfusion therapy? An optimal candidate?

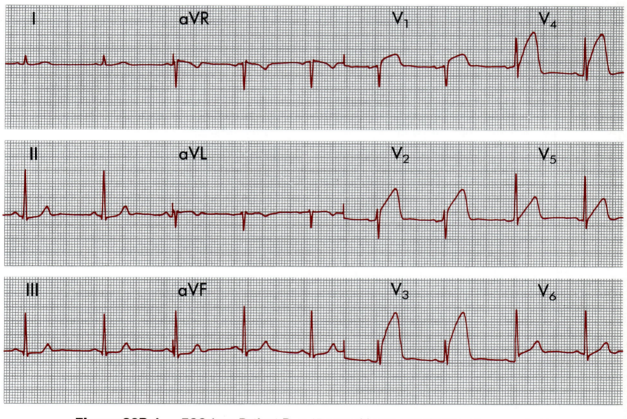

Figure 20D-1.   ECG from **Patient D,** a 45-year-old man complaining of severe chest pain that had begun 4 hours earlier. *Is the patient a candidate for reperfusion therapy? An optimal candidate?*

Interpretation of Figure 20D-1

Descriptive analysis. There is sinus arrhythmia. All intervals are normal. The axis is normal (and approximately $+75°$). There is no evidence of chamber enlargement.

Small q waves are present in the inferior leads. R wave progression is normal, with transition occurring between leads V_2 and V_3. There is coved ("frowny") ST segment elevation in leads V_1 through V_5 (which is almost "tombstone" in appearance in leads V_3 and V_4). Finally, there is ever so slight reciprocal ST segment depression in the inferior leads.

Clinical impression. Assuming that the changes in Figure 20D-1 do not represent coronary (Prinzmetal's) spasm, it is exceedingly likely that the acute injury current in Figure 20D-1 would evolve into a large anterior infarction.

Patient D is *definitely* a candidate for acute reperfusion therapy because he satisfies all of the criteria listed in Table 12-3 *(on pocket reference p. 35):*

1. He is young (45 years old).
2. The history is consistent with new-onset ischemic chest pain beginning within the "window of opportunity" (i.e., less than 6 hours ago)
3. There is definite ECG evidence of acute infarction.
4. There are no contraindications to thrombolytic therapy.

According to Table 12-4 *(on pocket reference p. 36),* Patient D is a good (but not optimal) candidate for thrombolytic therapy. Initial electrocardiographic findings are consistent with a large, potentially reversible infarction in progress (i.e., anterior location, marked ST segment elevation, absent Q waves). Unfortunately, because of the patient's own tardiness *(he waited at home for 4 hours before coming to the hospital!),* optimal benefit from thrombolytic therapy is unlikely to be achieved.

• • •

The patient's blood pressure remains stable. There is no clinical evidence of heart failure. As preparations are made to administer thrombolytic therapy, Patient D is treated with oxygen, aspirin, IV nitroglycerin, morphine sulfate, IV β-blockers, and prophylactic lidocaine. Despite these measures, chest pain persists. A change in the appearance of the QRS complex on telemetry prompts the order for a repeat ECG (Figure 20D-2). *What has happened?*

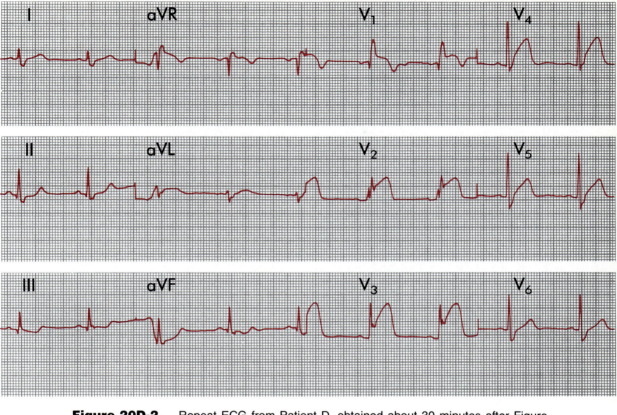

Figure 20D-2.   Repeat ECG from Patient D, obtained about 30 minutes after Figure 20D-1. The patient continues to have chest pain. *What has happened?*

Comparison of Figure 20D-2 with Figure 20D-1

There is a regular sinus rhythm at a rate of about 60 beats/minute. The QRS complex has widened. Inspection of the three key leads reveals a QR pattern in lead V_1, and wide, terminal S waves in leads I and V_6, indicating that the patient has developed *complete RBBB*. Otherwise, there has not really been any acute change.

• • •

Thrombolytic therapy is begun. One hour into the infusion, the ECG shown in Figure 20D-3 is obtained. How does this compare with Figure 20D-2?

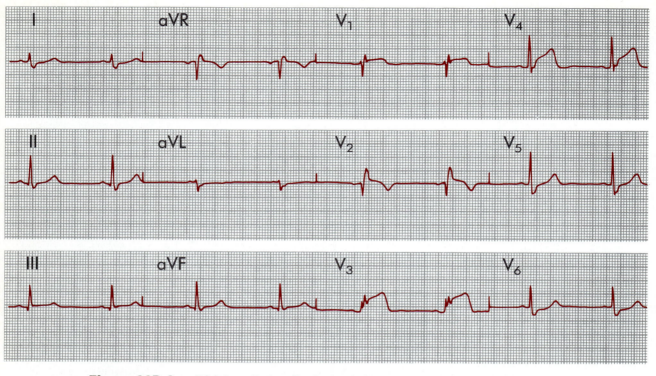

Figure 20D-3.   ECG from Patient D, obtained about 1 hour after Figure 20D-2. Chest pain is much less, but still present. *How would you interpret this tracing?*

Interpretation of Figure 20D-3/Comparison with Figure 20D-2

There is sinus bradycardia at a rate of about 50 beats/minute. The QRS complex remains widened with an RBBB pattern.

Lead-to-lead comparison with Figure 20D-2 suggests that the anterior precordial ST segment elevation is returning to the baseline. The pattern (sequence of tracings) is consistent with *acute, evolving anterior infarction.*

Note that when one interprets a sequence of ECGs from the same patient, it is not necessarily essential to describe each finding on each tracing! Doing so would be not only tedious but also inefficient. This is because there will almost always be minor changes in heart rate, axis, and QRST appearance that either defy description or are simply due to the fact that an ECG is being repeated at another instant in time and under slightly different conditions.

What is essential is that the interpreter systematically inspect and compare each lead in each tracing. One need only comment on changes that are likely to be clinically significant. Thus, in the case of acute infarction in progress, one may sometimes be able to summarize changes on sequential tracings as being consistent with *acute, evolving infarction* (as we have done for Figure 20D-3).

Shortly after the thrombolytic therapy is complete, the patient notes that his chest pain has disappeared. Another 12-lead ECG is recorded (Figure 20D-4). *What has happened?*

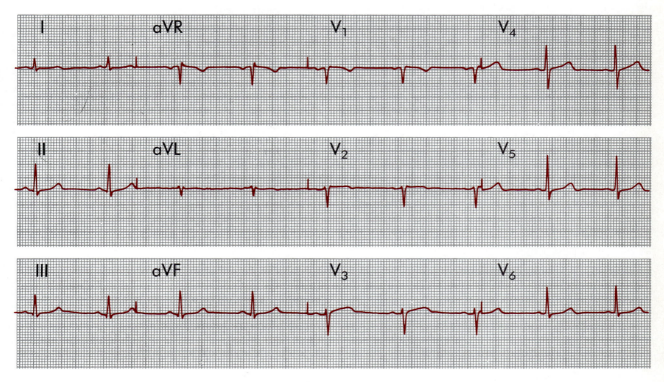

Figure 20D-4.   Repeat ECG from Patient D after completion of thrombolytic therapy. His chest pain has disappeared. *What has happened?*

Interpretation of Figure 20D-4/Comparison with Figure 20D-3

There is still sinus bradycardia (now at a rate of about 55 beats/minute). The QRS complex has narrowed!

Lead-to-lead comparison with Figure 20D-3 shows that all there is left from the complete RBBB is the trace of an s wave in leads I and V_6. In addition, ST segment and T wave changes seen on prior tracings have virtually normalized! Finally, except for the QS complex in lead V_1, anterior Q waves did not develop!

Three bedside parameters have been used clinically to suggest that thrombolytic therapy has successfully reperfused an infarct-related artery (Table 20-1):

Table 20-1
Bedside Parameters Suggesting Successful Reperfusion with Thrombolytic Therapy
1. Complete relief of chest pain 2. Resolution of acute ECG changes 3. Development of reperfusion arrhythmias

Patient D did develop frequent PVCs and AIVR during administration of thrombolytic therapy. These are the most common reperfusion arrhythmias seen. Considered in the context of the series of tracings we presented (Figures 20D-1 through 20D-4), and in light of the disappearance of his chest pain with completion of thrombolytic therapy, it is likely that Patient D ended up with a much smaller infarction than he would have had if he had not received this treatment.

Does the Computer Know Better?

Hospital use of computerized ECG analysis systems has increased tremendously in recent years. If the present trend continues, it is likely that the overwhelming majority of hospital-obtained ECGs will soon be accompanied automatically by a computer analysis of each tracing. Is this good? Does the computer know better? Or is the ever-increasing prevalence of computerized ECG analysis systems a potentially dangerous trend?

The answer to the first and third questions is yes. Computerized ECG analysis systems can be extremely helpful to medical care providers. However, if blind faith is placed in the computer report, the potential is there for them to do more harm than good. Thus, the answer to the second question must be a qualified one—the computer *may* know better under *certain* circumstances. The trick is knowing when and how the computer should be used.

The goal of this chapter is to emphasize the benefits and drawbacks of computerized ECG analysis systems. Many types of systems flood the market. Rather than focus on specific differences between the different brands of these devices, we'll limit our comments to general principles applicable to most of the currently available models.

BENEFITS AND DRAWBACKS OF COMPUTERIZED SYSTEMS

The most important point to stress about computerized ECG analysis systems is that they are not infallible. *Computerized systems are only as good as the information they are programmed with.* How helpful a particular system is depends directly on the user's appreciation of this fact.

Computerized ECG analysis systems are most accurate in computing values. This is logical, since computation is the forte of computers. Thus, computerized systems are usually extremely accurate in calculating heart rate, intervals (PR, QRS, and QT), and axis. Beginning interpreters can profit from knowing this by using the immediate feedback provided by the computer report to check their calculation of heart rate and axis.

In general, computerized ECG analysis systems are also reliable in recognizing normal sinus rhythm and normal tracings. As a result, they may be of tremendous assistance in saving the experienced interpreter time, especially if he or she is asked to interpret a large number of tracings from a generally healthy population.

Computerized systems do not fare as well with abnormal tracings (especially when complex abnormalities are present). In general, they are much less reliable in interpreting rhythms that do not have a sinus mechanism. They sometimes miss subtle infarctions. Equally disturbing is the fact that they may overinterpret early repolarization patterns and mislabel these normal variants as suggestive of acute infarction. Other drawbacks are that pacemaker spikes and WPW are not always picked up, and that most systems are not programmed to interpret pediatric tracings. Finally, comparison with prior tracings and correlation of an ECG with clinical history are rarely possible.

What then is the great attraction of computerized ECG analysis systems? We feel that the most important asset of these systems lies in their ability to provide a second opinion. They may suggest findings not initially thought of by the beginning interpreter. They may also suggest findings initially overlooked by the expert in a hurry.

We have listed these along with other potential benefits of computerized ECG analysis systems in Table 21-1. Note that benefits vary depending on the experience of the interpreter.

Table 21-1

Potential Benefits of Computerized ECG Analysis Systems

For the Expert/Experienced Interpreter

Saves time
Provides backup opinion that may help prevent the expert in a hurry from overlooking any findings

For Less Experienced Interpreters

Provides a second opinion
May suggest additional findings not initially thought of
Encourages more careful, targeted review of the tracing
Computer feedback may help educationally

For ALL Interpreters

Usually provides accurate calculation of heart rate, intervals, and mean QRS axis
Generally reliable reporting of normal tracings

The KEY for the less experienced electrocardiographer is to WRITE OUT an interpretation BEFORE looking at the computer analysis!

USE OF COMPUTERIZED SYSTEMS BY EXPERT INTERPRETERS

Realistically speaking, expert interpreters are unlikely to be taught by a computer report. Thus, for interpretation of any given tracing, the accuracy of an expert electrocardiographer will virtually always equal or surpass that of the computer analysis. However, in actual practice, experts are often called on to interpret a large number of tracings in a limited period of time. Under these circumstances, even the experts occasionally overlook potentially important findings. The extra opinion provided by the computer report may act as a backup to prevent this from happening.

Time saving may be an even more important practical benefit that computerized systems offer the experts. Instead of having to write out each finding, it suffices to place a check mark next to each computer statement that the expert agrees with. For example, imagine that the computer reported the following:

> Normal sinus rhythm. Heart rate = 75/minute.
>   PR interval = 0.18 seconds.
>   QRS interval = 0.09 seconds.
>   QTc = 0.40 seconds *(which is normal)*.
> Voltage for LVH.
> Otherwise normal ECG.

If you as the expert interpreter completely agreed with the computer, you would have no more to do than to check each computer statement, indicate your agreement, and sign your name:

> √Normal sinus rhythm. Heart rate = 75/minute.
>   √PR interval = 0.18 seconds.
>   √QRS interval = 0.09 seconds.
>   √QTc = 0.40 seconds *(which is normal)*.
> √Voltage for LVH.
> √Otherwise normal ECG.

Agree   *Ken Grauer*

If you agreed with everything except the statement about LVH, you could cross out this statement and indicate your *amended* agreement as follows:

> √Normal sinus rhythm. Heart rate = 75/minute.
>   √PR interval = 0.18 seconds.
>   √QRS interval = 0.09 seconds.
>   √QTc = 0.40 seconds (which is normal).
>   ~~Voltage for LVH.~~
> √Otherwise normal ECG.

Agree as corrected   *Ken Grauer*

In either case, considerable time would be saved because you would not have to hand write out each of your findings. Time might also be saved because the expert would not have to personally calculate values already determined by the computer. Little more than a glance would be needed to confirm that the rhythm is sinus, and that heart rate, intervals, and axis are all normal.

Overall, we estimate that familiarity with the computer system we use has cut the time it takes us to render an ECG interpretation by more than half. Obviously, the more abnormal and unusual the tracings are in the population you work with, the less impact this timesaving feature will have.

USE OF COMPUTERIZED SYSTEMS BY LESS EXPERIENCED INTERPRETERS

Saving time is much less of a concern among nonexpert interpreters (who are rarely called on to interpret more than a few tracings at any one time). For such individuals, improved accuracy of interpretation is a much more important consideration. We feel that the best way for the nonexpert to use the computer is to first *WRITE OUT* his or her interpretation without looking at the computer report. Doing so forces him or her to commit to an interpretation without being biased by the computer. The computer analysis can then be used as it was intended—to provide a backup (second) opinion that may also be informative and educational to the interpreting clinician.

If the computer comments on a finding you didn't list, ask yourself why. Is the computer correct? Did you overlook the finding? Or is the computer in error? In either case, analysis of the discrepancy between your interpretation and the computer report will have encouraged a much more targeted and productive review of the ECG, with improved accuracy as the end result.

CONCLUSION

We acknowledge that the issue of the utility of computerized ECG analysis systems remains controversial. Personally, we feel the benefits of these systems far outweigh their drawbacks, provided the user appreciates that computer systems are only as good as the information they are programmed with. The systems are not infallible. They are most helpful in calculating values and recognizing normal tracings. They may save experienced users a tremendous amount of time. The second opinion they provide may improve accuracy of interpretation, especially for less experienced electrocardiographers. However, computer statements should *never* be accepted at face value without first confirming accuracy by personal inspection of the tracing.

REFERENCES

Grauer K: Optimal use of computerized electrocardiogram interpretations, Phys Market Place 23:2, 1989.

Grauer K, Kravitz L, Ariet M, Curry RW, Nelson WP, and Marriott HJL: Potential benefits of a computer ECG interpretation system for primary care physicians in a community hospital, J Am Bd Fam Pract 1:17, 1989.

Grauer K, Kravitz L, Curry RW, and Ariet M: Computerized electrocardiogram interpretations: are they useful for the family physician? J Fam Pract 24:39, 1987.

Basic Review Tracings

It's time to apply what we've learned. Interpret the 20 tracings in this chapter according to the systematic approach. For each ECG, indicate the following parameters in your **descriptive analysis:** **R**ate, **R**hythm (and Intervals), **A**xis, **H**ypertrophy (= chamber enlargement), and **I**nfarct (= QRST changes), as suggested on pocket reference pp. 1 to 4. Then formulate your **clinical impression,** taking into account the information provided in the capsule summary below each tracing. *You will benefit most from this exercise by WRITING OUT your interpretation of each ECG BEFORE looking at our responses!*

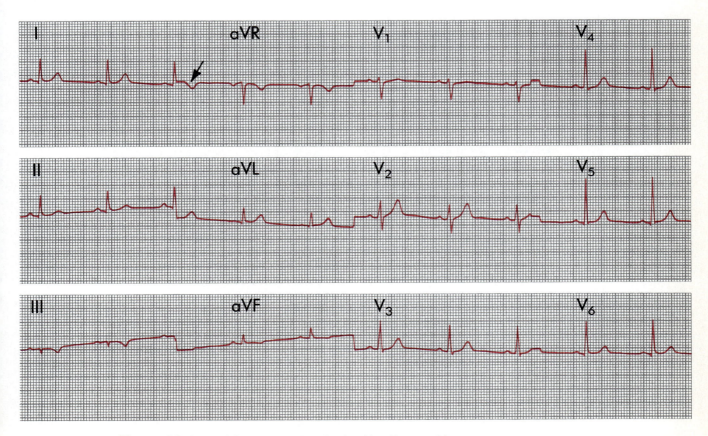

Figure 22-1. ECG from an otherwise healthy 40-year-old man.

Interpretation of Figure 22-1

Descriptive analysis. There is regular sinus rhythm, at a rate of about 65 beats/minute. All intervals are normal. The axis is normal (and approximately 20°). There is no evidence of chamber enlargement. There is a QS complex in lead III (and tiny septal q waves in several other leads). Transition is early (occurring between leads V_1 and V_2). The T wave is inverted in lead III and flat in lead aVF.

Clinical impression. This is a normal ECG.

Questions to Further Understanding

1. *Which leads may normally demonstrate Q waves?*

   Answer: Leads III, aVF, aVL, and V_1 may all normally demonstrate moderate- to large-sized Q waves as an isolated finding (*see Table 10-3,* on pocket reference p. 27). Thus the QS complex in lead III of Figure 22-1 should *not* be cause for alarm. In this otherwise healthy 40-year-old man, it is almost certainly a normal variant.

2. *Which leads may normally demonstrate T wave inversion?*

   Answer: The same leads that may normally demonstrate Q waves may also normally demonstrate T wave inversion (*Table 10-6, on pocket reference p. 28). Remember that the direction of T waves often tends to follow the direction of the QRS complex.* Thus, the fact that the QRS complex in lead III is negative in Figure 22-1 makes it even more likely that the T wave inversion in this lead reflects a normal variant rather than ischemia.

   The QRS complex and T wave in lead aVR are almost always negative. **For practical purposes, we can almost always ignore lead aVR in our interpretation process** (unless we are considering lead misplacement)!

3. *Why is the T wave of the third QRS complex in lead I inverted (arrow in Figure 22-1)?*

   Answer: It's not. Three QRS complexes appear in simultaneously recorded leads I, II, and III. Immediately after the third QRS complex was inscribed, the leads changed, so that the T wave indicated by the arrow is actually the T wave of the QRS complex from lead aVR.

4. *Is there "low voltage" in the limb leads?*

   Answer: No. Low voltage is said to be present when QRS amplitude in each of the limb leads (I, II, III, aVR, aVL, and aVF) is 5 mm or less. Although QRS amplitude is reduced in leads III, aVL, and aVF, it clearly exceeds 5 mm in leads I, II, and aVR.

   Low voltage is a descriptive finding that is most often seen in patients with COPD (who have large, emphysematous chests) or obese individuals (because of the greater distance between the heart and the recording electrodes).

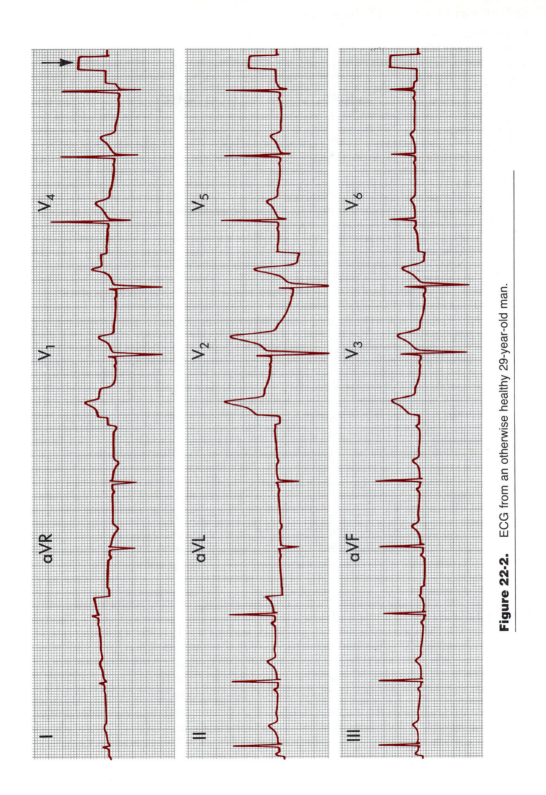

Figure 22-2. ECG from an otherwise healthy 29-year-old man.

Interpretation of Figure 22-2

Descriptive analysis. There is regular sinus rhythm, at a rate of about 65 beats/minute. All intervals are normal. The axis is normal (and approximately +80°). There is no evidence of chamber enlargement. There is a tiny q wave in lead III and possibly also in lead aVF. R wave progression is normal (with transition occurring normally between leads V_3 and V_4). ST segment elevation with an upward concavity (i.e., "smiley") is present in leads V_2 and V_3. T waves are prominent in the anterior precordial leads.

Clinical impression. This is probably also a normal ECG.

Questions to Further Understanding

1. *The sum of the S wave in lead V_2 plus the R wave in lead V_5 exceeds 35. Why is LVH not present?*

   Answer: Younger individuals often demonstrate increased QRS amplitude without necessarily having true chamber enlargement. As a result, the voltage criteria in Table 9-1 *(pocket reference p. 22)* are not valid for diagnosing LVH in individuals less than 35 years of age.

2. *If the patient in Figure 22-2 was 35 years old, would you say he had LVH?*

   Answer: No. If the patient in Figure 22-2 were 35, we would write **"voltage for LVH"** on our interpretation. This is our way of indicating that despite the increase in QRS amplitude, repolarization changes ("strain") are absent, and it is still quite likely that true chamber enlargement is not present.

3. *Which leads are most likely to demonstrate "normal septal q waves"?*

   Answer: Normal septal q waves are usually small (and narrow) and are commonly seen in lateral leads (I, aVL, V_4, V_5, and/or V_6). On occasion, they may also be seen in inferior leads (II, III, and/or aVF), especially in patients with a relatively vertical QRS axis (as is the case in Figure 22-2).

   Normal septal q waves can usually be differentiated from pathologic Q waves because they tend to be smaller and narrower, occur in otherwise healthy individuals, and are not accompanied by other ECG evidence of infarction.

4. *Why is the ST segment elevation seen in leads V_2 and V_3 most likely a normal variant?*

   Answer: ST segment elevation (of 1 to 3 mm) is very commonly seen in leads V_2 and V_3 in otherwise healthy individuals. The keys to recognizing such ST segment elevation as a benign normal variant are the clinical setting (usually occurring in an asymptomatic and otherwise healthy individual), the *shape* of the ST segment ("smiley," *as in Figure 10-15, A,* on pocket reference p. 28), and the otherwise normal ECG. All of these factors are present in Figure 22-2.

5. *Why are the prominent T waves seen in several of the precordial leads unlikely to be due to hyperkalemia?*

   Answer: Hyperkalemia typically produces tall, peaked (and pointed) T waves with a narrow base *(Figure 14-1, on pocket reference p. 44)*. Although prominent, the T waves in the anterior precordial leads in Figure 22-2 are not pointed, and they have a wide base. In addition, the ascending and descending limbs of the T wave are not symmetric as they usually are with hyperkalemia *(see Figure 10-16, B and C, on pocket reference p. 29)*.

   Another reason the prominent T waves in Figure 22-2 are unlikely to represent hyperkalemia is simply that this otherwise healthy 29-year-old man has no reason to be hyperkalemic. Hyperkaelmia is usually seen only in certain clinical settings, such as renal failure, acidosis, or dehydration, or in patients taking potassium-retaining diuretics or ACE-inhibitors *(Table 14-1, on pocket reference p. 44)*. It is a distinctly unusual occurrence in an otherwise healthy individual who is not on any medications.

6. *What is the rectangular mark at the very end of the tracing (arrow)?*

   Answer: This is the **standardization mark.** Ideally, it should appear at the beginning or end of every 12-lead ECG to verify that amplification of the machine is correctly set. Normally, the standardization mark will be 10 mm (= two large boxes) tall, as it is in Figure 22-2. If it is only 5 mm (= one large box) tall, the machine is set at *half standardization,* and QRS complexes will all be only half of their actual size. In patients with tremendously increased voltage, the ECG machine may have to be set at half standardization in one or more leads in order for QRS complexes to fit on the space allotted for the particular lead.

7. *Should the ECG machine have been set at half standardization for any lead in Figure 22-2?*

   Answer: Perhaps for lead V_2. Because of the descending baseline in this lead, the depth of the S wave of the second QRS complex in lead V_2 is unknown. The machine could have been adjusted to half standardization in order to accommodate the entire QRS complex within the space provided for the lead recording. It would have been even better to wait an extra moment (or redo the ECG) until the baseline leveled out.

8. *Is the T wave inversion in lead aVL normal?*

   Answer: Yes. Like Q waves, T waves may normally be inverted (as an isolated finding) in leads III, aVF, aVL, and V_1 *(Table 10-6, on pocket reference p. 28)*. Isolated T wave inversion is commonly seen in lead aVL as a normal variant when the QRS complex is predominantly negative (as it is in Figure 22-2).

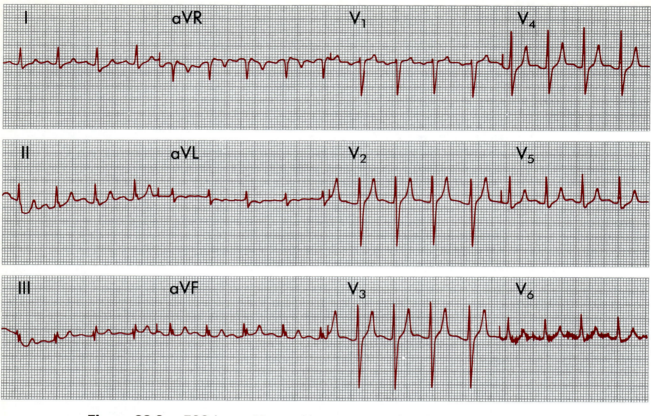

Figure 22-3.   ECG from a 90-year-old woman presenting with dehydration, renal failure, and acidosis.

Interpretation of Figure 22-3

Descriptive analysis. The rhythm is fairly regular, at a rate between 100 and 115 beats/minute. The mechanism is sinus. All intervals are normal. The axis is normal (and approximately 40° to 50°). There is no chamber enlargement. There are no Q waves. R wave progression is normal (with transition occurring between leads V_3 and V_4). There are minimal changes in the ST segments. The most remarkable finding on this tracing, however, is the alteration in T wave morphology.

Clinical impression. Sinus tachycardia. Tall, peaked T waves that strongly suggest hyperkalemia.

Questions to Further Understanding

1. *How do the T waves in the precordial leads in Figure 22-3 differ from those in Figure 22-2?*

   Answer: T waves are prominent in the precordial leads in both tracings. However, they are more pointed and have a much narrower base in Figure 22-3. Note that the ascending and descending limbs of the T waves are symmetric in Figure 22-3, compared with the more gradual ascending limb of the T wave in Figure 22-2.

2. *What other factors make it highly likely that the T wave alterations in Figure 22-3 truly reflect hyperkalemia?*

    Answer: The clinical history. Dehydration, renal failure, and acidosis may all predispose to hyperkalemia. *(See Table 14-1, on pocket reference p. 44)*.

3. *Could you hazard a guess as to the severity of hyperkalemia?*

    Answer: Because of the marked degree of T wave peaking, one might suspect that at least *moderate* hyperkalemia (serum $K^+ \approx 7.0$ mEq/L or higher) was present *(see Figure 14-1 on pocket reference p. 44)*. However, the fact that the QRS complex is not really widened, and P waves are still of reasonable amplitude, suggests that hyperkalemia is not yet severe (greater than 9.0 mEq/L).

4. *What happened in lead V_6?*

    Answer: The small, vertical spikes and undulations in the baseline in lead V_6 represent artifact.

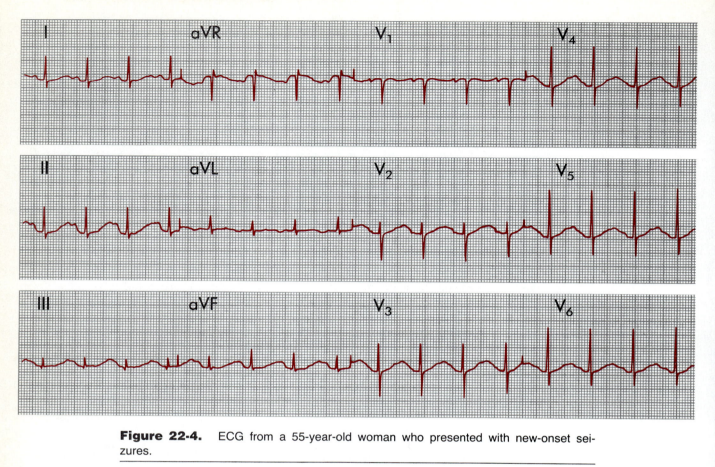

Figure 22-4.   ECG from a 55-year-old woman who presented with new-onset seizures.

Interpretation of Figure 22-4

Descriptive analysis. There is regular sinus rhythm, at a rate just under 100 beats/minute. The PR and QRS intervals are normal, but the QT interval is markedly prolonged! The axis is normal (and approximately 40° to 50°). There is no chamber enlargement. There is a small q wave in lead III. R wave progression is normal (with transition occurring between leads V_2 and V_3). There are diffuse nonspecific ST segment and T wave abnormalities.

Clinical impression. There is marked QT prolongation. This should suggest "Drugs/Lytes/CNS" as the cause (*see List #2 on pocket reference p. 38*).

Questions to Further Understanding

1. *If you were taking care of this patient, what clinical entities would you consider in your evaluation?*

   Answer: As suggested by List #2, QT prolongation should suggest ***Drugs*** (i.e., medication effect if the patient was taking quinidine, procainamide, disopyramide, tricyclic antidepressants, or a phenothiazine), ***Lytes*** (i.e., an electrolyte disorder such as hypokalemia/hypomagnesemia, or hypocalcemia), or a ***CNS*** *catastrophe* as possible underlying causes. Seizures in this patient may be contributory. More historical information and serum electrolyte values (including serum magnesium) would be needed to investigate "*Drugs*" and "*Lytes*."

2. *Are you sure that it is the QT interval that is prolonged in Figure 22-4? (Hint: What if hypokalemia was the cause of the QT prolongation?)*

   Answer: If hypokalemia was the cause of the QT prolongation, the apparent "QT" prolongation might actually reflect QU prolongation (*see Figure 14-2, on pocket reference p. 45*).

3. *Could the ST segment and T wave changes in Figure 22-4 also represent ischemia?*

   Answer: In addition to *"Drugs/Lytes/CNS,"* ischemia, infarction, and bundle branch block may all also prolong the QT interval. However, the presence of these other conditions will usually be obvious from inspection of the ECG. In Figure 22-4, the QRS complex is not widened, there are no signs of infarction, and T waves are not inverted. Thus, it is most probable that the marked QT prolongation reflects a problem with Drugs/Lytes/CNS.

4. *The terminal portion of the P wave in lead V_1 is negative. Is there LAA?*

   Answer: Maybe, although we would probably *not* call it. ECG criteria for diagnosing atrial abnormalities are poor. Echocardiography is a much better (albeit substantially more expensive) tool for this purpose. Because of the disappointing reliability of ECG criteria for diagnosing atrial abnormalities, we tend to *undercall* these diagnoses. Thus, we prefer the negative component of the P wave in lead V_1 to be clearly deeper and wider than one small box before calling LAA (*Figure 9-2, on pocket reference p. 24*).

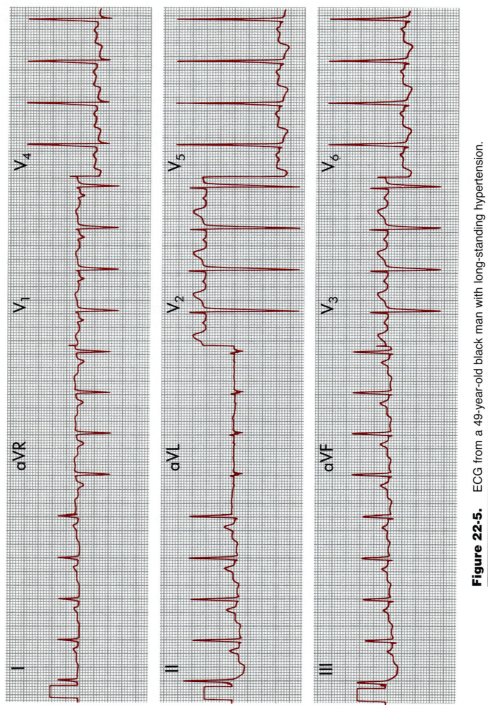

Figure 22-5.   ECG from a 49-year-old black man with long-standing hypertension.

Interpretation of Figure 22-5

Descriptive analysis. There is a regular sinus rhythm, at a rate just under 100 beats/minute. All intervals are normal. The axis is normal (and approximately $+70°$). There is RAA (tall, peaked P waves in the inferior leads, with P wave amplitude exceeding 2.5 mm in lead II), LAA (deep negative component of the P wave in lead V_1), and LVH (marked increase in voltage with "strain" in a patient over 35). There are small q waves in the inferior and lateral precordial leads. R wave progression is normal (with transition occurring between leads V_3 and V_4). There is ST segment flattening and depression in the inferolateral leads.

Clinical impression. Sinus rhythm. Biatrial abnormality (i.e., RAA and LAA). LVH and strain and/or ischemia.

Questions to Further Understanding

1. *Is the ST segment depression in leads V_5 and V_6 more suggestive of ischemia or "strain"?*

   Answer: Strain. (See *Figure 10-16, D and E, on pocket reference p. 29*). The gradual descent of the ST segment and more rapid terminal ascent of the T wave in leads V_5 and V_6, in association with the marked increase in voltage in these leads, present a classic picture of left ventricular strain.

2. *What is the likelihood that this patient has true chamber enlargement?*

   Answer: Exceedingly high (i.e., over 95%!). The patient is old enough (over 35), has the "right disease" (since long-standing hypertension very commonly predisposes to LVH, especially in blacks), and has tremendously increased QRS voltage, LAA, and classic strain.

3. *What is the ST segment depression in the inferior leads likely to be due to?*

   Answer: Strain, ischemia, or both (i.e., *"strain **and/or** ischemia"*), although it could be due to any of the common causes of ST segment depression listed in Table 13-4 *(List #3 on pocket reference p. 39)*. Morphologically, the inferior ST-T wave changes might best be described as "nonspecific" in nature *(similar to Figure 10-16, H, on pocket reference p. 29)*. If nothing else, one can at least say that the inferior ST-T wave changes do not appear to be acute (i.e., there is no ST segment elevation, the degree of ST segment depression is slight, and T waves are not deeply inverted).

4. *Are any of the q waves "significant"?*

   Answer: Probably not. The small q waves in leads V_5 and V_6 should be interpreted as *"normal septal q waves"* in these lateral leads. The q waves in the inferior leads (II, III, and aVF) are also small and narrow, and may also be "normal septal Q waves" in this patient who has a relatively vertical axis. Without knowing more about the patient, however, one could not absolutely rule out the possibility of prior inferior infarction (especially in view of the nonspecific ST-T wave changes in these leads.)

5. *What would be the best way to find out if the inferior q waves were new?*
   Answer: Look at an old tracing.

   Sometimes (all too often it seems), *no prior tracing* (i.e., **NPT**) is available for comparison. Our way of indicating on the interpretation that we saw the small q waves and don't think they are "significant" (but can't be sure) is to write either of the following in our descriptive analysis:

   > ***"small inferior q waves"***
   > or ***"small inferior q waves of ? significance"***

6. *Is the ECG in Figure 22-5 correctly standardized?*
   Answer: Yes. The standardization mark appears at the very beginning of the tracing and is 10 mm (two large boxes) in height (as it should be). If QRS amplitude in the precordial leads was any greater, one would have to reset the machine to half standardization in order to fit the QRS complex within the space provided.

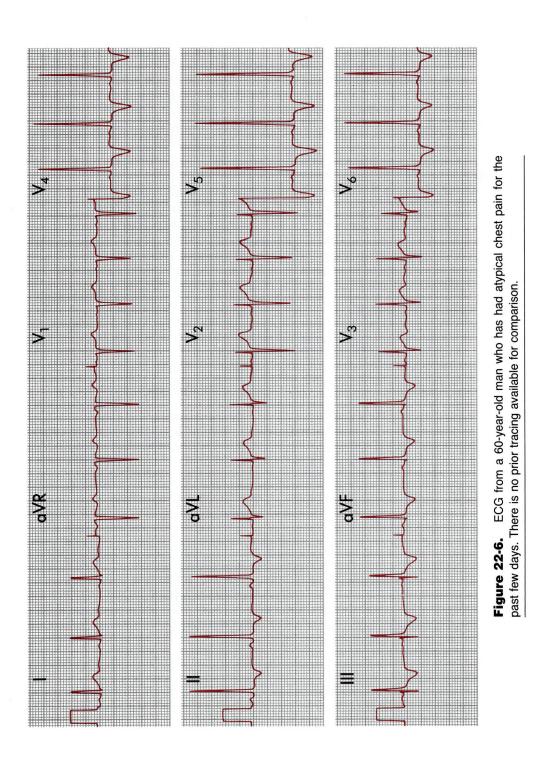

Figure 22-6.   ECG from a 60-year-old man who has had atypical chest pain for the past few days. There is no prior tracing available for comparison.

Interpretation of Figure 22-6

Descriptive analysis. The rhythm is slightly irregular, but the mechanism is sinus. All intervals are normal. The axis is normal (and approximately 50°). QRS amplitude is markedly increased in the lateral precordial leads, and easily satisfies voltage criteria for LVH. There is a small q wave in lead aVF. R wave progression is normal (with transition occurring between leads V_2 and V_3). The most remarkable finding on this tracing, however, is the deep, symmetric T wave inversion.

Clinical impression. Sinus arrhythmia. LVH and strain and/or ischemia. NPT. *Suggest clinical correlation.*

Questions to Further Understanding

1. *Why is the rhythm in Figure 22-6 slightly irregular?*

   Answer: It is often difficult to diagnose the rhythm with certainty from a 12-lead ECG when there is no accompanying rhythm strip. This is especially true when the rhythm is irregular. One never gets to look at more than a few complexes in any given lead. Since P wave morphology varies from lead to lead, and P waves are not always easily identifiable in each lead, it may be hard to tell if the site of impulse formation is changing. Nevertheless, one can be reasonably sure that the mechanism of the rhythm in Figure 22-6 is sinus, because the P wave is upright in lead II and "married" to the QRS. Variation of the rhythm from lead to lead is gradual, and P waves appear to be married to the QRS complex in virtually all leads with a similar PR interval. All of these factors strongly suggest sinus arrhythmia.

2. *What is the clinical significance of sinus arrhythmia?*

   Answer: The answer depends on the clinical setting and the age of the patient. Sinus arrhythmia is an extremely common normal phenomenon in children and young adults *(see Table 17-2, on pocket reference p. 50)*. While it may also be a normal variant in older individuals, it is sometimes a harbinger of sick sinus syndrome, especially when the sinus arrhythmia is accompanied by marked bradycardia.

3. *Is there a Q wave in lead III? (Why is this an important question?)*

   Answer: No. It appears that a tiny upward deflection *precedes* the negative deflection in the QRS complex in this lead. This defines the complex as having an rSR′ morphology. The lack of a Q wave in both leads II *and* III makes it much less likely that this patient has had a prior inferior infarction.

4. *Is the deep, symmetric T wave inversion more likely to reflect strain, ischemia, or both?*

   Answer: Deep, symmetric T wave inversion as seen in the inferior (II, III, and aVF) and lateral precordial (V_4, V_5, and V_6) leads in Figure 22-6 strongly suggests ischemia *(see Figure 10-16, D, on pocket reference p. 29)*. It is important to remember, however, that *ST-T wave changes of strain or ischemia may sometimes be masked by the pres-*

ence of the other condition! Considering the age of the patient and the tremendously increased voltage in the lateral precordial leads, there is an excellent chance that true left ventricular chamber enlargement (LVH) with strain is present in addition to ischemia. Our way of indicating these possibilities is to write the following on our interpretation:

"LVH and strain **and/or** ischemia"

5. *Should this patient be admitted to the hospital?*

   Answer: Yes. The ECG shown in Figure 22-6 is clearly abnormal and, viewed by itself, strongly suggests acute ischemia. Without the benefit of a prior tracing for comparison, there is absolutely no way to determine if the deep T wave inversion is a new finding. Thus, despite the history of atypical chest pain for several days, it would appear prudent to admit the patient to the hospital (at least to a telemetry unit) to rule out an acute ischemic event (i.e., unstable angina or infarction).

6. *If a prior ECG showing identical findings could be found, would the patient still need to be admitted to the hospital?*

   Answer: Not necessarily. If a prior ECG showed findings identical to those in the tracing in Figure 22-6, one could confidently say that these ECG changes are not acute. In this case, it might be appropriate to manage the patient on an ambulatory basis if the history was unconvincing for an acute ischemic event. *Remember that the onus always lies with the examining clinician to exclude acute infarction.* **If the slightest doubt exists, it is always better to err on the side of admission to the hospital, rather than take the chance of sending a patient with acute infarction home!** The value in having a prior tracing available to help make this decision is obvious.

7. *What if a patient presents with severe crushing chest pain but a totally normal ECG? Can such a patient be sent home because the ECG is normal?*

   Answer: No. History is an even more important parameter to assess than the initial ECG. This is because the initial ECG does not always show changes of acute infarction. Occasionally, no ECG changes at all ever develop, despite definite laboratory evidence of infarction (i.e., elevated CK isoenzymes). *Thus, a patient who presents with a convincing history of new-onset ischemic chest pain should always be admitted to the hospital, regardless of what an initial ECG shows!*

   A clinical point of interest is that the prognosis tends to be better and the likelihood of developing complications lower in patients with acute infarction if the initial ECG does not show acute changes. If hemodynamically stable, such patients do not necessarily require admission to a CCU, and often can be managed on a telemetry unit.

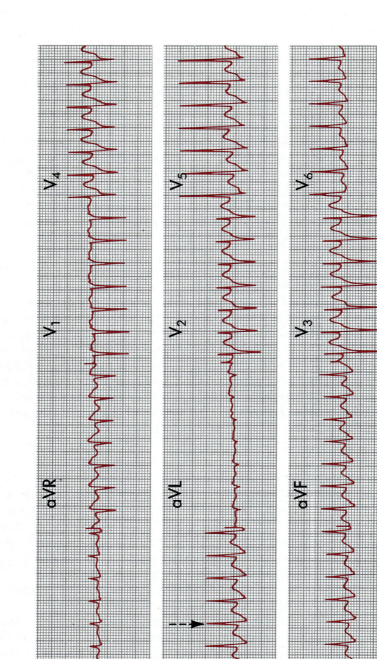
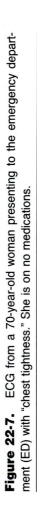

Figure 22-7.   ECG from a 70-year-old woman presenting to the emergency department (ED) with "chest tightness." She is on no medications.

Interpretation of Figure 22-7

Descriptive analysis. There is a regular, supraventricular tachycardia at a rate of about 180 beats/minute. It is impossible to tell from looking at lead II whether the upright deflection between QRS complexes represents a T wave, a P wave, or both.

The axis is normal (and approximately +70°). There is no evidence of ventricular enlargement. (One can't say anything about atrial abnormality, since there are no definite P waves on the tracing.) There is diffuse ST segment depression.

Preliminary *clinical impression.* SVT at 180 beats/minute. Nonspecific ST-T abnormalities (NS ST-T Abns).

Questions to Further Understanding

1. *What are the three main causes of a regular SVT that should be considered in Figure 22-7? Which of these three is the most likely diagnosis of the arrhythmia?*

    Answer: The three main entities to consider in the differential diagnosis for the regular SVT in Figure 22-7 are:

    a. Sinus tachycardia
    b. Atrial flutter
    c. PSVT

    Sinus tachycardia rarely exceeds 160 beats/minute in a nonambulatory adult. Heart rates of over 200 beats/minute may be seen with sinus tachycardia in children, and heart rates approaching 200 beats/minute are common in adults who are exercising—but for practical purposes, *if a regular SVT exceeds 160 beats/minute on the 12-lead ECG of an adult, it is highly unlikely that the mechanism is sinus!*

    As we emphasized on p. 8 in the pocket reference, the atrial rate of flutter is almost always close to 300 beats/minute. Most commonly there is 2:1 AV conduction—so that *the most common ventricular response to untreated* **atrial flutter** *in adults is a heart rate of about 150 beats/minute.*

    It is extremely easy to overlook atrial flutter. This is because characteristic (sawtooth) flutter waves are not always apparent in each lead of a 12-lead ECG, and sometimes they are not readily apparent in any of the leads! We have found the following two hints invaluable in helping to make the diagnosis:

    a. *Always maintain a high index of suspicion.*
    b. *Carefully calculate the heart rate of any SVT you encounter.*

    Practically speaking, **suspect atrial flutter until proven otherwise whenever you have a regular SVT at a rate of about 150 beats/minute, especially if you are uncertain about atrial activity.**

    Although atrial flutter has to be considered in the differential diagnosis of the regular SVT in Figure 22-7, it is not the mechanism of this arrhythmia. The ventricular response is 180 beats/minute. If atrial flutter with 2:1 AV conduction were present, this would mean that the atrial rate would have to be 360 beats/minute (i.e., 180 × 2), which is above the usual range for flutter. On the other hand, if the rhythm was atrial flutter with 1:1 AV conduction, the atrial rate would be 180 beats/minute—a much slower atrial rate than expected for flutter. (NOTE: The atrial rate of flutter may be reduced in patients treated with drugs such as quinidine or verapamil.)

By the process of elimination, the rhythm in Figure 22-7 is most likely to be **PSVT** (see pocket reference p. 8).

2. *Is there truly no sign of atrial activity in Figure 22-7?*

Answer: This is an extremely subtle point—but one that has incited a tremendous amount of interest in recent years among those with a passion for arrhythmias. *There IS evidence of atrial activity in this tracing!* Close inspection of the terminal portion of the QRS complex and the beginning of the ST segment in several leads (I, II, III, aVF, and especially V_1) reveals ever so subtle notching. This represents *retrograde* atrial activity, and proves AV nodal reentry as the mechanism for the arrhythmia. The retrograde atrial activity of AV nodal reentry with PSVT most often occurs at the same time as the QRS complex. As a result, it is usually completely hidden by (within) the QRS. Occasionally, however, retrograde P waves will be seen (if carefully looked for) to notch the end of the QRS or the beginning of the ST segment (as they do here). We emphasize that detection of retrograde atrial activity during PSVT is an *ADVANCED* concept that extends beyond the scope of this book. Nevertheless, we feel it worth mentioning to highlight how helpful the 12-lead ECG may be in elucidating the mechanism of an arrhythmia.

3. *What are the likely causes of the diffuse ST segment depression in this tracing?*

Answer: The common causes of ST segment depression are ischemia, strain, digitalis effect, hypokalemia (or hypomagnesemia), and rate-related changes *(List #3 on pocket reference p. 39)*. The history makes it unlikely that digitalis or an electrolyte disturbance is a factor. Voltage criteria for LVH are not satisfied in Figure 22-7. This leaves *ischemia* and/or *rate-related changes* as the most likely causes of ST segment depression.

Considering our discussion of these first three questions, we might amend our preliminary clinical impression to the following:

Clinical impression of Figure 22-7. PSVT at 180 beats/minute. Diffuse ST segment depression c/w (consistent with) ischemia and/or rate-related changes. *Suggest clinical correlation.*

4. *Should this patient be admitted to the hospital?*

Answer: Depends. If conversion of PSVT to sinus rhythm (by a vagal maneuver or medication) is easily accomplished in the ED and results in complete resolution of symptoms, the patient could probably be managed equally well on an ambulatory basis, provided the postconversion tracing did not show acute changes. This underscores the tremendous importance of *always* obtaining a **postconversion 12-lead ECG** after conversion of any cardiac arrhythmia. The postconversion tracing:

Confirms (and documents) that the patient is now in sinus rhythm

May clarify findings seen during the tachycardia

May elucidate the cause of the arrhythmia (i.e., acute infarction, WPW)

Thus, if the diffuse ST segment depression seen in Figure 22-7 completely resolved on the postconversion tracing, rate-related changes rather than ischemia were probably the cause. On the other hand, if ST segment depression persisted despite reduction of the heart rate and conversion to sinus rhythm, prudence would dictate admission to the hospital to rule out an acute ischemic event as the cause (or result) of the tachycardia.

5. *We emphasized the importance of accurate calculation of heart rate in diagnosing an arrhythmia. How can you be sure that the heart rate in Figure 22-7 is under 200 beats/minute? That it is significantly above 150 beats/ minute?*

Answer: The rhythm is regular, and the R-R interval is between one and two large boxes. This means that the heart rate must be between 300 and 150 beats/minute. **The easiest way to accurately calculate heart rate when the rhythm is fast and regular is to determine the rate for every other beat** (i.e., *half the rate*) **and then multiply this number by two.**

Pick a QRS complex that occurs on a heavy line (solid arrow in lead II of Figure 22-7). The R-R interval for every other beat (i.e., the interval from the solid arrow to the broken arrow) is just *over* three large boxes. Thus, *half* of the rate is about 90 beats/minute. The actual rate is 180 beats/minute (90 × 2).

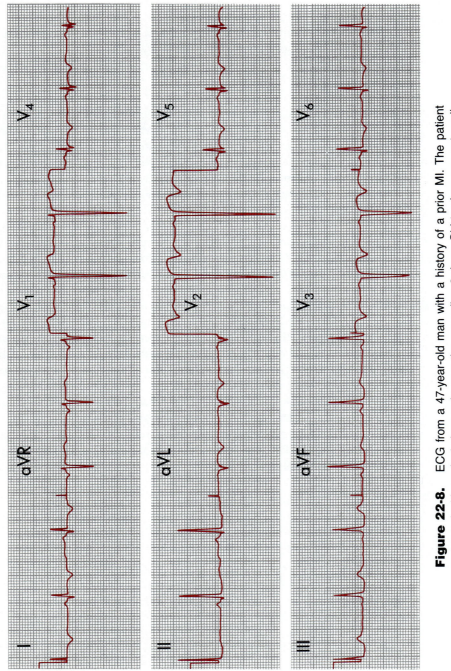

Figure 22-8. ECG from a 47-year-old man with a history of a prior MI. The patient presented with anginal chest pain over the preceding 2 days. Old tracings are not available for comparison.

Interpretation of Figure 22-8

Descriptive analysis. There is a regular sinus rhythm at a rate of about 65 beats/minute. All intervals are normal. The axis is normal (and approximately +70°). Voltage criteria for LVH are satisfied (because of the extremely deep S waves in leads V_1 and V_2). There is a QS complex in lead aVL, and Q waves in leads I, II, and V_2 through V_6. There is *loss of R wave* from lead V_1 to V_2. ST segments are coved and slightly elevated in many of the anterolateral leads, flat in lead II, and slightly depressed in leads III and aVF. T waves are symmetrically inverted in leads I, aVL, and V_2 through V_6.

Clinical impression. Sinus rhythm. Anterolateral infarction of ? age, possibly acute. NPT. *Suggest clinical correlation.*

Questions to Further Understanding

1. *Why did we label the infarction in Figure 22-8 as anterolateral instead of anteroseptal or isolated anterior?*

    Answer: The basic lead groups are listed in Table 10-2 (on pocket reference p. 27). As can be seen from this table, leads V_1 and V_2 are considered the septal leads. *Preservation of the initial small r wave in lead V_1 of Figure 22-8 therefore suggests* (at least electrocardiographically) *that the septum is intact.* Instead of the usual (expected) increase in R wave amplitude as one moves across the precordial leads, *R wave is lost* from lead V_1 to V_2 (with development of deep QS complexes in leads V_2 and V_3). This suggests *anterior* infarction. Infarction is not localized (limited) to the anterior wall, however, since Q waves persist in leads V_4 to V_6, and are also present in leads I and aVL. This means the infarction is *anterolateral*.

2. *Should this patient be admitted to the hospital?*

    Answer: The answer depends on three factors:
    a. How sick is the patient?
    b. How worrisome is the history?
    c. How sure can we be that the patient's ECG does not reflect an acute change?

    It is impossible to evaluate how sick the patient is from the capsule history provided in the legend to Figure 22-8. Our suspicion of acute ischemic heart disease is certainly heightened by knowledge of prior infarction, although it is lessened by the fact that chest pain has been ongoing for 2 days. Nevertheless, a number of findings on the ECG have to be viewed with concern *(see Figure 12-1, on pocket reference p. 34).* ST segments in several leads are coved, slightly elevated, and associated with fairly deep, symmetric T wave inversion; ST segment depression in leads III and aVF may reflect reciprocal changes. Without the benefit of a prior tracing, one has to consider the possibility of acute changes until proven otherwise.

3. *Is this patient a potential candidate for thrombolytic therapy?*

    Answer: No. By history, chest pain has been ongoing for the past 2 days. Even if the patient were infarcting, he is well beyond the "window of opportunity," and therefore should not be considered as a potential candidate for thrombolytic therapy (*see Table 12-3, on pocket reference p. 35).*

• • •

NOTE: Some clinicians extend the "window of opportunity" for thrombolytic therapy beyond 6 hours for selected patients with *ongoing,* severe ischemic chest pain if they feel that symptoms began with unstable angina and evolved into acute infarction. This is unlikely to be the case for a patient with 2 days of chest pain and an ECG showing as deep Q waves and as little ST segment elevation as are seen in Figure 22-8.

4. *How would you interpret the anterior ST segment elevation if you were told that the patient had an identical ECG in 1987?*

   Answer: If this patient's ECG had not changed since 1987, one could safely conclude that none of the electrocardiographic findings were acute. An interesting clinical point is that persistent (lasting more than 3 to 6 months) ST segment elevation over an area of infarction suggests development of a *ventricular aneurysm.*

5. *Can you think of an explanation for the deep S waves in lead V_1 and V_2 other than LVH?*

   Answer: The very deep S waves in leads V_1 and V_2 satisfy voltage criteria for LVH. That is, the sum of the deepest S wave in lead V_1 or V_2 PLUS the tallest R wave in lead V_5 or V_6 easily exceeds 35 mm. Technically speaking, however, true left ventricular chamber enlargement may not necessarily be present. This is because the anterior infarction itself may be responsible for the loss of anterior forces (i.e., for the loss of R wave in leads V_2 and V_3). Posterior (left ventricular) forces become more prominent because they are no longer opposed by anterior forces. BOTTOM LINE: ***Diagnosis of LVH is often extremely difficult in the presence of anterior infarction (and vice versa).***

• • •

It is important to realize that the ECG is far from being an infallible diagnostic tool. We do not feel you are wrong if you indicated LVH on your interpretation of Figure 22-8. We feel it is equally correct to avoid comment altogether regarding the possibility of LVH, in view of the presence of anterior infarction.

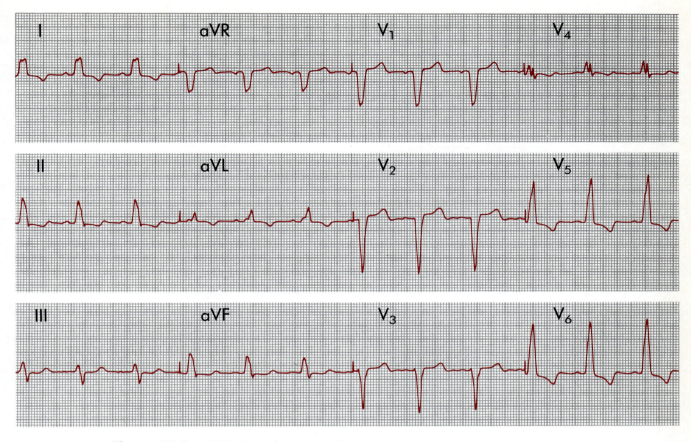

Figure 22-9.   ECG from a 70-year-old woman with new-onset chest pain. No prior tracing is available.

Interpretation of Figure 22-9

Descriptive analysis. There is a regular sinus rhythm at a rate of 75 beats/minute. The PR interval is normal, but the QRS complex is widened and the QT interval prolonged. QRS morphology is consistent with complete LBBB. The axis is normal. There is no chamber enlargement. Typical *secondary* ST segment and T wave changes of LBBB are present.

Clinical impression. Sinus rhythm. Complete LBBB. NPT.

Questions to Further Understanding

1. *Is there evidence of anterior infarction?*

    Answer: No. Diagnosis of anterior infarction is much more difficult in the presence of complete LBBB. Deep QS complexes in leads V_1 through V_3 or V_4 and/or poor R wave progression are a natural accompaniment of this conduction disorder. Thus, nothing can be said about the possibility of anterior infarction in Figure 22-9.

2. *Is there evidence of strain and/or ischemia?*

   Answer: No. Asymmetric ST segment depression and T wave inversion in the lateral leads are typical of the *secondary* ST-T wave changes expected with uncomplicated LBBB (*see Figure 5-9, on pocket reference p. 15*). Thus, because of the LBBB, nothing can be about the possibility of strain and/or ischemia in Figure 22-9.

3. *Why is it important to evaluate INTERVALS early in the process of your systematic interpretation?*

   Answer: Evaluating intervals early in the process of your systematic interpretation not only saves time but also improves diagnostic accuracy. We suggest that if the QRS complex is widened, you stop in your tracks and ask yourself why (*Figure 5-1, on pocket reference p. 13*). Does the patient have RBBB, LBBB, or IVCD? If so, diagnosis of ventricular enlargement, ischemia, and/or infarction will be much more difficult (if possible at all). If, in addition to QRS widening, the PR interval is short and there are delta waves, the patient has WPW (*Figure 5-14, on pocket reference p. 16*), and nothing more can be said about QRST morphology.

4. *Is QRST morphology in Figure 22-9 suggestive of "typical" LBBB?*

   Answer: As suggested by Figures 5-8 and 5-9 (*pocket reference pp. 14 and 15*), QRST morphology suggests "typical" LBBB because:

   a. The QRS complex is widened (to ≥ 0.12 second).

   b. QRS morphology in the three key leads (I, V_1, and V_6) is as expected for LBBB (monophasic R wave without a septal q in leads I and V_6, and predominantly negative complex in lead V_1).

   c. Typical secondary ST-T wave changes of LBBB are seen in these three key leads (i.e., orientation of the ST segment and T wave is opposite that of the last QRS deflection).

5. *Should the patient be admitted to the hospital?*

   Answer: Probably. The history of new-onset chest pain in a 70-year-old woman is by itself worrisome. Moreover, evaluation of the ECG shown in Figure 22-9 for acute ischemic changes is not possible, because of the presence of LBBB. Without the benefit of a prior tracing, there is therefore no way to know if the LBBB is new (i.e., if LBBB developed as the direct result of acute infarction). In the absence of this information, the wisest course of action may be to admit the patient until serial enzyme studies determine if acute infarction has occurred.

6. *Can you diagnose LVH in the presence of complete LBBB?*

   Answer: Sometimes. It is often impossible to comment on the likelihood of ventricular enlargement in the presence of LBBB. However, when there are exceedingly deep S waves (of at least 25 to 30 mm) in the anterior precordial leads (V_1, V_2, or V_3), one can say that LVH is probably also present in addition to LBBB. This is not the case in Figure 22-9, because S waves do not exceed 20 mm in the anterior precordial leads.

An interesting point about our clinical impression of Figure 22-9 is its brevity: "Complete LBBB." Nothing more need (or can) be said about this tracing.

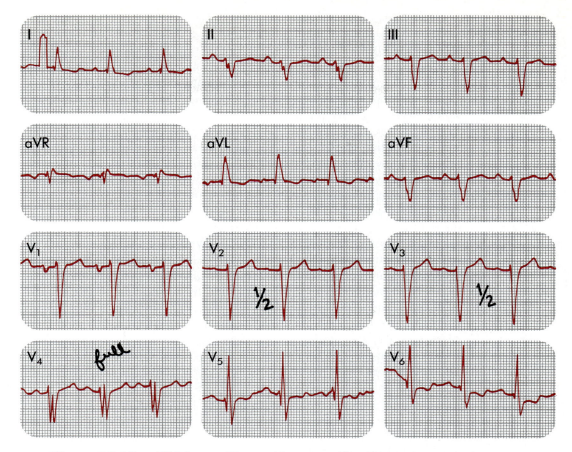

Figure 22-10.   ECG from a 67-year-old woman with a history of a congestive cardio-myopathy.

Interpretation of Figure 22-10

Descriptive analysis. There is a regular sinus rhythm at a rate of about 80 beats/minute. The PR interval is normal, but the QRS complex and QT interval are both prolonged. There is marked LAD. There is LAA (as judged by the deep, terminal negative component of the P wave in lead V_1), but no other definite evidence of chamber enlargement.

Clinical impression. Sinus rhythm. LAA. IVCD with LAD.

Questions to Further Understanding

1. *Note that the lead orientation in Figure 22-10 is different from that of the other tracings we have looked at so far in this chapter. Why might the simultaneous vertical lead orientation used throughout most of this book be preferable to the horizontal orientation shown here? Are there any advantages to the horizontal orientation?*

   Answer: A decided advantage of the vertical lead orientation is the *simultaneous* recording of three leads at any one moment in time. This allows comparison of a particular complex in three different leads at the same instant in time. It is particularly helpful in rhythm analysis when P waves may not be evident in all leads, or when it becomes important to evaluate QRS morphology in several key leads at once. ECGs that display the horizontal orientation have usually been recorded on a single-channel ECG machine, and often have to be mounted by hand. This introduces a considerable time factor compared with simultaneously recorded tracings, which are immediately available for interpretation.

The disadvantage of the vertical lead orientation is that simultaneous recording minimizes the number of beats displayed in any one tracing. Thus, there are a total of 36 beats in Figure 22-10, whereas there are only 12 in Figure 22-9. Despite this, the above stated advantages of simultaneous recording have led to the ever-increasing popularity of the vertical orientation.

2. *Why is IVCD the best descriptor for the QRS widening in Figure 22-10?*

   Answer: As emphasized in Figure 5-1 *(pocket reference p. 13)*, QRS widening is due to typical RBBB, typical LBBB, or IVCD. Determination of typical RBBB or LBBB is made by evaluation of QRS morphology in the three key leads (I, V_1, and V_6), as indicated in Figure 5-8 *(pocket reference p. 14)*. QRS widening in Figure 22-10 is not due to typical RBBB, because there is no rSR' or RBBB-equivalent in lead V_1. It is not due to typical LBBB, because QRS morphology in the key lateral leads (I and V_6) is not in the form of a monophasic R wave. WPW is not present, because the PR interval is normal. Therefore, by the process of elimination, QRS widening must be due to IVCD.

3. *In addition to IVCD, is there also LAHB?*

   Answer: We know at a glance that there is *pathologic* LAD (i.e., an axis more negative than $-30°$), because the QRS complex is more negative than positive in lead II. Under normal circumstances, we equate pathologic LAD with LAHB. In the presence of LBBB, however, it becomes redundant to say that there is also LAHB (since complete LBBB implies block in *both* anterior and posterior divisions of the left bundle branch). The same probably holds true for IVCD. As a result, we prefer to describe the conduction defect and axis deviation in Figure 22-10 as *"IVCD with LAD"* rather than to say "IVCD with LAHB." This point is mainly a semantic one.

4. *The PR interval measures 0.20 second in lead II. Should we have indicated "borderline 1° AV block"?*

   Answer: The upper limit of normal for the PR interval in adults is 0.20 to 0.21 second. Consequently, many clinicians have adopted the term "borderline 1° AV block" to signify a PR interval between 0.19 and 0.20 second. *We disagree with this practice.* Clinically, the isolated finding of 1° AV block (in the absence of other cardiac pathology) has virtually no significance (or impact on prognosis). Wouldn't a "borderline" call of a clinically insignificant finding be of even less importance? *Why bother?*

As indicated in Table 4-1 *(pocket reference p. 11)*, we prefer not to call 1° AV block unless the PR interval is 0.22 second or greater (although we realize other sources call a PR interval of 0.21 second prolonged). Practically speaking, **unless the PR interval is clearly GREATER than a large box, it is normal.**

5. *Can you explain the QT prolongation in Figure 22-10?*

    Answer: The common causes of QT prolongation are Drugs/Lytes/CNS *(List #2 on pocket reference p. 38)*. Ischemia, infarction, and/or conduction defects (such as bundle branch block or IVCD) can also prolong the QT interval. The presence of IVCD is therefore the most likely explanation for QT prolongation in Figure 22-10.

6. *Is there evidence of infarction in Figure 22-10?*

    Answer: As is the case with LBBB, detection of infarction is difficult in the presence of IVCD. Occasionally, deep Q waves in unexpected locations or dramatic ST-T wave changes (i.e., marked ST segment elevation or T wave inversion) may suggest infarction or ischemia. Little can be said about the possibility of infarction, however, from the small q wave in lead aVL and the nonspecific ST-T wave changes seen in Figure 22-10.

7. *What do you think the notation "½" means in leads V_2 and V_3? (Hint: What do you think the notation "full" in lead V_4 means?)*

    Answer: The notation "½" in leads V_2 and V_3 indicates *half standardization*. That is, the actual dimensions of all complexes in these leads have been reduced in half. Thus, the actual depth of the S wave in lead V_2 is not 18 mm as shown, but really twice that amount (36 mm). Similarly, all dimensions in lead V_3 must also be doubled (since this lead was also recorded at half standardization). Full (normal) standardization has resumed by lead V_4. Unless otherwise indicated, one can usually assume full standardization.

8. *Is the patient likely to have LVH?*

    Answer: Determination of LVH is generally extremely difficult in the presence of complete LBBB. As indicated in our answer to Question #6 for Figure 22-9, however, *LVH can be suspected despite the presence of LBBB if S waves are exceedingly deep (at least 25 mm) in the anterior precordial leads.* The same probably holds true for IVCD. Thus, marked deepening of S waves in leads V_2 and V_3 (which easily exceeds 30 mm when one accounts for half standardization in these leads) makes it likely that the patient in Figure 22-10 also has LVH.

•   •   •

We emphasize that the ECG in Figure 22-10 is not an easy tracing to interpret. However, recognition that the QRS complex is widened and does not fit the pattern of either typical RBBB or typical LBBB should lead to the diagnosis of IVCD. It is important to appreciate that interpretation of ST-T wave changes in the setting of a conduction defect is difficult. *If you got no further than this, you're doing well!*

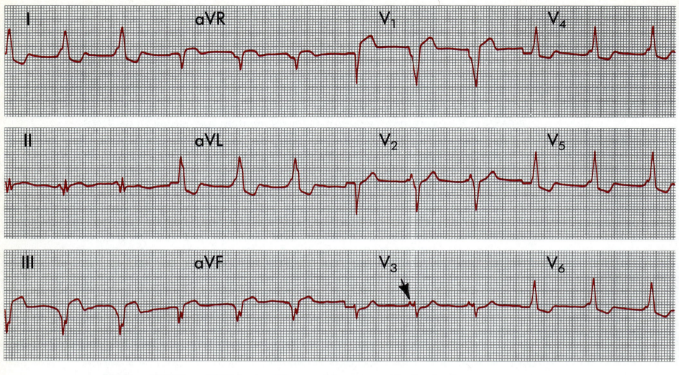

Figure 22-11.   ECG from a 50-year-old woman with chest pain.

Interpretation of Figure 22-11

Descriptive analysis. There is a fairly regular sinus rhythm at a heart rate of about 75 beats/minute. The PR interval is short. The QRS complex is prolonged and marked by an initial slurring.

Clinical impression. Sinus rhythm. WPW. *(See Addendum to Chapter 5.)*

Questions to Further Understanding

1. *What are the three characteristic findings of WPW?*
   Answer: The three characteristic findings of WPW are:
      a. QRS widening
      b. A delta wave
      c. A short PR interval
   (See Figure 5-14, on pocket reference p. 16)

2. *Are all three of these findings always present in patients with WPW?*
   Answer: No. Delta waves are not always present (or identifiable), and the QRS complex will not always appear widened in each of the 12 leads of an ECG taken from a patient with WPW. For example, in lead V₃ of Figure 22-11, the QRS complex does not appear to be widened at all and the delta wave simulates a P wave *(arrow).*

An even more difficult problem in diagnosis is that conduction down the accessory pathway with WPW may be intermittent. As a result, the QRS complex will be wide with conduction down the accessory pathway, but may appear entirely normal when conduction proceeds down the normal pathway (i.e., through the AV node, bundle of His, and bundle branches). Sometimes conduction may occur simultaneously down both the accessory pathway and the normal pathway. When this happens, the QRS complex may demonstrate characteristics of normal conduction as well as WPW. That is, the QRS complex may be only slightly widened, the PR interval may be almost normal, and the delta wave may be barely detectable. Obviously, recognition of WPW is more difficult when conduction occurs down both pathways, especially when it travels predominantly over the normal pathway.

In Figure 22-11, we can tell that conduction must be occurring predominantly over the accessory pathway, because the QRS complex is significantly widened and delta waves are present in virtually every lead.

3. *Will WPW be picked up by the systematic approach?*

Answer: It should be. There are *four* places in our systematic approach where WPW should be picked up:

When assessing *INTERVALS:*

If the PR interval is short

If the QRS complex is widened

When evaluating *QRST CHANGES:*

If there is a tall R wave in lead V_1 *(see List #4 on pocket reference p. 39)*

If delta waves are seen while you are systematically looking for q waves in each lead

4. *How common is WPW in the general population?*

Answer: The incidence of WPW in the general population is approximately 2 per 1000. This is common enough that most practitioners will encounter a couple of cases each year.

5. *Does the patient in Figure 22-11 have an inferior infarction?*

Answer: No. The patient has WPW. Delta waves with WPW may be negative or positive. They are negative in the inferior leads in this tracing, and simulate Q waves. Remember—***nothing can be said about the possibility of infarction in the presence of WPW.***

6. *What is the significance of the ST segment elevation in leads III, aVF, and V_1? of the ST segment depression in the lateral leads?*

Answer: None. The patient has WPW. ***For practical purposes, nothing can be said about the possibility of acute injury or ischemia in the presence of WPW.***

• • •

The most important aspect of recognizing WPW is to avoid misdiagnosing the patient as having a number of other ECG conditions. Other conditions may be recognized only if (when) conduction down the accessory pathway is intermittent.

The other important aspect of WPW is the propensity such patients have for certain cardiac arrhythmias. Antiarrhythmic treatment may have to be adjusted accordingly. For example, drugs such as verapamil and digoxin are extremely effective in slowing conduction down the normal pathway (through the AV node), but may paradoxically accelerate conduction of tachyarrhythmias that travel down the accessory pathway.

BOTTOM LINE: *Be aware of WPW. Remember how to recognize it, because you WILL see cases from time to time.*

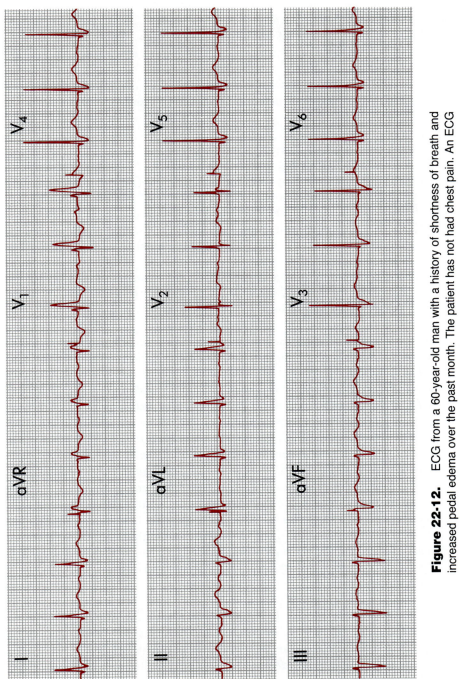

Figure 22-12. ECG from a 60-year-old man with a history of shortness of breath and increased pedal edema over the past month. The patient has not had chest pain. An ECG recorded a year ago was completely normal.

Interpretation of Figure 22-12

Descriptive analysis. Except for the eighth beat (which is early), there is a regular sinus rhythm at a rate of about 80 beats/minute. The PR interval is 0.24 second in duration. The QRS complex is widened and demonstrates an rSR′ in lead V_1 and S waves (albeit relatively narrow ones) in leads I and V_6. There is pathologic LAD. There is no evidence of chamber enlargement. There are Q waves in leads I, aVL, and V_3 through V_6. T waves are flattened in several leads.

Clinical impression. Sinus rhythm and a PAC. 1° AV block, RBBB, and LAHB. Possible old anterolateral infarction. NS ST-T Abns. *Changes do not appear acute.*

Questions to Further Understanding

1. *Is QRST morphology in Figure 22-12 suggestive of "typical" RBBB?*

    Answer: As suggested by Figures 5-8 and 5-9 *(pocket reference pp 14 and 15)*, QRST morphology suggests "typical" RBBB because:

    The QRS complex is widened (to ≥0.11 second).

    QRS morphology in the three key leads (I, V_1, and V_6) is as expected for RBBB (rSR′ in lead V_1, and a terminal S wave in leads I and V_6).

    There are typical secondary ST-T wave changes of RBBB in these three key leads (i.e., orientation of the ST segment and T wave is opposite that of the last QRS deflection).

2. *How can you tell at a glance that there is LAHB in addition to RBBB?*

    Answer: We define *pathologic* LAD as an axis more leftward than −30°. For practical purposes, we equate pathologic LAD with LAHB. *One can diagnose LAHB at a glance simply by looking at lead II:* **If lead II is more negative than positive, the patient has LAHB.**

    Our rationale for this statement is as follows: Lead II is located at +60° (see *Figure 7-14, on pocket reference p. 19*). We know that if the QRS complex is isoelectric (= equiphasic = equal parts positive and negative) in a particular lead, the axis must be perpendicular to (90° away from) this lead. Thus, if the QRS complex in lead II is isoelectric, the axis must be 90° away, or at −30° *(Table 7-2, on pocket reference p. 21)*. If the QRS complex in lead II is more negative than positive, then the axis must lie slightly *more* than 90° away from lead II—which puts it more leftward than −30°. *Since the QRS complex in lead II of Figure 22-12 is clearly more negative than positive, the patient has LAHB.*

3. *What is trifascicular block? Is it present in Figure 22-12?*

    Answer: The three basic conduction fascicles are the *right bundle branch,* the *left anterior hemidivision* of the left bundle branch, and the *left posterior hemidivision* of the left bundle branch. The term **trifascicular block** implies impaired conduction in each of these three fascicles. In Figure 22-12, there is block in *both* the right bundle branch (i.e., RBBB) and the left anterior hemidivision of the left bundle branch (i.e., LAHB). This means that the electrical impulse must travel down the posterior hemidivision of the left bundle branch (since this is the only one of the three conduction fascicles that isn't blocked). However, the fact that there is 1° AV block in addition to RBBB and LAHB means that conduction down this one remaining fascicle is delayed.

Thus, there is trifascicular block:
   a. RBBB
   b. LAHB
   c. Delayed conduction (manifested by 1° AV block) down the remaining fascicle

Clinically, the more fascicles with impaired conduction, the greater the chance a patient will develop complete AV block. This is especially true in patients with acute infarction.

4. *Is there evidence of infarction in Figure 22-12? of acute infarction?*

   Answer: Yes, there is evidence of infarction. As opposed to LBBB, Q waves can readily be seen with RBBB. Q waves are present in leads I, aVL, and V_3 through V_6 on this tracing. Although these Q waves could represent "normal septal depolarization," they are somewhat larger than normal septal q waves and are found in more leads than one might normally expect. Considering that the patient previously had a normal ECG and has had symptoms of heart failure over the past month, it is likely that he sustained a recent infarction (which would explain the trifascicular block and anterolateral Q waves). However, the lack of *acute* ST-T wave changes (absence of ST segment elevation or deep T wave inversion) suggests that the infarction took place some time ago, and is consistent with the history of symptom onset a month ago.

5. *Can you diagnose LVH in the presence of complete RBBB?*

   Answer: Sometimes, although it is generally much harder to do so than when there is no conduction defect. Because RBBB produces an R′ (terminal upright) deflection in lead V_1, criteria that use S wave deepening in leads V_1 or V_2 will not be helpful. However, if the R wave exceeds 12 mm in lead aVL, 25 mm in lead V_5, or 20 mm in lead V_6, LVH is probably present *(Tables 9-1 and 9-2, on pocket reference p. 22)*. This is not the case in Figure 22-12.

6. *Can you diagnose RVH in the presence of complete RBBB?*

   Answer: Maybe. Some clinicians feel that the presence of a right-sided conduction defect such as RBBB makes it impossible to diagnose concommitant RVH. Others believe that the presence of RVH can be suspected in patients with RBBB if the R′ (terminal upright) deflection in lead V_1 exceeds 15 mm, especially if there is also RAA. There is no RAA in Figure 22-12, and the R′ (terminal upright) deflection in lead V_1 is much less than 15 mm tall.

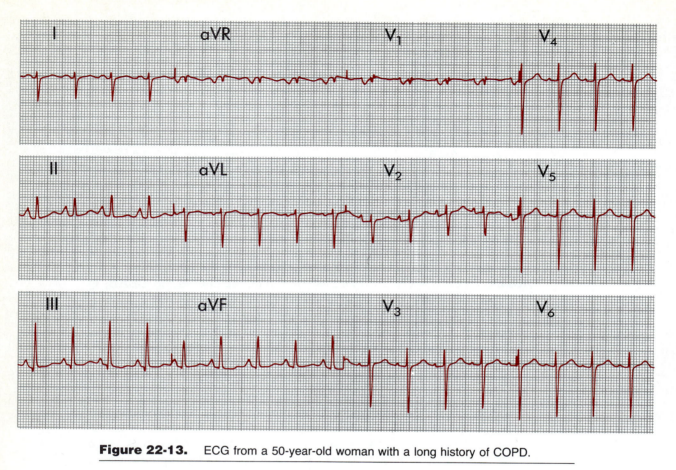

Figure 22-13.   ECG from a 50-year-old woman with a long history of COPD.

Interpretation of Figure 22-13

Descriptive analysis. The rhythm is sinus tachycardia, at a rate of about 115 beats/minute. PR and QRS intervals are normal. (The tachycardia makes it difficult to comment on QT interval duration.) There is definite RAD (since the QRS complex is markedly negative in lead I). P waves are tall and peaked in the pulmonary leads (II, III, and aVF), and there is a very deep terminal negative component to the P wave in lead V_1. There is an rSr' pattern in lead V_1, R wave progression is poor (i.e., transition never occurs), and S waves persist across the precordial leads (with deep S waves still present in leads V_5 and V_6). Finally, there is a small q wave in lead III, and nonspecific ST-T wave flattening in the inferior leads.

Clinical impression. Sinus tachycardia. Biatrial abnormality (RAA and LAA). Incomplete RBBB. Probable RVH. *Nonspecific ST-T wave abnormalities that do not appear acute.*

Questions to Further Understanding

1. *How does one diagnose RVH by ECG? Why is this a hard diagnosis to make electrocardiographically in adults?*

    Answer: Electrocardiographic diagnosis of RVH is often extremely difficult in adults. This is because the left ventricle is normally three times as thick as the right ventricle and has 10 times the electrical mass of the right ventricle. As a result, right ventricular forces must increase greatly before they ever make their presence known. One rarely sees RVH on an adult ECG unless the patient has marked pulmonary hypertension or long-standing (and end-stage) pulmonary disease.

    In contrast, RVH is much easier to diagnose in children. Because right ventricular electrical mass is comparable to left ventricular mass in young children, it is much easier to demonstrate a relative increase in ventricular chamber size at a much earlier stage in the process.

    The most definitive electrocardiographic findings of RVH are a predominant R wave in lead V_1 and right ventricular strain (i.e., asymmetric ST segment depression in the anterior and/or inferior leads). As we indicated above, in adults the predominance of left ventricular mass makes it unlikely that these two findings will be seen until late in the process. As a result, diagnosis of RVH in adults usually has to be made *indirectly* by detection of a constellation of other findings, including RAA, RAD or indeterminate axis, incomplete RBBB, low voltage, or persistent precordial S waves *(Table 9-3, on pocket reference p. 25)*. The collective appearance of most of these supportive findings in Figure 22-13, especially in view of the patient's history, strongly suggests RVH.

2. *Why do we say there is incomplete RBBB?*

    Answer: Complete RBBB is diagnosed by the finding of QRS widening (of ≥ 0.11 second) with appropriate QRS morphology (rSR′ or "RBBB equivalent" in lead V_1, wide terminal S wave in leads I and V_6) in the three key leads *(see Figure 5-8, on pocket reference p. 14)*. QRS morphology in Figure 22-13 is consistent with RBBB: there is an rsr′ in lead V_1 and definite S waves in leads I and V_6. However, the QRS complex is not widened enough to satisfy criteria for complete RBBB. Therefore, there is *incomplete RBBB*.

    In many patients, the right ventricular outflow tract is the last portion of the ventricles to depolarize. This is especially likely to be the case in patients with increased right ventricular forces, and explains why a terminal upright (r′ or R′) deflection is commonly seen in right-sided lead V_1 with RVH.

3. *Why do patients with pulmonary disease often have poor R wave progression?*

    Answer: Normally, the heart lies to the left and posteriorly in the thoracic cavity. With long-standing pulmonary disease, the heart's electrical axis tends to rotate posteriorly and to the right. As a result, the QRS complex no longer becomes taller (i.e., R waves no longer "progress") as one moves across the precordial leads. Instead, transition is often delayed, and deep S waves may persist in the lateral precordial leads. Thus, the deep S waves in leads V_5 and V_6 of Figure 22-13 suggest a large amount of electrical activity lying *away* from these left-sided leads (or toward the right), and are consistent with increased right ventricular forces.

4. *Why do patients with COPD often have low voltage? Is there low voltage in Figure 22-13?*

   Answer: Patients with emphysema tend to have large, "barrel-shaped" chests as a result of chronic air trapping because of their disease process. We think of the heart as being "insulated" by air, as well as being anatomically separated by a greater distance from the chest wall. As a result, QRS amplitude may decrease. Technically, **low voltage** is said to be present only if QRS amplitude does not exceed 5 mm (one large box) in any of the six limb leads (I, II, III, aVR, aVL, and aVF). This is clearly not the case in Figure 22-13.

   The other clinical condition in which low voltage is commonly seen is obesity. In this case, decreased QRS amplitude is thought to result from increased thickening of the chest wall.

5. *How does one diagnose RAA by ECG?*

   Answer: RAA (or **P-P**ulmonale) is diagnosed by the finding of **p**rominent ($\geq$2.5 mm tall) P waves in the **p**ulmonary leads (II, III, and aVF). *If the P wave looks uncomfortable to sit on in lead II, think of RAA (Figure 9-2, on pocket reference p. 24).*

6. *What is the difference between RAA and RAE? between LAA and LAE?*

   Answer: **RAA** and **LAA** stand for right and left atrial **a**bnormality. **RAE** and **LAE** stand for right and left atrial **e**nlargement. It is important to realize that conditions other than true atrial chamber enlargement may give rise to abnormal (or unusual) P wave morphology. The beauty of the terms RAA and LAA is that they allow for etiologies other than true atrial chamber enlargement as the cause of alterations in P wave morphology. Thus, it may be preferable to say that an otherwise healthy young adult with "funny looking P waves" has RAA (rather than RAE), because such P waves may have nothing to do with actual atrial chamber enlargement. *Practically speaking, the terms RAA and RAE (and LAA and LAE) are often used interchangeably.*

7. *How many clinical conditions produce right atrial enlargement (RAE) without also producing right ventricular enlargement (RVH)?*

   Answer: The only clinical condition likely to produce RAA without also producing RVH is triscuspid stenosis. Thus, the finding of RAE, especially in patients with pulmonary disease, provides indirect evidence that the patient also has RVH.

· · ·

We emphasize again that RVH is often an extremely difficult diagnosis to make electrocardiographically in adults. Unless there is marked pulmonary hypertension or long-standing (and end-stage) pulmonary disease, ECG diagnosis of RVH will usually have to be made *indirectly* by detection of a constellation of findings, rather than from any one particular finding.

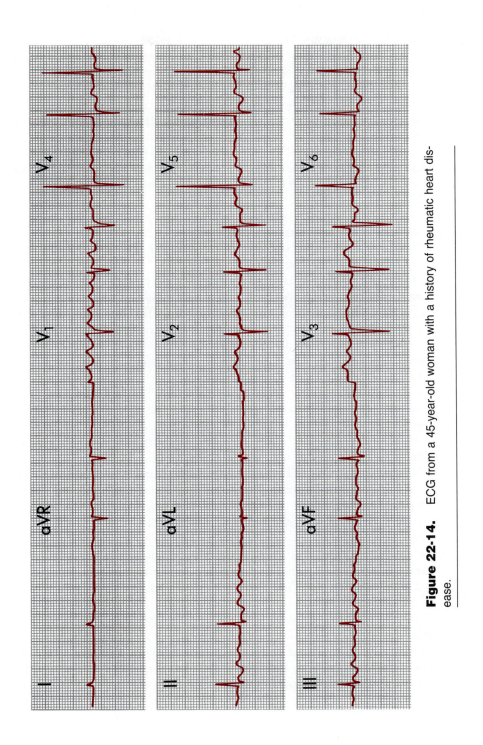

Figure 22-14.   ECG from a 45-year-old woman with a history of rheumatic heart disease.

Interpretation of Figure 22-14

Descriptive analysis. The rhythm is irregularly irregular. Although there are coarse undulations in the baseline in several leads, definite P waves are absent. The QRS interval is normal, and the QT interval does not appear to be prolonged. (There is no PR interval to speak of because of the rhythm.) The axis is normal (and approximately $+70°$). There is no chamber enlargement. There is an isolated Q wave in lead aVL. R wave progression is normal (with transition between leads V_3 and V_4). Interpretation of ST segments and T waves is difficult because of the variable baseline, but there appears to be ST segment depression and T wave inversion in several leads.

Clinical impression. Atrial fibrillation (or atrial "fib-flutter") with a controlled ventricular response. Nonspecific ST-T wave Abns, possibly ischemic. *Suggest clinical correlation.*

Questions to Further Understanding

1. *Atrial activity in lead V_1 suggests flutter. Is the rhythm in Figure 22-14 atrial fibrillation, atrial flutter, or "fib-flutter"?*

    Answer: Atrial flutter is an organized (reentry) atrial tachyarrhythmia that usually produces extremely regular atrial activity *(flutter waves)* at a rate of approximately 300 beats/minute in adults. In contrast, atrial fibrillation is a totally disorganized atrial rhythm with an even faster rate of atrial discharge (usually 400 to 600 atrial impulses/minute) that may produce coarse undulations in the baseline *(fib waves)* in one or more monitoring leads.

    Sometimes, coarse irregular "fib waves" and organized "flutter waves" occur in the same tracing. This is the case in Figure 22-14. It looks like the patient is in atrial fibrillation in all leads except in V_1, where fairly regular, sawtooth atrial activity suggests atrial flutter. Some clinicians have adopted the term "atrial fib-flutter" to acknowledge this pattern. Others insist that atrial fibrillation and atrial flutter can't coexist, and describe the pattern as atrial fibrillation (or "coarse" atrial fibrillation). We feel that both sides have a point. Clinically, the rhythm behaves as if it were atrial fibrillation.

2. *Is the Q wave in lead aVL likely to be of any significance?*

    Answer: No. The isolated occurrence of a Q wave in lead aVL is of no clinical significance. *(See Table 10-3, on pocket reference p. 27).*

3. *What can be said about the appearance of ST segments and T waves in this tracing?*

    Answer: Because of the coarse undulations in the baseline (from atrial activity), it is hard to interpret ST-T wave changes in Figure 22-14. Nevertheless, there appears to be some ST segment depression, which might reflect ischemia, strain, digitalis effect, or an electrolyte abnormality *(See List #3 on pocket reference p. 39).* Clinical correlation is needed.

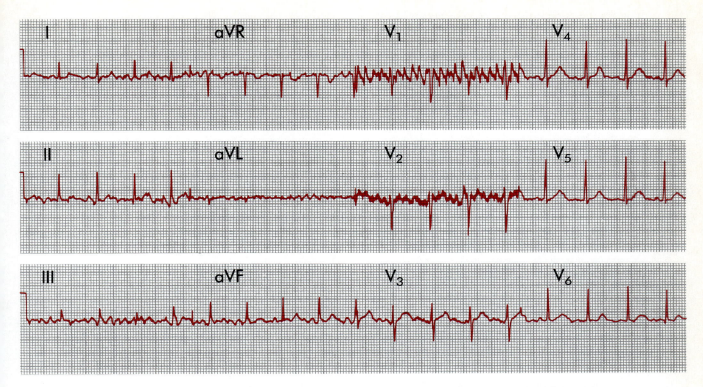

Figure 22-15. ECG from a 60-year-old man with a history of coronary artery disease.

Interpretation of Figure 22-15

Descriptive analysis. The ventricular response is regular, at a rate of about 110 beats/minute. The axis is normal. There is no evidence of LVH. *Nothing else can really be said!*

Clinical impression. Regular, supraventricular rhythm at 110 beats/minute. *MUCH ARTIFACT.* Suggest repeat ECG!

Questions to Further Understanding

1. *Is the patient in atrial fibrillation? Or did he go into ventricular tachycardia in lead V_1?*

   Answer: The gross undulations in the baseline of this tracing represent artifact. The regularity of the rhythm argues against atrial fibrillation. The fact that the QRS complex can be seen to march through the interference in lead V_1, and that a more normal pattern is seen in simultaneously recorded lead V_3, rules out ventricular tachycardia. However, the main point we want to illustrate (and the reason we chose to include this tracing) is that *very little useful clinical information can be obtained from an ECG distorted by this much artifact.* The course we recommend in such cases is to:

   a. ***Avoid trying to interpret a tracing filled with artifact.***
   b. Try to obtain another ECG with less artifact. This may or may not be possible, depending on the cause of the artifact.

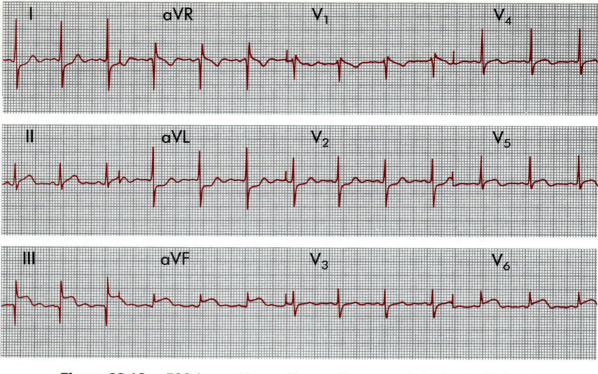

Figure 22-16.   ECG from a 45-year-old man with new-onset chest pain of 3 hours' duration.

Interpretation of Figure 22-16

Descriptive analysis. There is a regular sinus rhythm at 85 beats/minute. All intervals are normal. The axis is normal (and approximately 40° to 50°). There is no evidence of chamber enlargement. There is a Q wave in lead III. Transition is early (occurring between leads V_1 and V_2). There is an rSr' complex in lead V_1. The most remarkable finding on the tracing is the ST segment coving and elevation (especially in leads III, aVF, V_5, and V_6). Finally, there is ST segment depression in leads I and aVL, and to a smaller extent in lead V_2.

Clinical impression. Sinus rhythm. rSr' *(incomplete RBBB)* in lead V_1. Acute inferolateral infarction.

Questions to Further Understanding

1. *What is the most likely explanation for the ST segment depression seen in leads I, aVL, and V_2?*

    Answer: ST segment depression in leads I, aVL, and V_2 is likely to reflect *reciprocal* changes *(see Figure 12-1, D, on pocket reference p. 34)*. Considering ECG evidence of acute inferior infarction, two other possible causes of ST segment depression in lead V_2 are concomitant *anterior ischemia* and *posterior infarction (List #5 on pocket reference p. 41)*.

2. *Are the ST segments abnormal in leads II and V₄?*

> **Answer:** Viewed alone, the ST segments in leads II and V_4 do not appear all that abnormal. The key is to interpret the ST segments in these leads in context. ***View patterns of leads.*** The three inferior leads are II, III, and aVF. Considering obvious abnormalities in leads III and aVF, the straightening, slight coving, and elevation of the ST segment in lead II are likely to be significant and consistent with an acute injury current. Similarly, one should look at lead V_4 in the context of changes occurring in its neighboring leads. The ST segment is definitely coved *("frowny")* and elevated in leads V_5 and V_6. In this context, it is extremely likely that the ever-so-slight ST segment coving and shallow T wave inversion in lead V_4 are significant.

3. *Could you "date" the infarction?*

> **Answer:** Both the electrocardiographic picture and the clinical history (new-onset chest pain of 3 hours' duration) strongly suggest that the infarction is acute *(see Table 12-2, on pocket reference p. 33).* That is, there is coved ST segment elevation with "hyperacute" changes in leads aVF and V_6, as well as reciprocal ST segment depression in several leads. Although it often takes some time for Q waves as deep as the one in lead III to develop, the overall picture is most consistent with acute infarction, probably beginning at the time of symptom onset.

4. *Is the patient a candidate for thrombolytic therapy? an optimal candidate?*

> **Answer:** Assuming there were no contraindications to thrombolytic therapy, this patient would seem to be a good (if not excellent) candidate for such treatment *(Tables 12-3 and 12-4, on pocket reference pp. 35 and 36).* He is young (45 years old), symptom onset is recent (3 hours ago), and the initial ECG suggests a large, potentially reversible infarction (marked ST segment elevation with involvement of inferior *and* lateral walls, reciprocal changes, and Q waves in only one lead).

5. *Why do we say that the axis is between 40° and 50°?*

> **Answer:** Calculation of axis is made difficult when deep Q waves or deep S waves offset R wave deflections. This is the case in lead I of Figure 22-16. Nevertheless, the *net* QRS deflection in this lead is approximately 5 mm (R wave height of 15 mm minus the S wave depth of 10 mm). Since this net deflection is about the same as the net deflection of the QRS complex in lead aVF (which displays an R wave 4 mm tall), the axis must be almost midway between lead I (at 0°) and lead aVF (at 90°), or at about +40° to +50°.

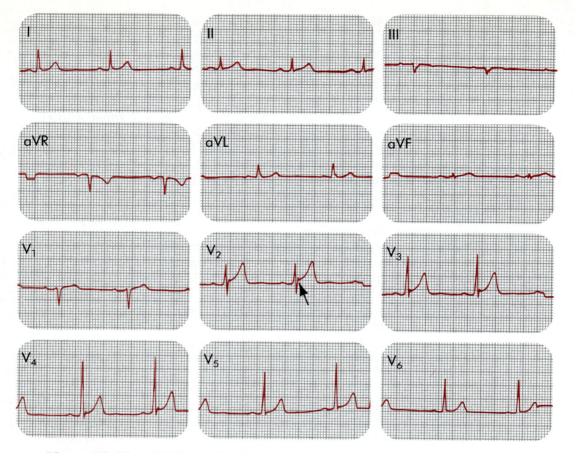

Figure 22-17.   ECG from a healthy 40-year-old man that was obtained during an employment physical. He is completely asymptomatic. Physical examination is normal. There is no prior tracing.

Interpretation of Figure 22-17

Descriptive analysis. The rhythm is slightly irregular, at a rate between 55 and 60 beats/minute. The mechanism is sinus. All intervals are normal. The axis is normal (and approximately $+10°$ to $+20°$). There is no evidence of chamber enlargement. There are no Q waves. Transition occurs early (between leads V_1 and V_2). The ST segment is almost flat in lead III, and slightly elevated with an upward concavity (i.e., "*smiley*") and J point notching in leads V_2 through V_5. There is no ST segment depression.

Clinical impression. Sinus arrhythmia. "J point" ST segment elevation and notching that probably reflects the normal variant of *early repolarization*. NPT. *Suggest clinical correlation.*

Questions to Further Understanding

1. *What is "J point" ST segment elevation? What is early repolarization?*

    Answer: The **J** point **j**oins the end of the S wave of the QRS complex with the beginning of the ST segment. ST segment elevation of the J point is an extremely common electrocardiographic finding. When J point elevation is associated with an upward concavity ("smiley" appearance) of the ST segment and occurs in an otherwise healthy, asymptomatic young adult, it almost always reflects the normal variant known as *early repolarization.* Diagnosis of early repolarization is virtually clinched in this clinical setting if there is also *notching* of the J point *(Figure 10-14, B, on pocket reference p. 31).*

2. *Why is the ST segment elevation in Figure 22-17 unlikely to reflect acute infarction? Can you be sure?*

    Answer: ST segment elevation in leads V_2 to V_5 of Figure 22-17 most likely represents early repolarization, because the patient is relatively young (40 years old), healthy, and asymptomatic, and the involved ST segments demonstrate an upward concavity ("smiley") with J point notching *(arrow in Figure 22-17).* It is extremely unlikely for an acute injury current to have this shape of ST segment elevation with J point notching. Moreover, Q waves and the reciprocal ST segment changes that commonly accompany acute infarction are absent. Nevertheless, if this patient had presented with new-onset chest pain and no prior tracing, one could not rule out the possibility that ST segment elevation might represent acute injury. In such a case, the patient might need to be admitted to the hospital until the picture could be clarified. *The importance of* **clinical correlation** *for interpreting the meaning of ECG findings is obvious from this example.*

3. *Could the patient have pericarditis?*

    Answer: Yes, although this would be extremely unlikely, considering the history in this case. The presentation of acute pericarditis is varied. Nevertheless, clinical history and physical examination usually provide the key clues to the diagnosis. Patients with pericarditis tend to be younger than those with acute infarction, and typically give a history of pleuritic chest pain in association with a viral illness. Detection of a pericardial friction rub solidifies the diagnosis.

    There are four electrocardiographic stages in pericarditis *(pocket reference p. 46).* The earliest stage is characterized by diffuse ST segment elevation in virtually all leads except aVR, V_1, and III *(Figure 15-1, on pocket reference p. 46).* Despite the fact that ST segment elevation is lacking in the limb leads in Figure 22-17, one would have to include pericarditis in the differential diagnosis if the history was suggestive. However, considering that this ECG comes from an otherwise healthy, asymptomatic 40-year-old man with a normal physical examination, the likelihood of pericarditis is exceedingly small. Finding a prior tracing with similar J point ST segment elevation in the anterior leads would rule it out.

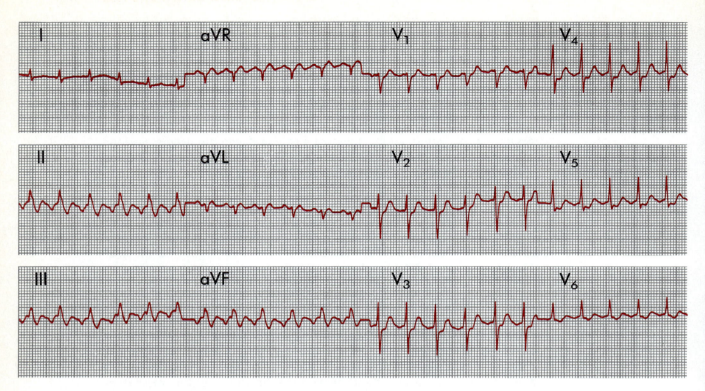

Figure 22-18.   ECG from a 60-year-old woman with "palpitations."

Interpretation of Figure 22-18

Descriptive analysis. There is a regular rhythm at a rate of 140 beats/minute. Atrial activity is not "normal" (since P waves are not upright in lead II). The QRS complex does not appear to be widened (since it is not *greater* than half a large box in any lead). Considering the rapid rate, measurement of the QT interval is not meaningful. The axis is normal (since the QRS complex is upright in leads I and aVF), but it is hard to accurately estimate because of the undulations in the baseline. There is no evidence of ventricular enlargement. (One can't comment on atrial abnormality, considering the lack of normal atrial activity.) There are no Q waves, R wave progression is normal (with transition occurring between leads V_3 and V_4), and there is ST segment depression in a number of leads.

Clinical impression. SVT at a rate of 140 beats/minute. NS ST-T Abns.

Questions to Further Understanding

1. *What is the rhythm most likely to be?*

   Answer: Our approach to arrhythmia diagnosis in this example is similar to the approach we suggested in our answer to Figure 22-7. Thus, the three main entities to consider in the differential diagnosis for this regular SVT are:

   a. Sinus tachycardia
   b. Atrial flutter
   c. PSVT

The rhythm in Figure 22-18 is not sinus tachycardia, because the P wave is not upright in lead II. PSVT should be considered as a possibility, but this is not the answer.

As we have previously emphasized, **suspect atrial flutter until proven otherwise whenever you have a regular SVT at a rate of about 150 beats/minute, especially if you are uncertain about atrial activity.** The heart rate in Figure 22-18 is 140 beats/minute. On close inspection, *flutter waves* can be seen in each of the inferior leads. There are two negative deflections (flutter waves) for each QRS complex. Thus, the rhythm is *atrial flutter with 2:1 AV conduction*.

NOTE: *We have already seen this arrhythmia!* We presented a rhythm strip of lead I from Figure 22-18 as an unknown in Figure 19A-1, and indicated atrial activity with arrows in a simultaneously recorded lead II rhythm strip (Figure 19A-2).

2. *Clinically, what could be done to verify your answer to Question #1?*

   Answer: A vagal maneuver could be performed at the bedside *(under constant ECG monitoring!)* in an attempt to slow AV conduction and bring out the flutter waves. *(Figure 3-31, B, shows the effect of carotid sinus massage on atrial flutter.)*

3. *What are the likely causes of the ST segment depression in this tracing?*

   Answer: Some of the ST segment depression in Figure 22-18 is likely to be due to superposition of the negative flutter waves on the ST segment. In addition, one needs to consider the common causes of ST segment depression. These are ischemia, strain, digitalis effect, hypokalemia (and/or hypomagnesemia), and rate-related changes *(List #3 on pocket reference p. 39)*. Voltage criteria for LVH are not satisfied in Figure 22-18. We don't know enough about the patient clinically to comment on the likelihood of the other causes listed. Comparison of a postconversion 12-lead ECG with this tracing would be helpful in determining how much of the ST segment depression was due to the rapid heart rate.

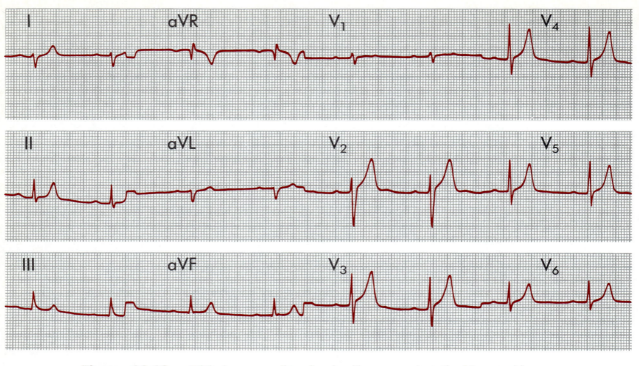

Figure 22-19. ECG from an otherwise healthy, asymptomatic 30-year-old man. Physical examination is normal. He is on no medications. There is no prior tracing.

Interpretation of Figure 22-19

Descriptive analysis. The rhythm is slightly irregular, at a rate of between 50 and 55 beats/minute. The mechanism is sinus. There is RAD (since the QRS complex is upright in lead aVF, but *negative* in lead I). There is no evidence of chamber enlargement. There are no Q waves. R wave progression is normal (with transition occurring between leads V_2 and V_3). There is some J point ST segment elevation in leads V_2 and V_3, and T waves are somewhat prominent. There is no ST segment depression.

Clinical impression. Sinus bradycardia and arrhythmia. RAD. Probable repolarization variant. *Suggest clinical correlation.*

Questions to Further Understanding

1. *What is the significance of the RAD in this clinical setting?*

   Answer: Although RAD is one of the ECG signs of RVH, there is no other evidence of RVH in this tracing *(Table 9-3, on pocket reference p. 25)*. That is, there is no RAA, right ventricular strain, or tall R wave in lead V_1. Low voltage is not present. S waves persist and are seen in leads V_5 and V_6, but they are not nearly deep enough to suggest RVH. Furthermore, RVH would be unexpected in an otherwise healthy, asymptomatic 30-year-old individual without a heart murmur. Thus, it is probable that the RAD in this tracing is of no clinical significance.

2. *Why is the ST segment elevation in leads V$_2$ and V$_3$ unlikely to represent acute infarction?*

> **Answer:** There are several reasons why the ST segment elevation in leads V$_2$ and V$_3$ is unlikely to represent acute infarction. First, 1 to 3 mm of ST segment elevation is commonly seen as a normal phenomenon in these leads. The upward concavity ("smiley" configuration) of the ST segment strongly suggests its benign nature *(Figure 10-15, on pocket reference p. 28)*. There are no Q waves or reciprocal ST segment changes on the tracing. Finally, the clinical history of the ECG, coming from an otherwise healthy, asymptomatic 30-year-old man, argues strongly against any pathology.

3. *Could the patient have hyperkalemia?*

> **Answer:** Possibly, but highly unlikely. Although T waves in Figure 22-19 are prominent, they are not pointed, and they have a wide base *(Figure 10-16, B and C, on pocket reference p. 29)*. In contrast, the T waves of hyperkalemia tend to be pointed, and have a narrow base with symmetric ascending and descending limbs *(Figure 14-1, on pocket reference p. 45)*. Moreover, there is no reason for an otherwise healthy, asymptomatic 30-year-old individual on no medications to be hyperkalemic *(Table 14-1, on pocket reference p. 44)*.

• • •

The importance of clinical correlation should be obvious from this example. If one were asked to interpret the identical ECG in a different clinical setting, the RAD might suggest RVH, and the ST segment elevation and T wave prominence might suggest acute anterior infarction/ischemia and/or hyperkalemia. In the setting of an otherwise healthy, asymptomatic 30-year-old man, the ECG probably reflects a normal variant.

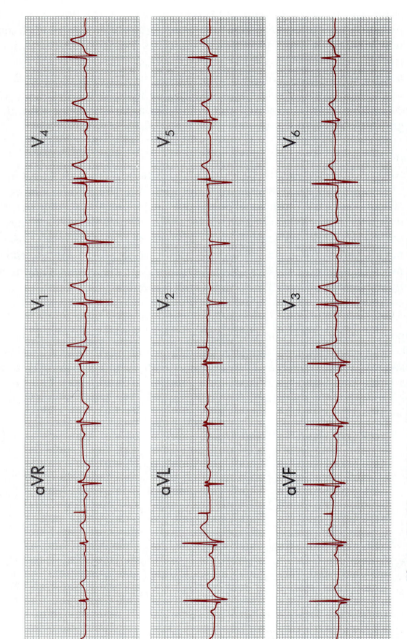

Figure 22-20.   ECG from a 60-year-old woman presenting with new-onset chest pain. She is on no medications. There is no prior tracing.

Interpretation of Figure 22-20

Descriptive analysis. There is a regular sinus rhythm at 70 beats/minute. All intervals are normal. The axis is normal (and approximately $+70°$ to $+80°$). There is no evidence of chamber enlargement. There are q waves in the inferior leads. R wave progression is unusual (i.e., the R wave is relatively tall in lead V_1, virtually disappears in lead V_2, and abruptly returns again in lead V_3). ST segments are slightly coved (but not elevated) in leads II, III, and aVF. There is ST segment flattening in lead V_2. T waves are somewhat prominent in leads V_1, V_3, and V_4.

Clinical impression. Sinus rhythm. Inferior infarction of ? age, possibly recent. Suspect precordial lead misplacement (vs posterior involvement). NPT. *Suggest clinical correlation.*

Questions to Further Understanding

1. *Should the patient be admitted to the hospital?*

    Answer: Yes, since this ECG is consistent with inferior infarction of unknown age. Although there is no ST segment elevation or reciprocal ST segment depression, subtle coving of the ST segments in the inferior leads could be an acute change. The finding of small q waves in each of these inferior leads should add to this concern. Considering the history (new-onset chest pain in a 60-year-old woman) and the absence of a prior tracing, it is impossible to tell if these changes are new. The patient should be admitted to rule out acute infarction.

2. *Is the patient a candidate for thrombolytic therapy?*

    Answer: Probably not. The patient does not demonstrate *definite* ECG evidence of acute infarction, since there is no ST segment elevation *(Table 12-3, on pocket reference p. 35).*

3. *Why should you suspect lead misplacement? How could you verify your suspicion?*

    Answer: There is no evidence of limb lead misplacement *(pocket reference p. 48).* However, R wave progression is highly suspect. Normally, the R wave becomes progressively taller as one moves across the precordial leads, at least until lead V_4 *(Figure 10-3, on pocket reference p. 30).* This is not the case in Figure 22-20, where the R wave abruptly loses amplitude from lead V_1 to V_2 before regaining it in lead V_3. In addition to the loss of R wave between leads V_1 and V_2, note how T wave amplitude is lost and then regained. *Wouldn't R wave (and T wave) progression look more natural if leads V_1 and V_2 were interchanged?* This is precisely what has happened: somehow precordial lead V_2 was placed in the V_1 recording position, and V_1 was placed in the V_2 recording position.

    It is easy to verify whether lead misplacement has occurred. Simply repeat the ECG and compare the leads in question on the two tracings. *(Ideally, the patient should not be charged for this repeat ECG if the mistake was ours.)*

4. *What is the likely cause of the prominent T waves in the anterior leads?*

Answer: Considering the error in precordial lead misplacement (i.e., that lead V_1 is really lead V_2), there are prominent T waves in leads V_2 through V_4. This finding should suggest three entities:

    a. Hyperkalemia
    b. Normal variant
    c. Ischemia

T wave prominence in several leads should always raise the possibility of hyperkalemia *(Figure 14-1, on pocket reference p. 44).* Although the clinical setting in this case would not be expected to produce hyperkalemia, we would still consider it worthwhile to check the patient's serum potassium value.

However, **all that produces tall, peaked T waves is NOT necessarily hyperkalemia!** T waves may appear prominent in certain normal (repolarization) variants *(Figure 10-16, C, on pocket reference p. 29).* The ECG in Figure 22-20, however, is not otherwise normal. Considering the possibility of recent inferior infarction, the most likely cause of the prominent anterior T waves would seem to be ischemia. As we discussed in "Potential Pitfalls in the ECG Diagnosis of Hyperkalemia" in Chapter 14, anterior T wave prominence may reflect a positive mirror test. *(If you flipped Figure 22-20 upside down, wouldn't the precordial T waves be deeply and symmetrically inverted?)*

Challenge Tracings

The ECGs in this chapter offer an additional opportunity to apply what you've learned. Approach these 25 tracings as you did the tracings in Chapter 22—*systematically*, and by *writing out* your interpretation *BEFORE* looking at our responses. Some of these tracings may be a bit more complex than those in the previous chapter. *Are you up to the challenge?*

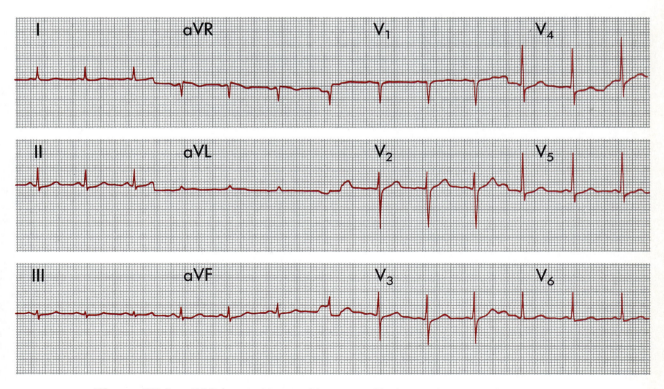

Figure 23-1. ECG from a 60-year-old woman with chest pain.

Interpretation of Figure 23-1

Descriptive analysis. There is a fairly regular sinus rhythm at a rate of 80 to 85 beats/minute. All intervals are normal. The axis is normal (and approximately 40° to 50°). There is no evidence of chamber enlargement. There are no q waves. R wave progression is normal (with transition occurring between leads V_2 and V_3). There are nonspecific ST segment and T wave abnormalities.

Clinical impression. Sinus rhythm. NS ST-T Abns. *Suggest clinical correlation.*

Questions to Further Understanding

1. *Why do we say that ST segment and T wave changes are "nonspecific"?*

   Answer: The reason we call these changes "nonspecific" is that although the ST segments and T waves are not normal in this tracing, they do not suggest any specific abnormality.

   Normally, T waves are upright in most leads of a 12-lead ECG, and the ST segment gradually slopes upward, blending inperceptibly into the T wave *(Figure 10-16, A, on pocket reference, p. 29)*. Although the change is subtle, T waves in Figure 23-1 are "flatter" than expected in virtually every lead except V_2.

2. *Are these changes new?*

   Answer: The only way to tell if these changes are new would be to compare this tracing with a prior ECG. No mention is made as to whether a prior tracing is available.

3. *Should this patient be admitted to the hospital?*

   Answer: Not because of this ECG. Even if a prior ECG could be found and was entirely normal, nothing definitive could be said about the cause of the nonspecific ST-T wave abnormalities in Figure 23-1. Whether this patient should be admitted to the hospital will depend on how suspicious the history is for an acute ischemic chest pain syndrome.

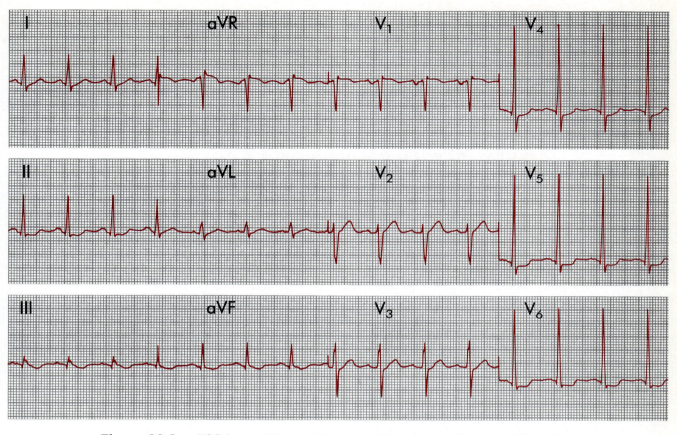

Figure 23-2.   ECG from a 65-year-old woman with new-onset chest pain. The patient is taking multiple medications, including several "heart pills." No prior tracing is available.

Interpretation of Figure 23-2

Descriptive analysis. There is a regular sinus rhythm at a rate of 90 beats/minute. All intervals are normal. The axis is normal (and approximately +40° to 50°). There is a deep, negative component to the P wave in lead V_1. QRS amplitude in the lateral precordial leads is greatly increased (*and measures over 30 mm in lead V_5!*). There are small q waves in the inferolateral leads. R wave progression is normal (with transition occurring between leads V_3 and V_4). There is an rSr′ complex in lead V_1 (with shallow s waves in leads I and V_6). There is ST segment depression in multiple leads.

Clinical impression. Sinus rhythm. rSr′ (or incomplete RBBB) in lead V_1. LAA. LVH and strain and/or ischemia. Possible inferior infarction of ? age. NPT. *Suggest clinical correlation.*

Questions to Further Understanding

1. *Are the q waves in the inferior leads "significant"? How about the q waves in the lateral leads?*

    Answer: The q waves in leads I and V_4 to V_6 should be interpreted as "normal septal q waves." They are small and narrow, and occur in the expected location for normal septal q waves *(see pocket reference p. 3).*

    It is harder to comment on the significance of the q waves in leads II, III, and aVF of this tracing. These inferior q waves are clearly neither wide nor deep. Nevertheless, *each* of these three inferior leads has a q wave, as well as associated ST-T wave changes. Specifically, there appears to be ST segment depression in leads II and aVF, and T wave inversion in lead III. There may also possibly be a small amount of residual ST segment elevation in lead III. *We emphasize that these inferior lead findings are subtle. If you simply noted "nonspecific ST-T wave changes," you're still doing fine!*

2. *Should this patient be admitted to the hospital?*

    Answer: Regardless of how you interpreted the ST-T wave changes in the inferior leads, the ST segment depression in the lateral precordial leads should be cause for concern, especially considering the history (i.e., new-onset chest pain in a 60-year-old woman). Any (or all) of the common causes of ST segment depression may be operative *(List #3 on pocket reference p. 39).* Without the benefit of a prior tracing for comparison, prudence suggests admission to the hospital to rule out an acute ischemic event as the wisest course of action.

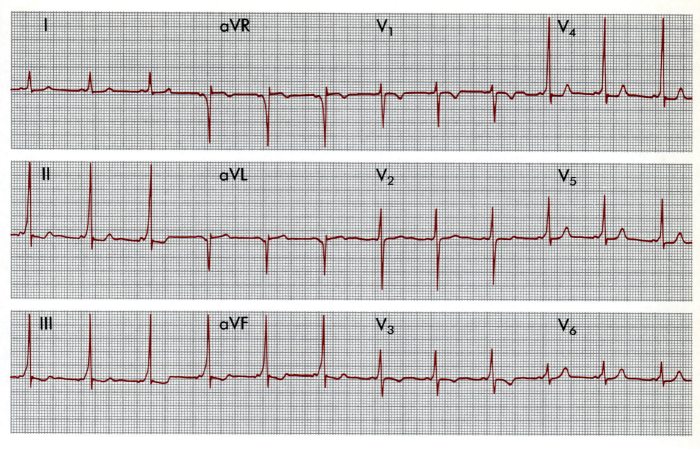

Figure 23-3. ECG from an otherwise healthy 30-year-old man.

Interpretation of Figure 23-3

Descriptive analysis. There is a sinus rhythm at a rate of between 70 to 75 beats/minute. The PR interval is short. The QRS interval is prolonged and marked by an initial slurring *(delta wave)* in many leads.

Clinical impression. Sinus rhythm. WPW *(see pocket reference p. 16)*.

Questions to Further Understanding

1. *Practically speaking, can anything other than "WPW" be said about this tracing?*
   Answer: No.

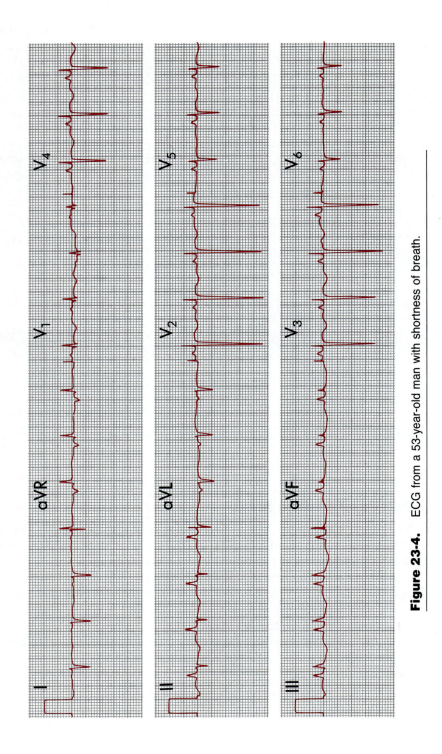

Figure 23-4. ECG from a 53-year-old man with shortness of breath.

Interpretation of Figure 23-4

Descriptive analysis. There is a regular sinus rhythm at a rate of 85 beats/minute. The PR and QRS intervals are normal, but the QT interval appears to be prolonged. There is marked RAD (since the QRS complex is markedly negative in lead I). There is RAA (i.e., very tall, peaked, and "uncomfortable to sit on" P waves in the inferior leads). There is a q wave and a predominant R wave in lead V_1. Deep S waves persist in leads V_5 and V_6. The ST segment is somewhat amorphous in many leads, with shallow (albeit symmetric) T wave inversion anteriorly and inferiorly.

Clinical impression. Sinus rhythm. RAD. RAA. RVH. Prolonged QT interval. Nonspecific ST-T wave changes, possibly ischemic (and/or reflective of right ventricular strain). *Suggest clinical correlation.*

Questions to Further Understanding

1. *List all of the findings on this tracing that support the diagnosis of RVH.*

   Answer: Findings on this tracing that support the diagnosis of RVH include RAA, RAD, relatively low voltage in the limb leads, persistent precordial S waves, a relatively tall R wave in lead V_1, and possible right ventricular strain (*Table 9-3,* on pocket reference p. 25).

2. *What one disease explains all of these findings?*

   Answer: Long-standing and/or severe **pulmonary disease** (i.e., pulmonary hypertension, pulmonary stenosis, end-stage COPD, etc.) is a unifying diagnosis that explains all of these findings.

3. *Why do you suspect that the QT interval is prolonged in this tracing?*

   Answer: Three common causes of QT prolongation to consider are "Drugs/Lytes/CNS" (*List #2 on pocket reference p. 38*). We are not told enough clinical history to know if any of these causes may be operative in this example. QT interval prolongation can also be seen with infarction or ischemia, which is another possibility to consider here.

4. *What is the most likely cause of the T wave inversion in the inferior and anterior leads?*

   Answer: T wave inversion in Figure 23-4 is associated with QT interval prolongation. Therefore, any (or all) of the entities listed in the answer to Question #3 (i.e., Drugs/Lytes/CNS and/or ischemia) should be considered. In addition, inferior and/or anterior T wave inversion could also reflect right ventricular strain, a likely possibility considering the other supportive findings of RVH seen in this example.

5. *What ECG changes are seen with pulmonary embolism?*

   Answer: Most of the time, the 12-lead ECG of a patient with acute **pulmonary embolism** is not diagnostic. The ECG may even be completely normal, especially if the embolus involves only a small portion of the pulmonary vasculature.

   With greater involvement of the pulmonary vasculature, the patient is more likely to be tachycardic and to demonstrate nonspecific ST-T wave abnormalities. Occasionally, there may be the acute onset of rapid atrial fibrillation and/or incomplete or complete RBBB. But the most characteristic ECG finding of acute pulmonary embolism is "acute right heart strain," manifested by rapid development of the findings of RVH. Thus, the ECG picture seen in Figure 23-4 would be consistent with acute pulmonary embolism if these findings were new and development of shortness of breath was sudden.

We emphasize that history plays an essential role in suspecting acute pulmonary embolism, and that the definitive diagnostic tests are a lung scan and/or a pulmonary angiogram. Most of the time, the ECG will be of little diagnostic help in evaluating such patients. Nevertheless, we feel that it should always be done for two reasons:

a. An ECG can rule out acute myocardial infarction as the cause of the sudden onset of shortness of breath.

b. Occasionally, the ECG will strongly suggest the diagnosis of pulmonary embolism (i.e., when there is ECG evidence of "acute right heart strain").

•   •   •

In summary, RVH is a neat diagnosis to make electrocardiographically because it often requires deductive reasoning on the part of the interpreter. It's gratifying to be able to explain virtually all of the abnormalities seen in Figure 23-4 by this one unifying diagnosis.

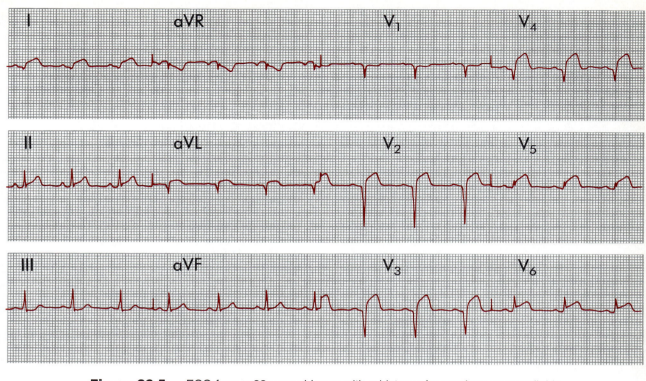

Figure 23-5. ECG from a 38-year-old man with a history of a previous myocardial infarction. He presents at this time after experiencing the sudden onset of severe chest pain 2 hours before. No prior tracing is available.

Interpretation of Figure 23-5

Descriptive analysis. There is a fairly regular sinus rhythm at a rate of between 80 and 85 beats/minute. All intervals are normal. The axis is probably normal (and approximately $+90°$, although it is hard to be sure of the amplitude of the R wave in lead I because of associated ST segment changes in this lead). There is no evidence of chamber enlargement. There are Q waves in leads I, aVL, and V_4, and a QS complex in leads V_1 through V_3 (although, admittedly, in some of these leads it is hard to determine if an R wave is present or if there is just marked ST segment elevation). Transition is delayed (and does not occur until V_4 to V_5). There is marked ST segment elevation with coving in many leads.

Clinical impression. Sinus rhythm. Acute anterolateral infarction.

Questions to Further Understanding

1. *What is the likely location of this patient's previous infarction?*

   Answer: Although it is impossible to answer this question with certainty without availability of a prior ECG, Q waves in the anterior leads are much deeper than one might expect from infarction of only 2 hours' duration. It is therefore quite likely that this patient's previous infarction was anterior. The history and the marked ST segment elevation seen in Figure 23-5 are consistent with a new (second) infarction in the same location.

2. *Is this patient a candidate for thrombolytic therapy? an optimal candidate?*

   Answer: Assuming there were no contraindications to thrombolytic therapy, this patient would be an excellent candidate for it. He is young (38 years old), symptom onset is recent (only 2 hours ago), and there is definite ECG evidence of a large, potentially reversible infarction *(Tables 12-3 and 12-4, pocket reference pp. 35 and 36)*. That is, the infarct is anterior, and there is marked ST segment elevation in multiple leads. Large Q waves are present, but as alluded to above, it is likely that these Q waves reflect the patient's previous anterior infarction.

3. *Is the ECG picture in Figure 23-5 consistent with acute pericarditis?*

   Answer: Stage I of pure, acute pericarditis is characterized by the absence of Q waves and by diffuse ST segment elevation in virtually all leads except aVR, V_1, and III *(Figure 15-1, on pocket reference p. 46)*. The presence of Q waves in multiple leads on this tracing is evidence of prior and/or ongoing infarction. While the clinical history is most consistent with new acute infarction, one could not rule out the possibility of superimposed acute pericarditis. Careful auscultation for the presence of a pericardial friction rub would be extremely helpful in clarifying the picture.

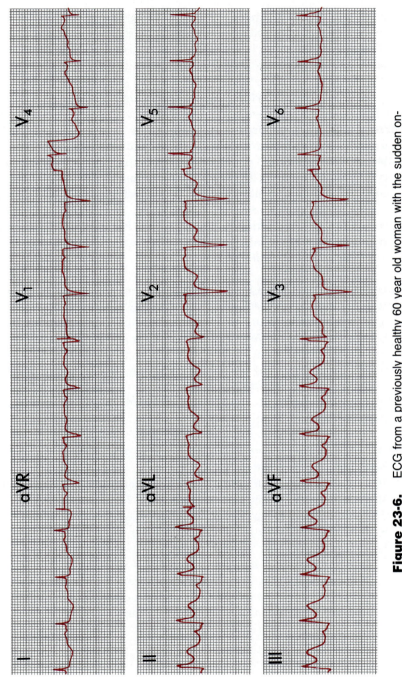
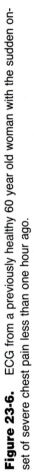

Figure 23-6. ECG from a previously healthy 60 year old woman with the sudden onset of severe chest pain less than one hour ago.

Interpretation of Figure 23-6

Descriptive analysis. There is a regular sinus rhythm at a rate of 85 beats/minute. The PR and QRS intervals are normal, but the QT interval appears to be prolonged. The axis is normal (and approximately +60° to +70°). There is no evidence of chamber enlargement. There are tiny q waves in the inferior leads. Transition is slightly delayed (and doesn't occur until leads V_4 to V_5). There is dramatic, *hyperacute* ST segment elevation in the inferior leads, and ST segment depression in the anterolateral leads, which is most marked in leads aVL, V_2, and V_3.

Clinical impression. Sinus rhythm. Acute inferior infarction.

Questions to Further Understanding

1. *Are the q waves in the inferior leads likely to be significant?*

    Answer: Yes. Although exceedingly small, the inferior q waves are associated with dramatic, hyperacute ST segment elevation that is highly suggestive of acute infarction at its earliest stage *(Figure 12-1, A, on pocket reference p. 34)*. In this context, it is likely that inferior Q waves are just beginning to develop, and that a repeat ECG in several hours (or the next day) will show more established Q waves *(Figure 12-1, C, on pocket reference p. 34)*.

2. *Is this patient a candidate for thrombolytic therapy? an optimal candidate?*

    Answer: Assuming there were no contraindications to thrombolytic therapy, this patient would seem to be an excellent candidate for thrombolytic therapy *(Tables 12-3 and 12-4, on pocket reference pp. 35 and 36)*. She is less than 75 years of age, symptom onset is recent (less than 1 hour ago), and her initial ECG suggests a large, potentially reversible infarction. Despite the infarction's inferior location, there is marked ST segment elevation, diffuse reciprocal changes, and only minimal q wave development.

3. *Which coronary artery would be most likely to demonstrate complete occlusion on acute cardiac catheterization?*

    Answer: Acute inferior infarction is most commonly due to acute occlusion of the right coronary artery *(Figure 12-3, on pocket reference p. 35)*. In addition to supplying the inferior wall of the left ventricle, the right coronary artery usually supplies the right ventricle and the posterior wall of the left ventricle.

    In contrast, acute anterior infarction is most often due to acute occlusion of the left anterior descending branch of the left coronary artery. Acute lateral infarction is most often due to acute occlusion of the circumflex branch of the left coronary artery.

4. *In addition to reciprocal changes, what else might account for the ST segment depression in leads V_2 and V_3 of Figure 23-6?*

Answer: In the setting of acute inferior infarction, there are three common causes of anterior ST segment depression:

   a. Reciprocal changes

   b. Concomitant anterior ischemia (from coronary disease in the left anterior descending branch of the left coronary artery)

   c. Posterior infarction

Any (or all) of these causes may account for the anterior ST segment depression in Figure 23-6 *(List #5 on pocket reference p. 41).*

5. *If the patient was having an infero**posterior** infarction, what might you see in the anterior leads on subsequent ECGs?*

Answer: Posterior infarction often causes an increase in R wave amplitude in the anterior leads. Because of the loss of posterior forces (from the infarction), anterior forces are unopposed. This may result in early transition and/or a tall R wave in lead V_1 *(List #4 on pocket reference p. 39).* Thus, if the patient in Figure 23-6 was having an inferoposterior infarction, R wave amplitude in the anterior leads might be expected to increase on subsequent tracings.

6. *Is this patient also having an acute right ventricular infarction? (How could you verify your answer?)*

Answer: It is hard to detect right ventricular infarction from inspection of the standard leads of a 12-lead ECG. This is because none of the standard leads directly view the right ventricle. The only one that comes close is the right-sided lead V_1 *(Figure 12-8).* To truly be able to view the right ventricle's electrical activity, right-sided precordial leads have to be used. The best lead for this purpose is V_4R. With acute right ventricular infarction, lead V_4R will show a Q wave and ST segment elevation *(Figure 12-11).*

Anatomic landmarks for positioning right-sided chest leads are the same as the ones described in Chapter 1 for left-sided leads. The only difference is that they are mounted on the other side of the chest. Thus, the V_4R recording electrode is placed in the midclavicular line in the fifth *right* interspace *(Figure 12-9).*

We summarize the key electrocardiographic factors to look for with acute right ventricular infarction as follows:

   a. Evidence of acute inferior infarction (since the right coronary artery supplies both the inferior wall of the left ventricle and the right ventricle). *Right ventricular infarction rarely occurs unless there is also inferior infarction.*

   b. ST segment elevation in lead V_1, but in none of the other anterior leads. *Acute anterior or anteroseptal infarction generally produces ST segment elevation in more than one lead.*

   c. *A Q wave and ST segment elevation in lead V_4R.*

In Figure 23-6 there is evidence of acute inferior infarction, but the ST segment is not elevated in lead V_1. If clinically indicated, one could ask the ECG technician to obtain an extra tracing with right-sided leads to see if acute changes were present in lead V_4R.

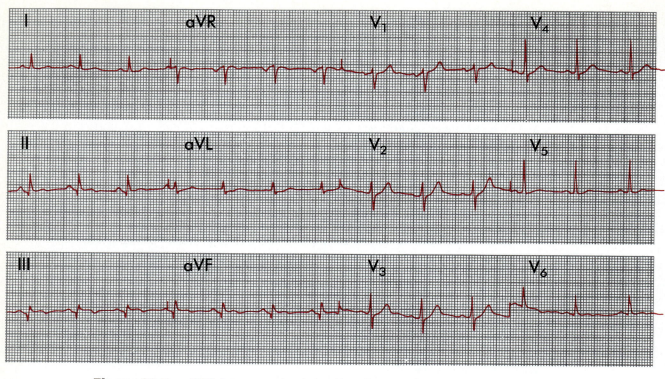

Figure 23-7.   ECG from a previously healthy 50-year-old man with "indigestion." Antacids seemed to relieve his symptoms. There is no prior tracing available.

Interpretation of Figure 23-7

Descriptive analysis. The rhythm is sinus at a fairly regular rate of between 80 and 85 beats/minute. All intervals are normal. The axis is normal (and approximately +15° to +30°). There is no evidence of chamber enlargement. There are small q waves in leads II and aVF, and a deeper (although still narrow) Q wave in lead III. R wave progression is normal (with transition occurring between leads V_2 and V_3). There is subtle ST segment elevation and coving (with a hint of T wave inversion) in *each* of the three inferior leads. There is also a hint of ST segment depression in lead aVL, and relative flattening of the T wave in leads I, V_5, and V_6.

Clinical impression. Sinus rhythm. Possible acute inferior infarction. NPT. *Strongly suggest clinical correlation!*

Questions to Further Understanding

1. *Which findings favor acute infarction in Figure 23-7?*

    Answer: The findings favoring acute infarction in this tracing are subtle, but definitely there! Despite the fact that q waves are small (and seemingly "insignificant") in leads II and aVF, and deeper but still narrow in lead III, *the fact remains that q waves are present in each of the three inferior leads!* Moreover, ST segments are slightly elevated in each of these leads. Even more important than the ST elevation itself, however, is the *shape* of these ST segments (coved), and the hint that the T wave is about to invert (especially in leads III and aVF). Non-specific ST segment depression and T wave flattening in other leads should add further to your suspicion.

It is important to remember that ECG changes of acute infarction may at times be subtle. This is especially true in the inferior leads, where QRS amplitude is often quite low (as it is here). Thus, the q wave in lead aVF is neither deep nor wide, but compared to the re-duced R wave amplitude in this lead, it is *relatively* deep. Similarly, the Q wave in lead III is only 3 mm deep, but this at least equals R wave height in lead III.

Another important reason why ECG changes of acute infarction are often subtle may relate to the timing of the ECG. Initially with infarc-tion, ST segments are elevated. With T wave inversion, ST segments tend to return to the baseline. *(Think of the T wave as "pulling" the ST segment back to the baseline as it inverts).* An ECG obtained dur-ing the period of transition (between the stage of ST segment elevation and the stage of T wave inversion) may therefore appear relatively "normal." This could be the case in Figure 23-7. ***Clinically, it is probably best to play it safe. Always maintain a high index of suspicion for any patient over 35 who presents with a history that may be consistent with acute ischemic heart disease.***

2. *Should this patient's history of "indigestion" increase our index of suspi-cion?*

   Answer: Yes. The inferior wall of the heart sits on the diaphragm. The diaphragm lies just above the stomach. "Indigestion" is a common manifestation of inferior infarction, especially when it occurs in a mid-dle-aged adult with cardiac risk factors and no previous history of gas-trointestinal problems. *Partial or even complete relief with a "GI cock-tail" should never dissuade you from obtaining an ECG in such indi-viduals!*

3. *Is this patient a candidate for thrombolytic therapy? An optimal candidate?*

   Answer: Assuming that there were no contraindications to thrombolytic therapy, and depending on the time of symptom onset, this patient could be a candidate for thrombolytic therapy. He is less likely to be an optimal candidate, however, since his infarction is inferior and the degree of ST segment elevation is small *(Tables 12-3 and 12-4, on pocket reference pp. 35 and 36).*

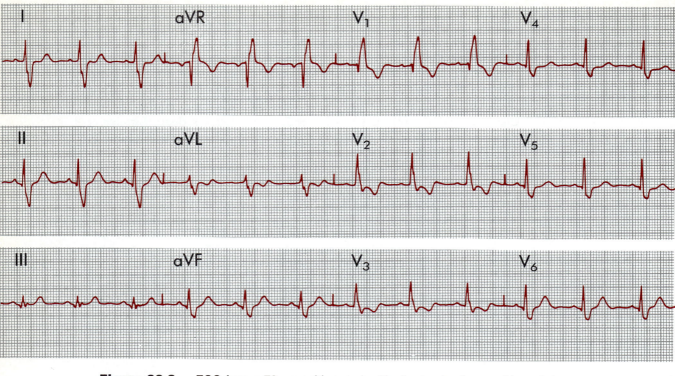

Figure 23-8.   ECG from a 70-year-old woman with chest pain of several hours' duration. No prior tracing is available.

Interpretation of Figure 23-8

Descriptive analysis. There is a regular sinus rhythm at a rate of 75 beats/minute. The PR interval is normal, but the QRS complex is wide. Morphology in the three key leads shows an rSR′ complex in lead V_1, and wide terminal S waves in leads I and V_6. (The QT interval also appears to be long, but this is likely to be due to the conduction defect, and need not necessarily be commented on.) There is no evidence of chamber enlargement. There are small q waves in the inferior and lateral precordial leads.

Clinical impression. Sinus rhythm. Complete RBBB. NPT. *Suggest clinical correlation.*

Questions to Further Understanding

1. *Is there any evidence of infarction in Figure 23-8?*

   Answer: Although there is no definite evidence of infarction, there are some unanswered questions. *Is the RBBB new?* New development of a conduction defect by itself (especially in an older adult with chest pain) suggests that the patient may have infarcted. Unfortunately, no prior tracing is available to help provide an answer.

   Two other findings on this tracing deserve comment. First, small q waves are present in the inferior and lateral precordial leads. While it is extremely likely that the small, narrow q waves in leads V_4 through V_6 represent normal septal q waves, the inferior q waves *could* reflect infarction. *Are these q waves new?* In addition, the ST segments in leads V_2 and V_3 look somewhat suspicious in that they are coved ("frowny") in appearance. This could reflect a primary ST-T wave change, although the presence of complete RBBB and the absence of a prior tracing make it extremely difficult to know for sure. *Let us emphasize that these findings are subtle, and if you said no more than "complete RBBB" for your analysis of Figure 23-8, you're doing fine!*

2. *Need we comment on the QRS axis in Figure 23-8?*

   Answer: No. As we discussed in Chapter 7, calculation of axis is often extremely difficult in the setting of complete RBBB. This is because we never know how much of the wide terminal S wave in lead I is due to an axis shift, and how much is due to the conduction defect itself. Practically speaking, all we need to be concerned about in a patient with complete RBBB is whether the axis is normal, markedly leftward (i.e., LAHB), or markedly rightward (i.e., LPHB).

   A glance at lead II tells us if a patient with complete RBBB has a marked left axis shift. If the QRS complex in lead II is decidedly more negative, the patient also has LAHB *(as discussed in answer to Figure 7-18).*

   A glance at lead I tells us if a patient with complete RBBB has a marked right axis shift. If the S wave in lead I is much, much deeper than the R wave in this lead, the patient also has LPBH *(as discussed in answer to Figure 7-20).*

   The patient in Figure 23-8 has neither LAHB nor LPHB.

•   •   •

The next day, the ECG shown in Figure 23-8A is obtained for this patient. Does this follow-up tracing help answer question # 1 above?

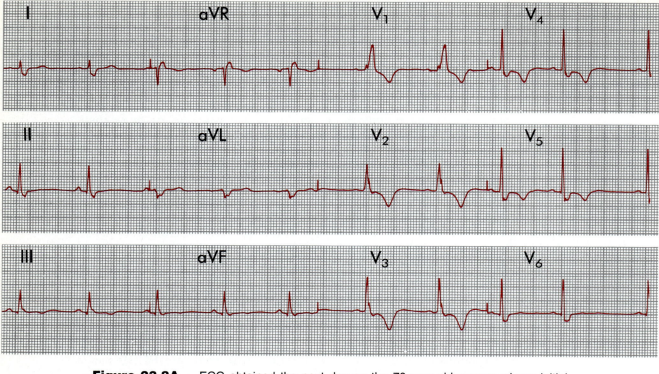

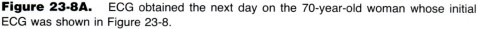

Figure 23-8A.   ECG obtained the next day on the 70-year-old woman whose initial ECG was shown in Figure 23-8.

Interpretation

Comparison of Figure 23-8A with Figure 23-8. The rhythm is now somewhat irregular, although the mechanism is still sinus. The PR interval is normal. The QRS complex is again widened in the pattern of complete RBBB. Small q waves are still present in the inferolateral leads. Lead-to-lead comparison now shows ST segment flattening in the inferior leads, with deepening and persistence of T wave inversion across the precordial leads and ST segment flattening in lead V_6. Although not elevated, the ST segment clearly appears coved in leads V_2 through V_5.

Clinical impression. Sinus arrhythmia. Complete RBBB. Diffuse ST-T wave changes since the day before, suggestive of ischemia and/or ongoing infarction. *Much more important than the ECG itself is the sequential change between the initial tracing (Figure 23-8) and the ECG obtained the next day (Figure 23-8A).*

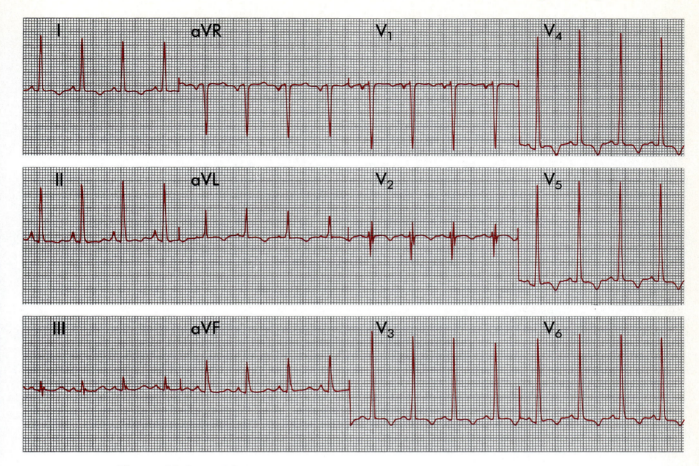

Figure 23-9. ECG from a 60-year-old woman with a history of heart failure who presents with shortness of breath and marked hypertension. She is not having chest pain. There is no prior tracing available.

Interpretation of Figure 23-9

Descriptive analysis. There is a regular sinus rhythm at a rate of about 100 beats/minute. The PR and QRS intervals are normal, but the QT interval appears to be slightly prolonged. The axis is normal (and approximately +40°). The P wave in lead II is tall and peaked, and there is a deep, negative component to the P wave in lead V_1. There may be a tiny q wave in lead II. Transition occurs normally between leads V_2 and V_3. The S wave is markedly deepened in lead V_1, and R wave amplitude is markedly increased in the lateral precordial leads. There is symmetric T wave inversion in many leads.

Clinical impression. Sinus tachycardia. Biatrial abnormality (i.e., RAA and LAA). LVH and ischemia and/or strain. *Suggest clinical correlation.*

Questions to Further Understanding

1. *Are the ST segment and T wave changes more suggestive of ischemia or strain?*

    Answer: Both. The age of the patient, the clinical history, and the markedly increased QRS amplitude all strongly suggest that she has LVH. The appearance of the ST segment in leads I, II, and V_6 is consistent with this diagnosis. T wave inversion becomes deeper and seems more symmetric in leads V_4 and V_5. It continues all the way over to lead V_1. Pure left ventricular strain is usually seen only in lateral leads. This strongly suggests that ST-T wave changes in Figure 23-9 are also due to ischemia. *ST-T wave changes of ischemia may sometimes mask ST-T wave changes of strain, and vice versa.* Our way of reflecting the likelihood that both processes are present in Figure 23-9 is to write the following in our interpretation:

    ### "LVH and strain and/or ischemia"

2. *There is an rSR's' complex in lead V_2. Does this reflect bundle branch block?*

    Answer: No. Bundle branch block is not present, because the QRS complex is not widened and QRS morphology is not consistent with either RBBB or LBBB in the three key leads (I, V_1, and V_6). Alterations in QRS morphology (such as notching, squiggles, etc.) in other leads are not of concern.

    The reason for the rSR's' complex in lead V_2 is probably that this lead is one of *transition* between the markedly negative complex in lead V_1 and the markedly positive complexes in the remaining precordial leads.

3. *Comment on the apparent QT interval prolongation.*

    Answer: The QT interval appears to be prolonged because it exceeds half the R-R interval. However, the presence of tachycardia makes it much more difficult to evaluate the meaning of QT prolongation. If the QT interval was truly prolonged (despite the heart rate), we would suspect ischemia as well as possible "Drugs/Lytes/CNS" effects as the cause (*pocket reference p. 38*).

4. *Note the slight but definite change that occurs in QRS morphology in lead III. What might account for this?*

    Answer: An S wave is present in the first two complexes in lead III, but not in the last two. The R-R and PR intervals remain constant throughout, and the QRS complex does not change appreciably in the other two simultaneously recorded leads. This suggests that the change is not due to a change in the rhythm or development of a conduction defect. The most likely explanation for the slight beat-to-beat variability in QRS morphology is respiratory variation. We think of leads III and aVF as "diaphragmatic leads" because of their anatomic proximity to this structure. As a result, some patients occasionally show slight variation in QRS morphology in these leads during deep inspiration.

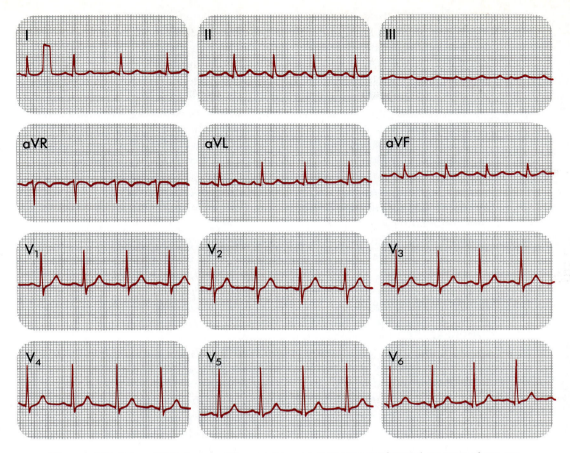

Figure 23-10.   ECG from a 50-year-old man that was performed as part of an employment physical. The patient is otherwise healthy, and completely asymptomatic. Physical examination is normal. There is no prior tracing.

Interpretation of Figure 23-10

Descriptive analysis. The rhythm is slightly irregular, but the mechanism is sinus. All intervals are normal. The axis is normal (and approximately +30 to +40°). There is no evidence of atrial abnormality or LVH. There are small q waves in the inferolateral leads. There is a tall R wave in lead V_1. ST segments and T waves appear to be normal.

Clinical impression. Sinus arrhythmia. *Tall R wave in lead V_1.* No acute changes. NPT. *Suggest clinical correlation.*

Questions to Further Understanding

1. *Comment on the tall R wave in lead V_1.*

   Answer: Recognition of the tall R wave in lead V_1 should prompt you to consider the common causes of this finding (*List #4 and Table 13-6, on pocket reference pp. 39 and 40*):

   a. WPW

   b. RBBB

   c. RVH

   d. Posterior infarction

   e. Normal variant

Normal QRS duration and the absence of delta waves rule out *WPW*. Normal QRS duration also rules out *RBBB*. None of the other findings suggestive of *RVH* are present (i.e., the axis is normal and there is no RAA, S wave persistence, or right ventricular strain). Clinical history (the patient is asymptomatic and otherwise healthy) and lack of evidence for inferior infarction argue against *posterior infarction*. By the process of elimination, this leaves *normal variant* as the most likely explanation for the tall R wave in lead V_1 of Figure 23-10, a logical deduction considering the patient is asymptomatic and otherwise healthy. One final possibility should be considered (Question #2):

2. *Is there anything unusual about R wave progression from V_1 to V_2 to V_3?* (**Hint:** *Would R wave progression look "more natural" if leads V_1 and V_2 were interchanged?*)

    Answer: Yes. Thus, another possible explanation for the unusually tall R wave in lead V_1 might be lead misplacement (mislabeling) of these precordial leads.

3. *Clinically, how might you proceed in your evaluation of this otherwise healthy and asymptomatic 50-year-old man?*

    Answer: Several things might be done:
    a. Verify that the tall R wave in lead V_1 is not due to lead misplacement. This can easily be done by repeating the ECG.
    b. Determine if a prior ECG has ever been performed on this patient. If so, comparison with this tracing would be invaluable in determining whether the tall R wave in lead V_1 is a new finding.
    c. Question the patient carefully. Is there truly no historical indication of prior infarction? (i.e., *Could the tall R in V_1 possibly reflect prior posterior infarction?*)
    d. Examine the patient carefully. In particular, is there any heart murmur that might suggest a cause for RVH?
    e. Consider obtaining additional information in the form of a chest x-ray, an echocardiogram, and/or a vectorcardiogram to help clarify the picture.
    f. *If all of the above are negative, reassure the patient and describe the tall R wave in lead V_1 as a "Normal Variant" finding!*

• • •

Without application of a systematic approach to ECG interpretation, it is all too easy to overlook the principal abnormal finding on this tracing. Simply including evaluation of **QRST Changes** makes it virtually *impossible* to miss the tall R wave in lead V_1, as this finding represents the extreme example of early transition. Review of the common causes for a tall R wave in lead V_1 (List #4) then allows the interpreter to arrive at a logical explanation.

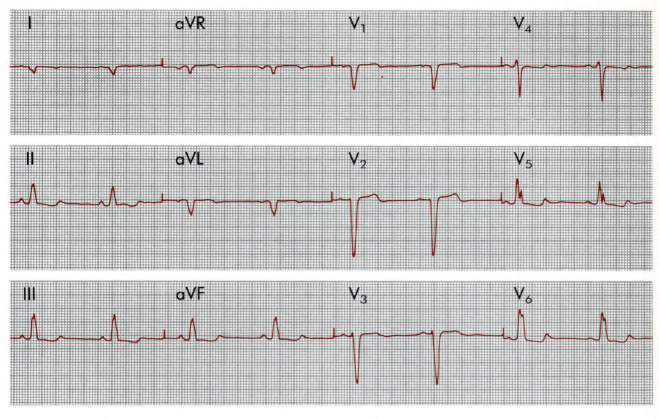

Figure 23-11.   ECG from a 57-year-old man with new-onset chest pain. There is no prior tracing available.

Interpretation of Figure 23-11

Descriptive analysis. The rhythm is slightly irregular, at a heart rate of between 50 and 55 beats/minute. The PR interval is normal, but the QRS complex is wide. QRS morphology is consistent with complete LBBB in leads V_1 and V_6, but not in lead I. There is RAD (since the QRS complex is completely negative in lead I). There is no evidence of atrial abnormality.

Clinical impression. Sinus bradycardia and arrhythmia. IVCD with RAD. NPT. *Suggest clinical correlation.*

Questions to Further Understanding

1. *Why did we label the conduction defect in Figure 23-11 IVCD instead of LBBB?*

    Answer: The key to diagnosis of bundle branch block in patients with QRS widening is to assess QRS morphology in the three key leads (I, V_1, and V_6). If QRS morphology is not typical for RBBB or LBBB in each of these three leads, the patient has IVCD *(Figure 5-1, on pocket reference p. 13).* As we have already noted, QRS morphology is consistent with typical complete LBBB in leads V_1 and V_6, but not in lead I. The patient certainly does not have RBBB. Therefore the patient has IVCD *(Figure 5-8, on pocket reference p. 14).*

2. *Is there evidence of infarction on this tracing?*

   Answer: At first glance it may appear that the patient has had a lateral infarction (QS complex in leads I and aVL) and anterior infarction (QS complex in lead V_1, tiny r waves in V_2 and V_3 with poor R wave progression). However, the presence of a conduction defect complicates matters. Although diagnosis of prior or ongoing infarction is often possible with complete RBBB, it is usually much more difficult with complete LBBB. Diagnosis of prior or ongoing infarction may be equally difficult with IVCD. Thus, despite QS complexes in leads I and aVL, the hint of ST segment coving and T wave inversion in lead aVL, and the upright T wave in lead V_6, we don't feel one can say for sure that this patient has had (or is having) a myocardial infarction. Nevertheless, the wisest course of action may still be to admit this 57-year-old man with new-onset chest pain because we also can't exclude the possibility of prior or ongoing infarction from inspection of this tracing.

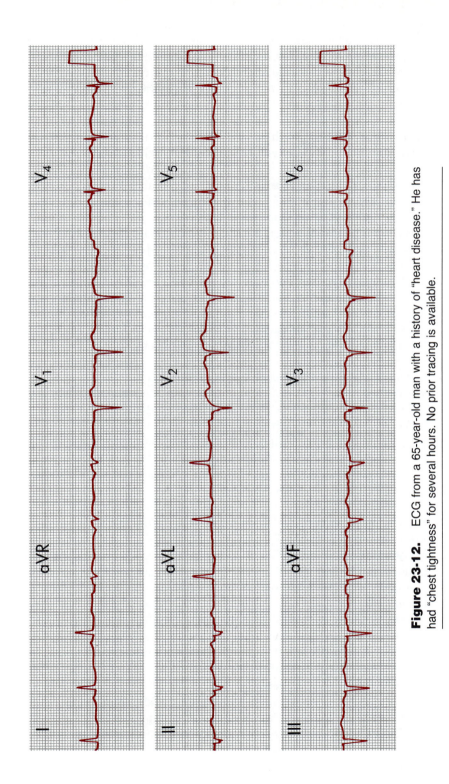

Figure 23-12.   ECG from a 65-year-old man with a history of "heart disease." He has had "chest tightness" for several hours. No prior tracing is available.

Interpretation of Figure 23-12

Descriptive analysis. There is a regular sinus rhythm at a rate of 75 beats/ minute. All intervals are normal. There is pathologic LAD (since the QRS complex is decidedly more negative in lead II). There is no evidence of chamber enlargement. There are QS complexes in leads V_1 to V_3, and a q wave in lead V_4. Transition is delayed until leads V_4 to V_5. There is ST segment and T wave flattening in multiple leads.

Clinical impression. Sinus rhythm. LAHB. Anterior infarction of unknown age. NS ST-T Abns, but changes do not appear acute. NPT. *Suggest clinical correlation.*

Questions to Further Understanding

1. *Could the changes in the anterior precordial leads be due to a lead placement error instead of anterior infarction?*

    Answer: The changes in leads V_1 to V_4 could be the result of lead placement error instead of anterior infarction. However, the lack of any r wave at all in leads V_1, V_2, and V_3, slurring of the downslope of the QS complex in leads V_2 and V_3, and the small but definite q wave in lead V_4 all support the diagnosis of anterior infarction. *R wave progression (and transition) is commonly delayed by lead placement error,* **but r waves are usually not totally lost in leads V_1, V_2, and V_3, unless there has been anterior infarction!**

2. *Why do we say that changes do not appear acute?*

    Answer: The reason we feel the infarction is unlikely to be acute is that there is really no ST segment elevation or depression in Figure 23-12. We do hedge our interpretation, however, by indicating anterior infarction "of unknown age," since ST segments are not normal and almost take on a coved appearance in leads V_2 and V_3. *Sometimes it is simply impossible to tell from examination of the 12-lead ECG whether infarction is new or not.*

3. *Clinically, what should be done when the initial ECG does not tell us whether changes are acute?*

    Answer: If the initial ECG does not provide definitive answers, depend more on the history. If the history is at all suggestive of an acute ischemic event, admit the patient to the hospital. *Better to admit a patient who does not have acute infarction than to send one home who does.*

    Sometimes comparison of the initial ECG with a previous tracing will provide insight into whether something acute is going on. If the patient is admitted, follow-up ECGs may similarly demonstrate subsequent changes that confirm an acute event.

    We tend *not* to depend on the results of cardiac enzymes drawn in the emergency department to help us decide whether to admit a patient with chest pain to the hospital. At the present state of technology, CK and LDH isoenzyme results cannot be obtained on a stat basis. Many conditions other than acute ischemic heart disease elevate CK and LDH values, including musculoskeletal conditions, intramuscular injections, hypothyroidism, blood disorders, and seizures. Thus, the finding of an elevated CK or LDH value in the ED in no way proves acute infarction. Furthermore, finding a normal CK or LDH value in the ED in no way disproves acute infarction, because it often takes hours (or more) for cardiac enzymes to go up. *If either the history or the initial ECG is at all suggestive of an acute ischemic event, we tend to admit the patient to the hospital.*

4. *Is there ECG evidence of inferior infarction in Figure 23-12?*

   Answer: No. Although small, r waves *are* present in each of the three inferior leads. Thus, the patient has LAHB (since the QRS complex is predominantly negative in lead II), but there is no definitive evidence of inferior infarction.

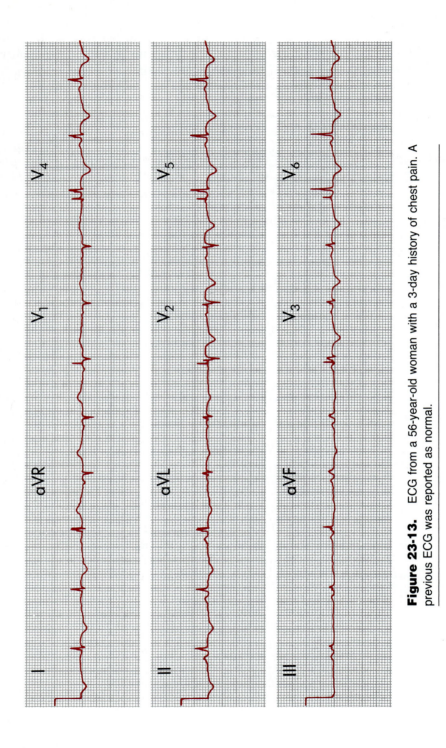

Figure 23-13.   ECG from a 56-year-old woman with a 3-day history of chest pain. A previous ECG was reported as normal.

Interpretation of Figure 23-13

Descriptive analysis. There is a regular sinus rhythm at a rate of 70 beats/minute. The PR and QRS intervals are normal, and the QT interval is borderline. The axis is normal (and approximately $+30°$ to $+40°$). There is no evidence of chamber enlargement. There is low voltage in virtually all leads. There appears to be a tiny q wave in lead aVL. R wave progression is normal (with transition occurring between leads V_2 and V_3). The most remarkable finding on this tracing is ST segment coving with fairly deep, symmetric T wave inversion in multiple leads. There may also be slight ST segment elevation in leads V_2 and V_3.

Clinical impression. Sinus rhythm. Generalized low voltage. ST segment coving and deep, symmetric T wave inversion, which may indicate ischemia (and/or ongoing infarction). *Strongly suggest clinical correlation.*

Questions to Further Understanding

1. *Should this patient be admitted to the hospital?*

    Answer: Yes. The diffuse ST segment coving ("frowny" appearance), slight ST segment elevation, and fairly deep, symmetric T wave inversion in Figure 23-13 paint a worrisome picture. Considering the clinical history (3 days of chest pain in a 56-year-old woman) and the fact that a prior ECG was reported as normal, these findings strongly suggest ischemia and/or ongoing infarction *(Figure 10-15 and Figure 10-16, D, on pocket reference pp. 28 and 29).*

2. *Is the patient a candidate for thrombolytic therapy? An optimal candidate?*

    Answer: This patient is not a good candidate for thrombolytic therapy because of the prolonged duration of symptoms (3 days) and the predominant T wave inversion rather than ST segment elevation on her admission ECG *(Tables 12-3 and 12-4, on pocket reference pp. 35 and 36).*

3. *What is a "non-Q-wave infarction"? Is the ECG shown in Figure 23-13 consistent with a non-Q-wave infarction?*

    Answer: Not all infarctions result in development of Q waves on ECG. A ***non-Q-wave infarction*** is one in which Q waves never develop.

    In the past, such infarctions were called *subendocardial* because it was thought that they involved only the subendocardial (or most vulnerable) layer of myocardium. In contrast, development of Q waves was thought to signal *transmural* (full-thickness) involvement of the myocardium. We now know that development of Q waves does not necessarily guarantee transmural involvement, and that transmural involvement does not always result in Q wave development. It is really much simpler (and technically more accurate) to classify infarctions as "Q-wave infarctions" and "non-Q-wave infarctions."

    Non-Q-wave infarctions are diagnosed by serial ST segment and T wave changes in a patient with a suggestive clinical history and laboratory evidence of infarction (i.e., acute CK isoenzyme elevation). Definite Q waves have not developed in the ECG shown in Figure 23-13. This tracing could therefore reflect a non-Q-wave infarction if cardiac isoenzymes were positive and serial tracings showed evolutionary ST-T wave changes without development of Q waves.

Clinically, non-Q-wave infarctions tend to be somewhat smaller and have a better short-term prognosis than Q wave infarctions. However, non-Q-wave infarctions also tend to be "incomplete." Recurrence (i.e., "completion" of the infarction) is common, and the long-term prognosis is identical to the prognosis for patients with Q-wave infarctions.

4. *What might explain the low voltage in Figure 23-13?*

   Answer: The term ***low voltage*** is used descriptively when QRS amplitude is less than expected. Technically, we say that there is *low voltage in the limb leads* when QRS amplitude does not exceed 5 mm (one large box) in any of the six limb leads (I, II, III, aVR, aVL, or aVF). We use the term *generalized low voltage* if in addition to low voltage in the limb leads, QRS amplitude in the precordial leads is also less than expected (i.e., less than 10 mm in most precordial leads).

   Low voltage might be expected in conditions in which the heart is either "insulated" or situated at an increased distance from recording electrodes on the chest. It is most commonly seen with COPD and obesity, although it may also occur with pericardial effusion or tension pneumothorax. Sometimes it occurs *without* any of these underlying causes (as is probably the case in Figure 23-13).

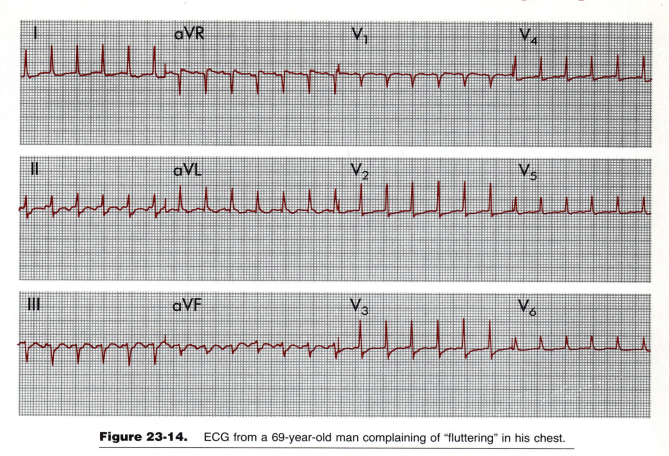

Figure 23-14. ECG from a 69-year-old man complaining of "fluttering" in his chest.

Interpretation of Figure 23-14

Descriptive analysis. There is a regular, supraventricular tachycardia at a rate of about 160 beats/minute. Normal atrial activity is absent (since the P wave is not upright in lead II). Considering the rapid rate, measurement of the QT interval is not meaningful. The axis is leftward (since the QRS complex is negative in lead aVF), but not pathologically so (since the QRS complex is still more positive than negative in lead II). We estimate the axis to be approximately −10° to −20°. There is no evidence of ventricular enlargement. (One can't say anything about atrial abnormality, since normal atrial activity is absent.) There is a tiny q wave in lead aVL, transition is early (occurring between leads V_1 and V_2), and there is diffuse ST-T wave flattening.

Clinical impression. Regular SVT at 160 beats/minute. Early transition. NS ST-T Abns.

Questions to Further Understanding

1. *What is the rhythm most likely to be?*

> **Answer:** Our approach to arrhythmia diagnosis is similar to the one suggested in our answer to Figures 22-7 and 22-18. Thus, the three main entities to consider in the differential diagnosis for this regular SVT are:
>
> a. Sinus tachycardia
> b. Atrial flutter
> c. PSVT
>
> The rhythm in Figure 23-14 is not sinus tachycardia because the P wave is not upright in lead II. PSVT should be considered as a possibility, but this is probably not the answer. ***Always suspect atrial flutter until proven otherwise whenever you have a regular SVT at a rate of about 150 beats/minute, especially if you are uncertain about atrial activity.*** Since the heart rate in Figure 23-14 is about 160 beats/minute, atrial flutter should therefore be strongly considered. The rhythm strip shown in Figure 23-14A indicates what probably is happening.

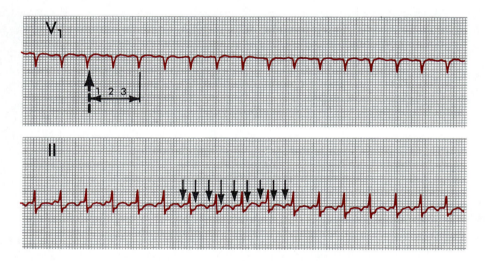

Figure 23-14A. Rhythm strip with simultaneous recording of leads V₁ and II from the 60-year-old man whose 12-lead ECG was shown in Figure 23-14.

Let's first review how we came up with a heart rate of 160 beats/minute. The easiest way to accurately calculate heart rate when the rhythm is fast and regular is to determine the rate of every other beat. The dotted arrow in lead V₁ of Figure 23-14A indicates a QRS complex that falls right on a heavy line. From this point it can be seen that the R-R interval of every other beat is just under four large boxes. Thus, half the ventricular rate is a little bit faster than 75 beats/minute, or about 80 beats/minute. *If half the rate is 80 beats/minute, the actual ventricular rate must be twice that, or 160 beats/minute.*

Now, let's look for atrial activity. Solid arrows in lead II of Figure 23-14A indicate probable atrial activity. Note that there are two solid arrows for each QRS complex. This would be consistent with 2:1 AV conduction, and an atrial rate of 320 beats/minute (i.e., 160 × 2). The only organized rhythm that could have an atrial rate this fast is atrial flutter.

2. *Clinically, what could be done to verify your answer to Question #1?*
   Answer: A vagal maneuver could be performed at the bedside *(under constant ECG monitoring!)* in an attempt to slow AV conduction to better bring out the flutter waves. *(The illustration on p. 53 shows the effect of carotid sinus massage on atrial flutter.)*

• • •

We emphasize that it is exceedingly easy to overlook the diagnosis of atrial flutter. We intentionally selected the ECG shown in Figure 23-14 because flutter waves are not readily apparent in any of the 12 leads on this tracing. Definitive diagnosis is not possible from inspection of this tracing alone. All one can say is that there is a regular SVT at a rate of about 160 beats/minute, and that the rhythm is not sinus tachycardia. We suspect atrial flutter, and indicate probable atrial activity by the solid arrows in lead II of Figure 23-14A, *but we can't be sure.* Maintaining a high index of suspicion for flutter (and appropriate use of vagal maneuvers) is the key to correct diagnosis.

Thus, we would amend our clinical impression as follows:

Clinical impression. Regular SVT at 160 beats/minute. **Suspect atrial flutter.** *Suggest clinical correlation.*

(NOTE: We have already seen this 12-lead ECG in Figure 11-4!)

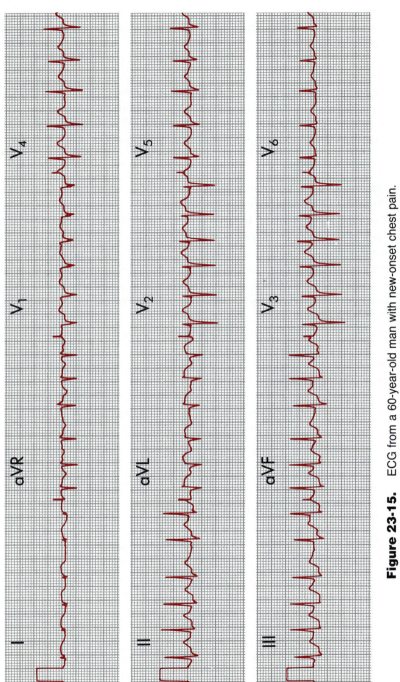

Figure 23-15. ECG from a 60-year-old man with new-onset chest pain.

Interpretation of Figure 23-15

Descriptive analysis. The rhythm is rapid and irregularly irregular. Definite atrial activity is absent. The QRS complex is of normal duration. (Considering the rapid rate, measurement of the QT interval is not meaningful.) The axis is normal (and approximately +80° to +85°, since the QRS complex is almost isoelectric in lead I). There is no evidence of ventricular enlargement. (One can't say anything about atrial abnormality, since atrial activity is absent.) There is a Q wave in lead aVL. R wave progression is normal (with transition occurring between leads V_3 and V_4). There is definite ST segment coving and elevation in the high lateral leads (I and aVL), and ST segment depression inferiorly and in lead V_1.

Clinical impression. Atrial fibrillation with a rapid ventricular response. Acute (high) lateral infarction.

Questions to Further Understanding

1. *Do leads I and aVL look at the same area of the heart as leads V_4 to V_6?*

   Answer: Leads I and aVL, and leads V_4 to V_6 all look at the lateral wall of the heart. However, they do *not* view the same area of the lateral wall. Leads I and aVL are termed "high lateral leads" because they look *down* at the heart from the left shoulder. In contrast, leads V_4 to V_6 are lateral precordial leads that view the heart's electrical activity at a slightly lower level. *We find it easy to remember that leads I and aVL are the "high lateral" leads because the left shoulder (aVL's viewpoint) is at a higher location than the precordium (which is the viewpoint of leads V_4 to V_6).*

2. *Is this patient a candidate for thrombolytic therapy? an optimal candidate?*

   Answer: Assuming there were no contraindications to thrombolytic therapy, and depending on the time of symptom onset, this patient should be a candidate for thrombolytic therapy because the initial ECG shows definite ECG evidence of acute infarction. That is, there is ≥1 mm of ST segment elevation in two contiguous leads *(leads I and aVL)*. Because of the localized (small) area of the infarction, however, the potential benefit from thrombolytic therapy is less and the patient may not be an optimal candidate.

3. *Could the supraventricular tachycardia in Figure 23-15 be atrial flutter? PSVT?*

   Answer: No. Although clearly supraventricular (since the QRS complex is definitely narrow), the rhythm in Figure 23-15 can't be PSVT because it is irregular. The rhythm is also unlikely to be atrial flutter, because the ventricular response to atrial flutter is usually (although admittedly not always) regular. More important than the lack of regularity, however, is the absence of flutter activity in any of the 12 leads.

   The point we wish to emphasize is that atrial fibrillation may sometimes look regular (and simulate these other rhythms) when the rate is rapid (as it is in Figure 23-15). Close inspection (and use of calipers) may be needed in such cases to verify the irregularity.

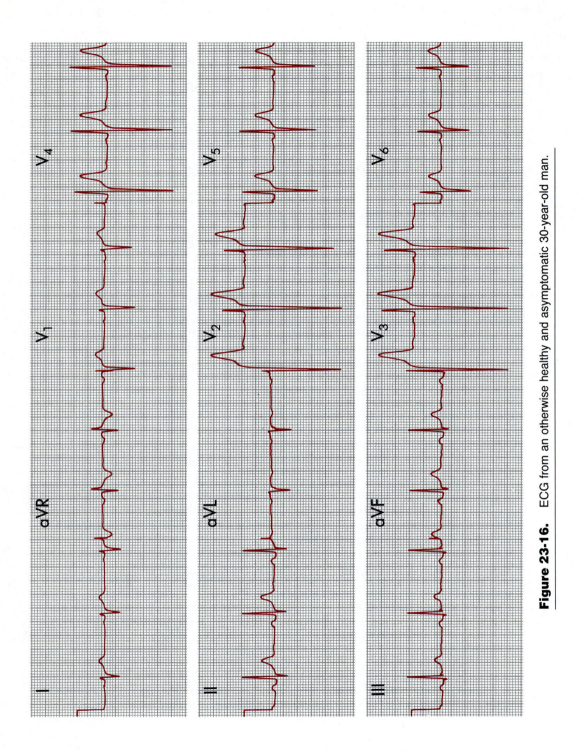

Figure 23-16.   ECG from an otherwise healthy and asymptomatic 30-year-old man.

Interpretation of Figure 23-16

Descriptive analysis. The rhythm is fairly regular, at a rate of between 65 and 70 beats/minute. All intervals are normal. There is marked RAD (since the QRS complex is predominantly negative in lead I). There is a small q wave in lead III. There is poor R wave progression (and transition never occurs). The T waves are prominent in the precordial leads.

Clinical impression. Sinus rhythm. RAD. Persistent S waves in the precordial leads. Prominent T waves. *These findings may be a normal variant. Suggest clinical correlation.*

Questions to Further Understanding

1. *Note the very deep S wave in lead V_2. Does the patient have LVH?*

   Answer: No. Voltage criteria for LVH would be met if the patient were 35 years of age or older *(Tables 9-1 and 9-2, on pocket reference p. 22)*. Since he is not, QRS amplitude falls within the normal limits for the patient's age.

   Even if the patient were 35 years of age, true chamber enlargement would be less likely because of the absence of ST-T wave changes of strain *(Figure 9-4, on pocket reference p. 23)*.

2. *Note the RAD and persistent S waves across the precordial leads. Does the patient have RVH?*

   Answer: Probably not, although it is hard to be sure from inspection of this ECG alone. Evidence against RVH is the *absence* of RAA, low voltage, right ventricular strain, and a tall R wave in lead V_1 *(Table 9-3, on pocket reference p. 25)*. Attention to the history, careful cardiac auscultation (listening for a murmur that might suggest a cause for RVH), and/or consideration of additional diagnostic tests (such as a chest x-ray or an echocardiogram) may all be helpful in clarifying the issue.

3. *Note the tall, pointed T waves in the precordial leads. Does the patient have hyperkalemia?*

   Answer: Probably not, although it is impossible to be sure from inspection of this tracing alone. It is important to remember that hyperkalemia is far more likely to occur in the presence of certain clinical conditions than in an otherwise healthy, asymptomatic 30-year-old man *(Table 14-1, on pocket reference p. 44)*. Thus despite an ECG appearance that closely simulates hyperkalemia, the precordial lead T waves in Figure 23-16 are much more likely to reflect a normal repolarization variant. Clinically, if doubt remains, it would be perfectly reasonable to check the patient's serum potassium.

• • •

We emphasize that if this same ECG was obtained from a patient with renal failure, acidosis, or dehydration, or from a patient taking a medication such as an ACE inhibitor or a potassium-retaining diuretic, we would definitely check the serum potassium level!

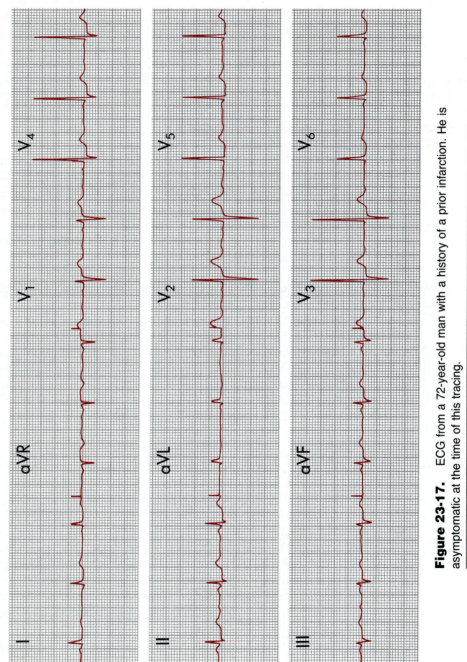

Figure 23-17. ECG from a 72-year-old man with a history of a prior infarction. He is asymptomatic at the time of this tracing.

Interpretation of Figure 23-17

Descriptive analysis. There is a regular sinus rhythm at a rate of 70 beats/minute. All intervals are normal. The axis is normal (and approximately +20° to +30°). There is no evidence of chamber enlargement. There is a q wave in lead aVL. R wave progression is normal (with transition occurring between leads V_2 and V_3). There is ST segment flattening in many leads. The T wave is flattened in lead aVL (and to a lesser extent in lead V_6), but is otherwise essentially normal.

Clinical impression. Sinus rhythm. Minimal NS ST-T Abns. *Changes do not appear acute. Suggest clinical correlation.*

Questions to Further Understanding

1. *Is the ECG shown in Figure 23-17 normal?*

   Answer: No. Although at first glance it may appear that this tracing is normal, this is not the case. Normally, there is a gradual upsloping of the ST segment as it blends imperceptibly into the T wave *(Figure 10-16, A, on pocket reference p. 29).* In Figure 23-17, the ST segments are horizontal (flat) in several leads, especially leads II, III, aVF, and V_3 through V_5. In addition, the T wave is flat in lead aVL, and relatively flat in lead V_6. Considering this patient's past medical history (that he has had a prior infarction), it is likely that these ST-T wave changes reflect coronary artery disease, although they may also be due to a host of other causes.

   •   •   •

The take-home message from this tracing is that the ST segments and T waves are *not* entirely normal. This type of ST-T wave abnormality is nonspecific and may or may not be due to coronary disease. Clinical correlation and comparison with prior tracings are invaluable in determining whether such changes are acute.

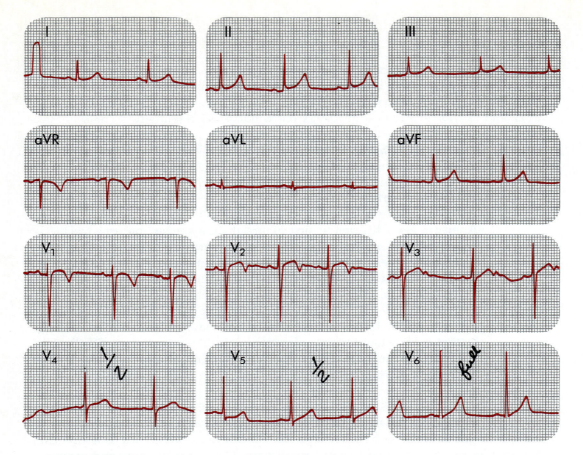

Figure 23-18. ECG from an otherwise healthy 12-year-old child. The "½" in leads V_4 and V_5 indicates that these leads were recorded at half standardization.

Interpretation of Figure 23-18

Descriptive analysis. There is sinus arrhythmia. All intervals are normal. The axis is normal (and approximately +50°). There is no evidence of chamber enlargement. There is a small q wave in lead I. R wave progression is normal (with transition occurring between leads V_3 and V_4). There is T wave inversion in leads V_1 and V_2, and T wave notching in lead V_3.

Clinical impression. Sinus arrhythmia. *ECG is normal for age.*

Questions to Further Understanding

1. *Comment on the significance of sinus arrhythmia in this age group.*

    Answer: As indicated in Table 17-2 *(pocket reference p. 50),* sinus arrhythmia is an exceedingly common, normal phenomenon in children.

2. *Comment on the significance of the anterior T wave change in this age group.*

> **Answer:** T wave inversion in several of the anterior precordial leads is also a common, normal phenomenon in childhood. Thus, the T wave may normally be inverted in leads V_1 through V_3 (or even V_4) throughout the teen-age years (and even into the early twenties). To emphasize that this phenomenon is a normal finding in this age group, anterior precordial T wave inversion is called a ***juvenile T wave variant*** when it occurs in children.

3. *How would you interpret the anterior T wave change if the patient was an adult complaining of new-onset chest pain?*

> **Answer:** If the ECG shown in Figure 23-18 was from an adult complaining of new-onset chest pain, one would have to be concerned that the anterior T wave inversion was due to ischemia.

4. *What is the actual amplitude of the R wave in lead V_5? Is this abnormal in this age group?*

> **Answer:** The lead V_4 and V_5 recordings in Figure 23-18 were obtained at half standardization. This means that the *actual* R wave amplitude in lead V_5 is twice the 14 mm seen in this tracing, or 28 mm (14×2). This is less than the maximum allowable R wave amplitude in lead V_5 for this age group *(Table 17-3, on pocket reference p. 52)*.
>
> We emphasize that Table 17-3 displays *greatly simplified voltage criteria for diagnosing RVH and LVH in children*. Values that slightly exceed the norms allowed for in the table are not infallible indicators of chamber enlargement, but merely suggest which children may require further evaluation.

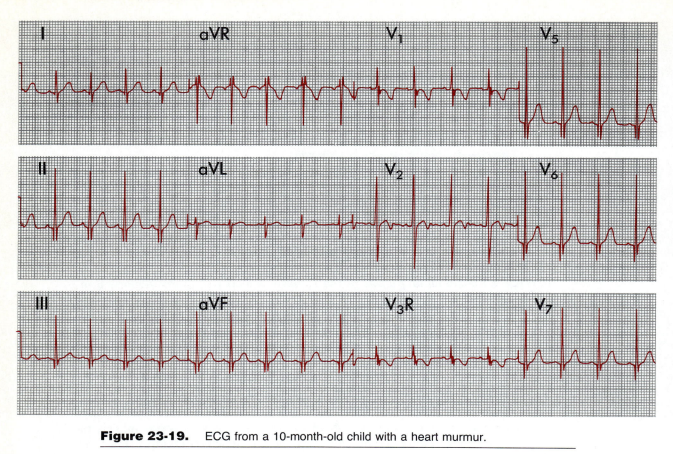

Figure 23-19.   ECG from a 10-month-old child with a heart murmur.

Interpretation of Figure 23-19

Descriptive analysis. Sinus rhythm at a rate of 110 beats/minute. The PR and QRS intervals are normal. (Considering the rate, measurement of the QT interval is not meaningful.) The axis is normal (and approximately +70°). R wave amplitude is relatively increased in lead V_6.

Clinical impression. Sinus rhythm. Borderline voltage for LVH. *Suggest clinical correlation.*

Questions to Further Understanding

1. *Note that the heart rate in Figure 23-19 exceeds 100 beats/minute. Why is this not "sinus tachycardia"?*

    Answer: As indicated in Table 17-1 *(on pocket reference, p. 51)*, a heart rate of 110 beats/minute is well within the accepted norm for this age group.

2. *Note that the R wave is relatively tall in lead V_1. Does the child have RVH?*

    Answer: Probably not. As indicated in Table 17-3 *(on pocket reference p. 52)*, the maximum allowable R wave in lead V_1 in this age group is 20 mm. Thus, the 8 mm amplitude of the R wave in lead V_1 of Figure

23-19 is not excessive. Furthermore, there is no other evidence for RVH on this tracing. That is, there is no RAD or RAA, S waves in leads V_5 and V_6 are not deepened, and T wave inversion in leads V_1 and V_2 is normal in this age group (juvenile T wave variant).

3. *Does the child have LVH? (Is there a way to be more certain of your answer?)*

    Answer: Maybe. According to Table 17-3 *(on pocket reference p. 52)*, the maximum allowable R wave amplitudes in leads V_5 and V_6 for a child less than a year old are 30 mm and 20 mm (respectively). The R wave in lead V_5 of Figure 23-19 is within this limit (it measures 28 mm). However, it exceeds the maximum allowable R wave limit in lead V_6 (where it measures 27 mm). Thus, the child may have LVH.

    As we emphasized in answer to Figure 23-18, Table 17-3 displays *greatly simplified voltage criteria for diagnosing RVH and LVH in children*. Values that slightly exceed the norms allowed in the table are not infallible indicators of chamber enlargement, and merely indicate which children may require further evaluation. In this particular case, the increased R wave amplitude in lead V_6 should prompt consideration for obtaining a chest x-ray and/or echocardiogram to further evaluate the significance of the heart murmur.

4. *Note that several additional leads have been recorded on this child. Why do you think some clinicians favor recording additional leads such as V_3R and V_7 on their very young pediatric patients?*

    Answer: Standard chest leads will not always provide an optimal view of the heart in pediatric patients. For example, in Figure 23-19, lead V_3R has been added because it provides another (perhaps better) vantage point for evaluating the child for RVH. Similarly, one can often better judge the likelihood of LVH in the small pediatric patient by addition of a more lateral precordial lead such as V_7. For practical purposes, we omit the norms for these special leads on pocket reference p. 52 so as not to complicate criteria for chamber enlargement in children.

5. *Why did we not even mention the T wave inversion in leads V_1, V_2, V_3R in our interpretation?*

    Answer: As we have already indicated, T wave inversion in leads V_1, V_2, and V_3R is a completely normal finding in the pediatric age group. As such, it need not even be mentioned.

6. *What do you think is the most common reason for obtaining an ECG on a pediatric patient in an ambulatory setting?*

    Answer: The need for obtaining an ECG on a child in a nonspecialized ambulatory care setting is quite limited. The most common reason for ordering an ECG is probably to help in evaluation of a heart murmur (i.e., for assessment of chamber enlargement). In general, a heart murmur in a pediatric patient is likely to be benign if neither an ECG nor a chest x-ray suggests chamber enlargement. When doubt remains, obtaining an echocardiogram and/or referral to a specialist should help resolve the issue.

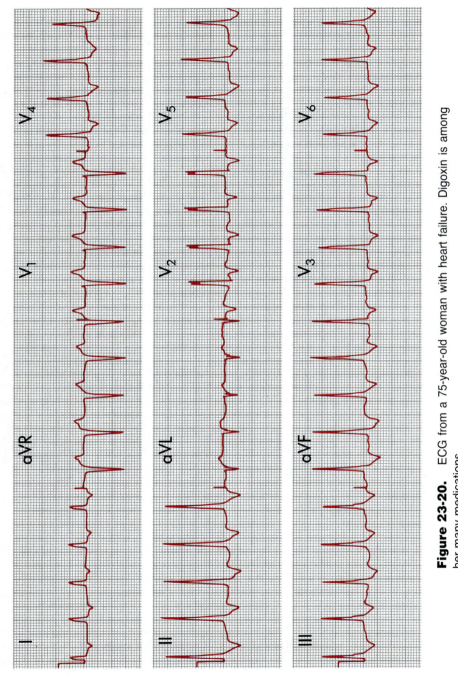
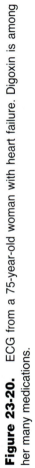

Figure 23-20. ECG from a 75-year-old woman with heart failure. Digoxin is among her many medications.

Interpretation of Figure 23-20

Descriptive analysis. There is a regular, supraventricular rhythm at a rate of 105 beats/minute. Atrial activity is absent!

Clinical impression. Junctional tachycardia.

Questions to Further Understanding

1. *Why is the rhythm junctional tachycardia?*

    Answer: The rhythm is regular and clearly supraventricular, since the QRS complex is of normal duration (i.e., it is not more than half a large box) in all 12 leads. Atrial activity is absent. The rate is too slow to be PSVT. This leaves junctional tachycardia as the most likely mechanism of the rhythm *(pocket reference p. 8).*

2. *In what two clinical settings is junctional tachycardia most likely to occur?*

    Answer: The two clinical settings in which accelerated junctional rhythms or junctional tachycardia most commonly occur are digitalis toxicity and inferior infarction. *The digitalis level definitely should be checked in this patient!*

3. *Can one comment on QRS morphology with junctional rhythms?*

    Answer: Yes, although there may be small differences between QRS morphology with junctional rhythm and QRS morphology with sinus rhythm. Thus, we could amend our clinical impression of Figure 23-20 to the following:

Clinical impression. *Junctional tachycardia.* Normal axis. Early transition. Probable LVH (based on voltage criteria for lead II in Table 9-2, on pocket reference p. 22) and strain and/or ischemia.

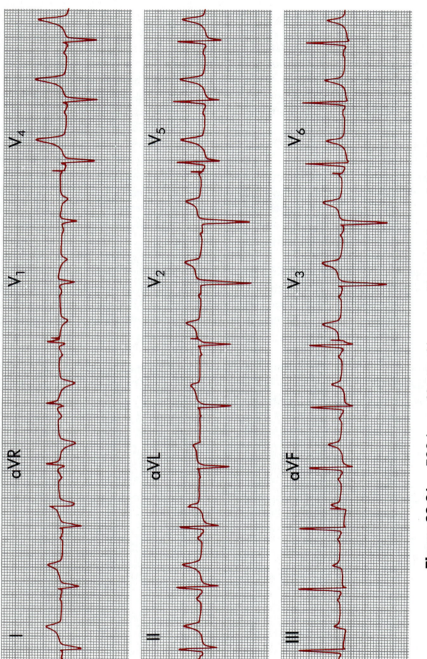

Figure 23-21.   ECG from a 60-year-old woman with renal failure and dehydration.

Interpretation of Figure 23-21

Descriptive analysis. There is a regular sinus rhythm at a rate of 65 beats/minute. The PR and QRS intervals are normal. The QT interval is borderline prolonged. There is marked RAD (since the QRS complex is predominantly negative in lead I). There appears to be a P-mitrale (i.e., notched and prolonged P wave) in lead II. There are QS complexes in lead V_1 and V_2, and a small r wave in lead V_3. Transition is delayed (to between leads V_4 and V_5). The most remarkable finding on this tracing is T wave prominence and peaking in multiple leads.

Clinical impression. Sinus rhythm. RAD. LAA. Tall, peaked T waves in multiple leads, suggestive of hyperkalemia. *Suggest clinical correlation.*

Questions to Further Understanding

1. *What factors make it highly likely that the T wave alterations in Figure 23-21 truly reflect hyperkalemia?*

   Answer: T wave morphology and the clinical history. Dehydration and renal failure both predispose to hyperkalemia *(see Table 14-1, on pocket reference p. 44).*

2. *Could you hazard a guess as to the severity of hyperkalemia?*

   Answer: Because of the marked degree of T wave peaking, one might suspect that at least moderate hyperkalemia (serum $K^+ \approx 7.0$ mEq/L or higher) was present *(see Fig. 14-1, on pocket reference p. 44).* However, the fact that the QRS complex is not really widened, and P waves are still of normal amplitude, suggests that hyperkalemia is not yet severe (greater than 9.0 mEq/L).

3. *Has this patient at some time had an anterior infarction? a lateral infarction?*

   Answer: The QS complex in leads V_1 and V_2 and the small r wave in leads V_3 and V_4 are certainly consistent with a possible anterior infarction of unknown age. In addition, the predominantly negative QRS complexes in leads I and aVL could reflect lateral infarction. However, the wisest course of action may be to repeat the ECG after serum potassium has been corrected rather than speculate on possible abnormalities from the ECG shown in Figure 23-21.

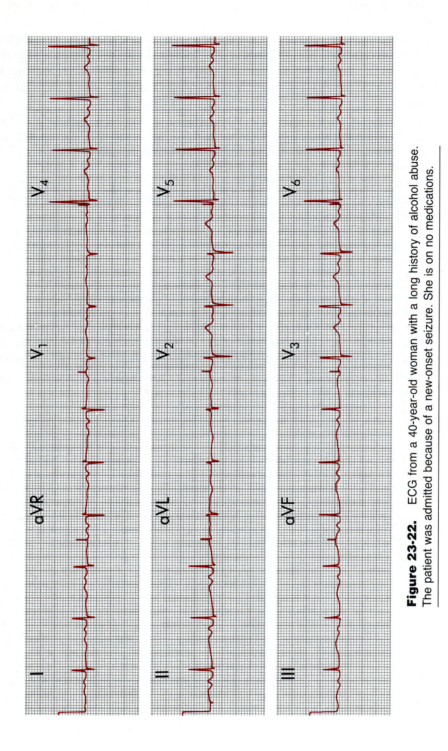

Figure 23-22.   ECG from a 40-year-old woman with a long history of alcohol abuse. The patient was admitted because of a new-onset seizure. She is on no medications.

Interpretation of Figure 23-22

Descriptive analysis. There is a regular sinus rhythm at a rate of 80 beats/ minute. The PR and QRS intervals are normal, but the QT interval is markedly prolonged! The axis is normal (and approximately +70°). There is no evidence of chamber enlargement. There is a QS complex in lead V_1. R wave progression is normal (with transition occurring between leads V_2 and V_3). The most remarkable finding on this tracing is the markedly prolonged QT interval.

Clinical impression. Sinus rhythm. Marked QT prolongation. *Consider Drugs/ Lytes/CNS as possible causes.*

Questions to Further Understanding

1. *Considering the clinical history in this example (new-onset seizure in a 40- year-old woman with alcohol abuse), what are the most likely causes of QT prolongation?*

   Answer: The common causes of QT prolongation are "Drugs/Lytes/ CNS" *(List #2 on pocket reference p. 38)*. The patient is not on any medications. Thus, the most likely causes for QT prolongation in this case are *"Lytes"* (i.e., hypokalemia, hypomagnesemia, and/or hypocalcemia) and/or *"CNS"* (especially CNS bleeding from an unsuspected fall or trauma).

   In this particular case, the patient had a normal CT scan (i.e., she did not have CNS bleeding), but had moderate hypokalemia and hypomagnesemia, severe hypocalcemia, and a seizure disorder as contributing causes of her markedly prolonged QT interval.

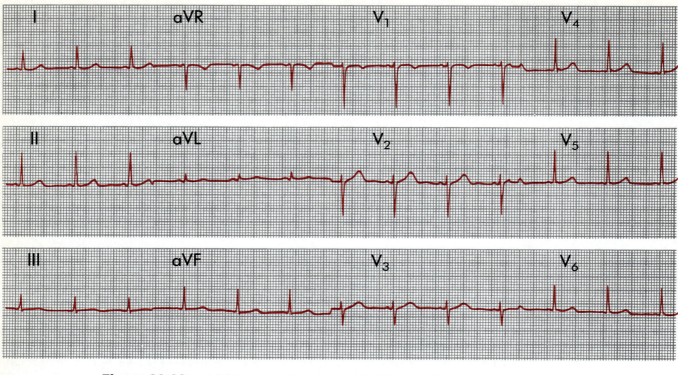

Figure 23-23.   ECG from an otherwise healthy 34-year-old woman.

Interpretation of Figure 23-23

Descriptive analysis. There is a regular sinus rhythm at a rate of 80 beats/ minute. The PR interval is short (0.10 second). The QRS and QT intervals are normal. The axis is normal (and approximately +40 to +50°). There is no evidence of chamber enlargement. Q waves are absent, R wave progression is normal (with transition occurring between leads V_3 and V_4), and ST segments and T waves are normal.

Clinical impression. Sinus rhythm. Short PR interval. Otherwise normal tracing.

Questions to Further Understanding

1. *Why do we say the PR interval is "short" in Figure 23-25?*

    Answer: The PR interval is defined as the period from the onset of atrial depolarization until the onset of ventricular depolarization. Normally in adults, it measures between 0.12 and 0.21 second. The PR interval in Figure 23-23 is short because it measures only 0.10 second (*Table 4-1, on pocket reference p. 11*).

Normally the electrical impulse originates in the SA node and travels down intraatrial pathways until it arrives at the AV node. The impulse is then momentarily delayed at the AV node, before entering the ventricular conduction system. As emphasized in Chapter 1, a large portion of the PR interval is normally made up of the delay of the electrical impulse at the AV node. The PR interval should therefore measure at least 0.12 second if the impulse has traveled down the normal conduction pathway and been delayed the usual amount of time at the AV node before being conducted further.

2. *Clinically, what is the significance of a "short PR interval"?*

   Answer: There are several reasons why the PR interval may be short. In some individuals, conduction of the electrical impulse may simply be faster and the impulse may thus require less time to arrive at the AV node. In others, the AV node itself may be smaller, and consequently delay the electrical impulse for a shorter period of time. The cause that brings about most concern, however, is PR interval shortening that results from the presence of an accessory pathway. Such individuals have a marked predisposition to developing certain cardiac arrhythmias (especially PSVT) because of the "built-in" reentry pathway they have (in which the impulse travels down the normal conduction pathway and back up the accessory pathway).

   When PR interval shortening is associated with delta waves and QRS widening, the patient is said to have WPW *(Figure 5-14, on pocket reference p. 16)*. Sometimes, however, the accessory pathway bypasses the AV node completely but still inserts directly into the ventricular conduction system. In such cases, the PR interval will be short, but the QRS complex may be entirely normal (i.e., narrow without a delta wave).

   Practically speaking, a majority of otherwise healthy individuals who have a slightly shortened PR interval (of between 0.10 and 0.11 second) but no history of cardiac arrhythmias do not have an accessory pathway. In such individuals, the short PR interval is of absolutely no clinical significance. Our way of acknowledging that the PR interval is short but probably of no clinical significance is to say, ***"Short PR interval. Otherwise normal tracing."***

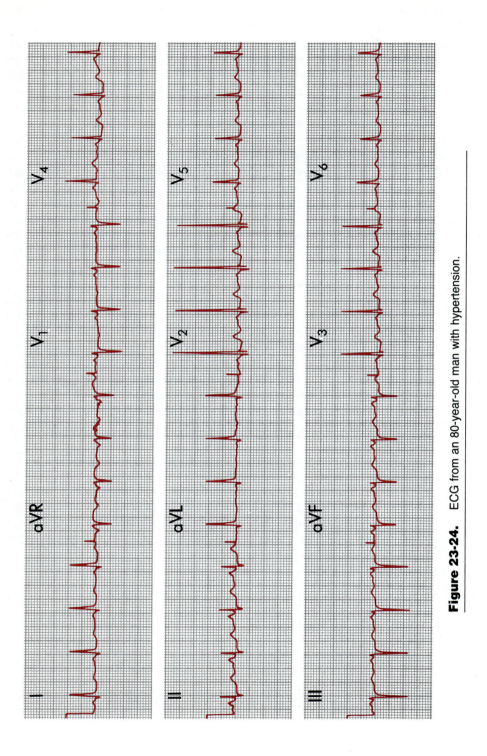

Figure 23-24. ECG from an 80-year-old man with hypertension.

Interpretation of Figure 23-24

Descriptive analysis. There is a regular sinus rhythm at 90 beats/minute. All intervals are normal. The axis is leftward, but not pathologically so (since the QRS complex is negative in lead aVF, but not in lead II). We estimate the axis to be between $-10°$ and $-20°$. There is no evidence of chamber enlargement. There are q waves in leads I, aVL, and V_2 through V_6. Transition is early (and occurs between leads V_1 and V_2). There is ST segment flattening and slight depression in many leads.

Clinical impression. Sinus rhythm. LAD. Early transition. Small q waves in the anterolateral leads of unknown significance *(possible prior anterior infarction?)*. Nonspecific ST segment flattening and depression that does not appear acute. *Suggest clinical correlation.*

Questions to Further Understanding

1. *What is the clinical significance of the small q waves in leads V_2 to V_6?*

   Answer: Small q waves in one or more of the anterior leads is a common finding in older individuals. In many cases, this finding is of little or no clinical significance, and probably reflects normal changes of aging (such as increased tortuosity of the aorta). Sometimes, however, small anterior q waves may be the marker of prior anterior infarction. There is no way to tell for sure from simple inspection of the tracing.

• • •

Our reason for including this tracing is admittedly to see whether you are still using a systematic approach. Unless you are, you may have found how easy it is to overlook the small q waves in leads V_2 through V_6 of this tracing.

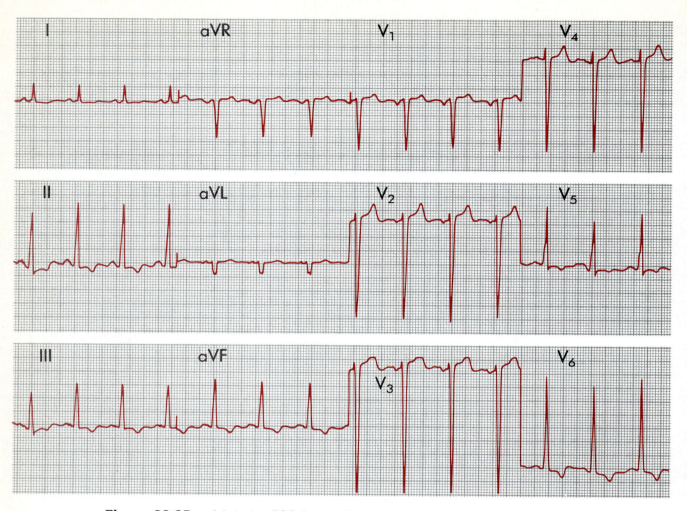

Figure 23-25.   Admission ECG from a 70-year-old woman with an exacerbation of heart failure. She denies chest pain. No prior tracing is available.

Interpretation of Figure 23-25

Descriptive analysis. There is a regular sinus rhythm at 85 beats/minute. The PR interval is normal. The QRS and QT intervals are at the upper limit of normal. The axis is normal (and approximately +70° to +80°). There is a deep negative component to the P wave in lead V_1. QRS amplitude is tremendously increased. There are no Q waves (i.e., a small r wave is present in both leads aVL and V_1). Transition is slightly delayed (and occurs between leads V_4 and V_5). There is ST segment depression and T wave inversion in the inferolateral leads.

Clinical impression. Sinus rhythm. LAA. LVH and strain and/or ischemia. NPT. *Suggest clinical correlation.*

Questions to Further Understanding

1. *Should this patient be admitted to the hospital?*

   Answer: The ECG shown in Figure 23-25 is not really helpful in answering this question. Although it is likely that the ST segment depression and T wave inversion in the inferolateral leads of this tracing reflect repolarization changes ("strain") resulting from the patient's LVH, they could also reflect ischemia. In particular, without the benefit of a prior tracing, it is impossible to tell if the inferior changes are new.

   • • •

The patient is admitted to the hospital because of her heart failure. The ECG shown in Figure 23-25A was obtained the next day. *Has there been any change?*

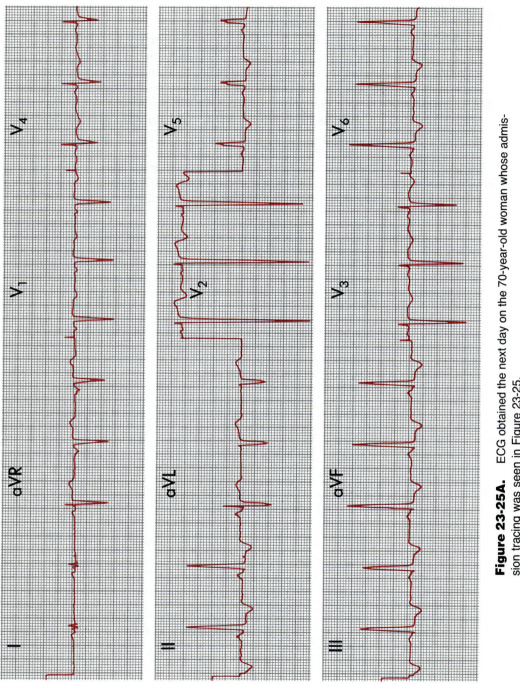

Figure 23-25A.   ECG obtained the next day on the 70-year-old woman whose admission tracing was seen in Figure 23-25.

Interpretation

Comparison of Figures 23-25 and 23-25A. The rhythm is again sinus, at a rate of 65 beats/minute. The terminal negative component of the P wave in lead V_1 is not as deep as it was in Figure 23-25. QRS amplitude is still greatly increased, although not quite to the extent it was in the earlier tracing. Lead-to-lead comparison reveals similar ST-T wave changes in the inferior leads, but new symmetric T wave inversion in leads V_3 and V_4. T wave inversion in lead V_5 is deeper, and there also appears to be beginning T wave inversion in leads V_1 and V_2.

Questions to Further Understanding

2. *What is the likely clinical significance of these serial ST-T wave changes?*

    Answer: T wave deepening and development of new T wave inversion in several precordial leads strongly suggest an ischemic process (and/or ongoing infarction).

3. *What might account for the change in P wave morphology in lead V_1 and the difference in QRS amplitude in the precordial leads?*

    Answer: Two possible explanations for these changes are patient positioning and lead placement. Although a 12-lead ECG should ideally be recorded with the patient completely supine, this is not always possible with acutely ill patients (especially when they are dyspneic). Small changes in the angle of the bed or in patient positioning may sometimes produce fairly significant differences in QRS morphology and/or amplitude. Whenever possible, it is best to indicate on the ECG the position the patient was in if he or she was not completely supine at the time the ECG was recorded.

    The other common reason for changes in QRS morphology and amplitude between serial ECGs is lead placement alterations. Awareness of the fact that even slight variation in lead placement may produce substantial changes in QRS amplitude or morphology is essential. Despite the difference in QRS amplitude between Figures 23-25 and 23-25A, we feel it unlikely that the T wave changes are simply the result of patient positioning.

Where Do We Go From Here?

Although we have reached the end of our text, we are really only at the beginning of mastering the exciting field of electrocardiography! All the tools needed to approach any 12-lead ECG you may encounter are now at your disposal. How accomplished you choose to become in ECG interpretation now depends on only one person—YOU!

The only way to retain what you have learned and to build on this knowledge is to *apply* it on a continuing basis. *No one can do this for you.* Failure to regularly practice ECG interpretation as soon as possible after completing this book is *guaranteed* to result in forgetting 99% of what you have read.

We suggest the following:

1. Make an attempt to look at the 12-lead ECGs of *ALL* patients you take care of.

2. If time permits, try to SYSTEMATICALLY interpret as many of these ECGs as you can *(WRITING OUT your findings if at all possible!).*

3. Be sure to interpret *at least* three ECGs each week (and, ideally, many more than this).

4. Always compare your interpretation with that of the interpreting physician. *(Realize that the interpreting physician will not necessarily be right all of the time. Realize also that there may be more than one "correct" interpretation to any given tracing.)*

5. Try to acquire one or more **"ECG mentors"** who will be happy to provide you with continual feedback on your interpretations.

6. Always use a systematic approach to interpretation.

7. Feel free to refer to the ECG pocket reference to refresh your memory as needed on the various ECG diagnostic criteria. Use this book as a reference when questions about ECGs arise in your everyday practice.

8. Remember how helpful careful comparison with prior tracings can be in determining whether ECG findings are likely to be new or old.

9. Remember how helpful the 12-lead ECG can be in arrhythmia interpretation.

10. Don't let yourself become discouraged.

A wealth of electrocardiographic information on each of your patients awaits you. Whether you choose to incorporate this information into your diagnostic armamentarium is up to you. *We hope you have enjoyed this book.*

Index